International Perspectives Series: Psychiatry, Psychology, and Neurosciences

Series Editors: A. Kales and C.N. Stefanis

A. Kales   C.N. Stefanis   J.A. Talbott
Editors

Recent Advances in Schizophrenia

With a Foreword by Lewis L. Judd

With 23 Figures in 33 Parts

Springer-Verlag New York Berlin Heidelberg
London Paris Tokyo Hong Kong

ANTHONY KALES, M.D.
Professor and Chairman, Department of Psychiatry and Director, Central Penn-
sylvania Psychiatric Institute, Pennsylvania State University College of Medicine,
Hershey, Pennsylvania, U.S.A.

COSTAS N. STEFANIS, M.D.
Professor and Chairman, Department of Psychiatry, Athens University Medical
School, Athens, Greece and President, World Psychiatric Association.

JOHN A. TALBOTT, M.D.
Professor and Chairman, Department of Psychiatry, University of Maryland,
School of Medicine, Baltimore, Maryland, U.S.A. and Director, Institute of Psychiatry and Human Behavior, University of Maryland Medical System, Baltimore, Maryland.

Library of Congress Cataloging-in-Publication Data
Recent advances in schizophrenia / editors, Anthony Kales, Costas N.
  Stefanis, John A. Talbott.
     p. cm.
    ISBN 0-387-97024-X (alk. paper)
    1. Schizophrenia. I. Kales, Anthony. II. Stefanis, C.N.
  (Costas N.) III. Talbott, John A.
    [DNLM: 1. Schizophrenia. WM 203 R2946]
  RC514.R37 1990
  616.89′82—dc20
  DNLM/DLC
  for Library of Congress   89-21928

Printed on acid-free paper

RC514
R37
1990

Typeset by David E. Seham Associates, Inc., Metuchen, New Jersey.
Printed and bound by R. R. Donnelley & Sons, Harrisonburg, Virginia.
Printed in the United States of America.

9 8 7 6 5 4 3 2 1

ISBN 0-387-97024-X Springer-Verlag New York Berlin Heidelberg (hard cover)
ISBN 3-540-97024-X Springer-Verlag Berlin Heidelberg New York
ISBN 0-387-97221-8 Springer-Verlag New York Berlin Heidelberg (soft cover)
ISBN 3-540-97221-8 Springer-Verlag Berlin Heidelberg New York

Foreword

I am honored to introduce readers to this extraordinary volume, the first in the annual *International Perspectives Series: Psychiatry, Psychology, and Neurosciences*. This particular volume on the *Recent Advances In Schizophrenia* stems from the Third Annual Pennsylvania Conference on Schizophrenia, held in March, 1988. At that international meeting, some of the most esteemed researchers in the field surveyed our current understanding of schizophrenia. Collectively, their presentations capture the excitement of a research field launching into a stage of rapid worldwide advancement.

The last decade has seen an enormous refocusing of scientific effort on schizophrenia, directed, in large measure, by the National Institute of Mental Health (NIMH). Our understanding of this mysterious, disabling disorder in all its diversity has been enhanced by a host of technologies, including new neuroimaging techniques, cognitive psychology, molecular genetics, and anatomical, biochemical, and molecular neuropathology. The resulting growth spurt in our knowledge constitutes the essence of the conference and of this volume. As the following pages amply document, it has been a decade of great progress, one in which we can take great pride. The science of our field has matured to the point that a major research thrust is now feasible—one likely to have enormous benefits for schizophrenic patients and their families. It is a very exciting time to be in this field and to participate in accelerating its advances.

The NIMH is prepared to take the lead in stimulating our next decade of progress. Research on schizophrenia—together with research in the neurosciences, with which it is synergistic—is a focal point of the Institute's current research program and will continue to have the highest priority at NIMH as long as I am director.

In 1988, the NIMH completed development of a National Plan for Schizophrenia Research, based on the contributions of eighty leading scientists in the United States and abroad, with an additional seventy scientists serving as advisors and consultants. The plan outlines an intensive national research effort to identify the causes of schizophrenia and develop effective treatment. It represents, I believe, a very solid, rational, and, most importantly, achievable scientific attack on what we recognize is one of mankind's most baffling and crippling disorders.

We are now in the process of implementing that plan in conjunction with a complementary plan termed "The Decade of the Brain," which is focused on ways to accelerate even further the pace of research advances in the neurosciences of mental illness. Both plans deal with the basic and clinical aspects of their respective topical areas; together, they constitute "A National Plan for Research on Schizophrenia and the Brain." Activities stemming from this combined plan span all aspects of the Institute's activities, as illustrated by the following examples: building upon the recent phenomenal growth in the neurosciences, NIMH is establishing a variety of research centers that focus on the neuroscience of schizophrenia and other serious mental disorders. All four Centers for Neuroscience and Schizophrenia established in fiscal years 1988 and 1989 are designed to integrate basic and clinical approaches by taking basic findings from the research laboratory into clinical research settings in order to improve the diagnosis and treatment of schizophrenia.

Other centers will focus explicitly on molecular neurobiology, a research area which, during the past decade, has: spurred the development of highly detailed understanding of neuronal and synaptic function; offered the promise of very accurate diagnosis using genetic markers; advanced the production of new biologic therapeutic compounds; promoted the development of new animal models for research; and stimulated the investigation of the structure/function relationships of CNS proteins. These scientific and technological advances offer many exciting opportunities for understanding normal and abnormal brain function. Thus, the new molecular neurobiology centers will stimulate the application of these important experimental strategies to the problems of the mentally ill, including those with schizophrenia.

The National Plan for Research on Schizophrenia and the Brain also includes a major Institute-wide initiative on the molecular genetics of mental illness. This initiative is spurred both by the recent advances in molecular genetics technology and by the identification of strong genetic linkages to schizophrenia, among other specific mental disorders. NIMH will develop a national "bank" of cell lines from individuals and families with high prevalence of schizophrenia, manic-depressive illness, or Alzheimer's disease. It will also create a network of centers functioning under rigorous, standardized research protocols to identify and meticulously study informative families and, ultimately, to identify the gene(s) involved.

Other aspects of the molecular genetics initiative include a National Pedigree Research Service, which will gather data on large families with many mentally ill members. This service is expected to provide technical assistance and financial support for the careful study of families affected by mental illness and identified by investigators who are not a part of the center network described above. Finally, the Institute is considering establishing a National Genotyping Laboratory. Collectively, these activities and programs will provide the foundation for a coordinated national effort to understand the genetic aspects of many mental disorders, including schizophrenia.

The study groups for the National Plan for Schizophrenia Research stressed the great need to improve the knowledge base underpinning the diagnosis, care, and treatment of people with severe and persistent mental disorders. For the severely mentally ill, for example, the U.S. service delivery system appears to be too fragmented to provide accessible, coordinated, long-term care. Furthermore, because the financial burden for these conditions is often substantial, efforts are needed to identify reimbursement mechanisms to support coordinated services. Therefore, the NIMH is mounting a major program to analyze and frame an agenda for both clinical services and service systems research for the long-term severely mentally ill.

Recognizing that such an effort can only be achieved by linking clinical research with service systems research, NIMH recently mounted an initiative to enhance research conducted in public mental health care settings. In September, 1988, the Institute first invited applications from prospective participants in the newly developed Public-Academic Liaison (PAL) program, designed to foster real partnerships between academic researchers and administrators working in public mental health systems. The PAL program's goals are both to enrich the questions researchers ask by having them conduct their studies in actual service settings and to foster knowledge transfer to the public service sector through the presence of academic and other researchers. This effort is expected to increase and improve the usefulness of services and clinical research in such important populations as the homeless mentally ill, children and adolescents, and the severely mentally ill with AIDS.

The initiatives I have just described are built on a foundation of expert assessments of research progress and needs. That foundation, in turn, is established as leading researchers meet periodically with their scientific peers, review and exchange developments in their field, identify unanswered questions old and new, and attempt to redirect their field through constructive criticism and leadership.

This book, the first in the International Perspectives Series, is drawn from one such seminal meeting—the Third Annual Pennsylvania Conference on Schizophrenia—and provides an enduring record of what is likely to be an important turning point in the field of schizophrenia research. I hope and am working my best to assure that by the Thirteenth Annual Pennsylvania Conference on Schizophrenia, we will reread this volume and say: "That was when the real revolution in schizophrenia research began."

LEWIS L. JUDD, MD
Director
National Institute of Mental Health

Preface

This volume, the first in the *International Perspectives Series: Psychiatry, Psychology and Neurosciences,* is devoted to *Recent Advances in Schizophrenia.* The series is dedicated to addressing mental health problems that are global in their occurrence, have far-reaching consequences and require international efforts for their effective solution. Up-to-date basic science findings and current, relevant clinical observations and approaches are integrated into a unified presentation of these mental health issues.

The symptoms of schizophrenia have interested and perplexed philosophers, clergy, and physicians for many years. Over the centuries the victims of this illness have been regarded as witches and demons or as possessing unique powers. Consequently, they have been mistreated, imprisoned, or regarded with special awe. In 1896, Emil Kraepelin brought together a variety of psychiatric syndromes under the term "dementia praecox," a term originally used by Benedict Morel in 1860. The term "schizophrenia" was coined in 1911 by Eugen Bleuler who conceptualized the condition both as a disease entity and as a psychopathological reaction to the consequences of the illness. In his 1924 textbook of psychiatry, Bleuler anticipated today's emphasis on community treatment for schizophrenia, which highlights assessment of areas of healthy functioning while minimizing the effects of the deficits caused by the illness.

With a lifetime prevalence of about 1%, more than twenty million people in the world are estimated to suffer from schizophrenia. It is primarily a disorder of the young that interrupts the years of productivity and, in many cases, results in life-long impairments with an enormous burden placed upon families and communities. The shame and stigma still attached to the term "schizophrenia" ensures that, even today in our enlightened age, the disorder is often hidden from society. While it is a major public health problem that demands sufficient resources for effective research and treatment, prior to the NIMH programs outlined by Dr. Judd there has been no significant national campaign mounted for its eradication.

The Annual Pennsylvania Conference on Schizophrenia provides a forum to discuss the efforts of researchers and clinicians who strive toward better methods of identifying and diagnosing this devastating illness, clarifying its etiology, and developing more effective treatment methods. The Arthur P. Noyes Award is presented annually at this conference and is named in honor of a man who was the long time superintendent of Norristown State Hospital and a recognized authority in the treatment of schizophrenia. Dr. Noyes foresaw mental health increasingly becoming a public health responsibility and believed the public hospital should represent only a small part of a network of community services, all designed to forestall or prevent hospitalization.

The Third Annual Pennsylvania Conference on Schizophrenia held in Harrisburg, Pennsylvania, brought together a distinguished group of scientists from around the world to address schizophrenia from an international perspective. The conference was sponsored by the Central Pennsylvania Psychiatric Institute, and the program was co-chaired by Drs. Kales, Stefanis, and Talbott. The Noyes award was presented to Dr. Timothy Crow under the auspices of: the Central Pennsylvania Psychiatric Institute; the seven medical school departments of psychiatry in Pennsylvania; the departments of psychiatry of the Albert Einstein Medical Center/Philadelphia Psychiatric Center and the Institute of Pennsylvania Hospital; and the Office of Mental Health, Department of Public Welfare, Commonwealth of Pennsylvania. Following the conference, an invitation to contribute to this volume was extended to other international researchers and clinicians in order to develop a comprehensive update on schizophrenia that would integrate the rapid advances in both clinical and basic science areas regarding this baffling disorder.

Dr. Lewis Judd, Director of the National Institute of Mental Health (NIMH), who welcomed participants to the conference, has written the foreword to this book. In his piece, Dr. Judd emphasizes the resurgence of interest in schizophrenia and the commitment of the NIMH through its "National Plan for Research on Schizophrenia and the Brain" to press forward with the study of brain mechanisms and their relationship to the most serious and persistent mental disorders, in particular, schizophrenia. He details the various current research initiatives ongoing at the NIMH as well as those that are planned. He also discusses an important new NIMH initiative, the liaison between the public sector and academic institutions (Public-Academic Liaison program), to provide the needed collaboration between clinical and research sectors in furthering an understanding of the etiology of schizophrenia and development of effective treatments for this disorder.

Within the body of the book there are three major sections. The first, "Conceptualization of Schizophrenia," brings together both a longitudinal and a cross-sectional approach to understanding this complex disorder. In the first chapter, "Schizophrenia: Historical Perspectives," Drs.

Anthony and Joyce Kales and Dr. Vela-Bueno trace the thread of understanding of bizarre and psychotic behaviors from prehistoric times through the dawn of civilization and Ancient, Medieval, and Renaissance periods to the era of Enlightenment. In addition, they focus on the contributions by Kraepelin and Bleuler leading to the emergence of the concept of schizophrenia as we know it today. Dr. Stefanis of Greece continues with a chapter on the "On the Concept of Schizophrenia." He traces the definition of the concept of schizophrenia over time, beginning with its ancient roots and culminating in the French and German schools, in which the syndromal, nosological, and theoretical approaches were more clearly delineated, providing the framework for our modern diagnostic and classificatory systems. He also considers the issue of the universality of schizophrenia as well as its incidence, morbidity, and outcome in various countries with emphasis on findings obtained from the World Health Organization studies. Finally, he concludes the chapter by reviewing the available evidence supporting the currently prevailing hypotheses on the etiology and pathogenesis of schizophrenia. Continuing in the section on conceptualization are three more contributions: Drs. Cleghorn and Albert of Canada contribute a chapter on "Modular Disjunction: A Framework for Pathological Psychophysiology." In this chapter, they detail how psychotic symptoms are related to a disjunction of functional units (cognitive modules) of the brain, hypothesizing a desynchronization of widely distributed neurocognitive systems. They proceed to support this theory of modular disjunction with relevant neurophysiological, neuroanatomical, and neuropharmacological data. In his chapter on "Meaning of Structural Changes in the Brain in Schizophrenia," Dr. Crow, the Noyes awardee from the United Kingdom, challenges the definition of schizophrenia as a "functional" psychosis and discusses work on brain alterations and their clinical correlates, arriving at the two-syndrome (positive and negative symptoms) concept for schizophrenia. Noting the asymmetry of certain structural brain changes such as left temporal horn enlargement, Dr. Crow also discusses genetic influences and the possible existence of a virogene to account for the developmental and episodic nature of the illness. From the United States, Drs. Carpenter, Kirkpatrick, and Buchanan offer their "Conceptual Approaches to the Study of Schizophrenia" with an emphasis on an integrated medical understanding and delineation of the domains of psychopathology that can be observed with schizophrenia, a heterogeneous clinical syndrome. In addition, they detail the variable course of the illness, from a long-term as well as a short-term standpoint and describe what is known about the prevention of relapse, such as the recognition of early warning signs and the use of interpersonal and pharmacologic treatment strategies.

In the second major section, "Recent Advances in the Diagnosis and Treatment of Schizophrenia," there are seven chapters. These important contributions give evidence to the fact that we are rapidly advancing our knowledge in the neurosciences and are standing at the threshold of a greater understanding of schizophrenia. Addressing the issue of "Risk Factors in Schizophrenia: Interaction between Genetic Liability and Environmental Factors," Drs. Schulsinger and Parnas from Denmark review the historical perspectives of genetic studies and discuss premorbid behavioral correlates and a high rate of pregnancy and birth complications associated with the schizophrenia spectrum. They also describe the findings of their longitudinal prospective study, which showed that with an increased level of stress, psychopathology increased in the high-risk group but not in the low-risk group. Next, Drs. DeLisi and Lovett from the United States discuss "The Role of Molecular Genetics in Psychiatry: Unraveling the Etiology for Schizophrenia." In their chapter, they offer evidence for a genetic cause for psychosis and discuss the promising and exciting new searches for biologic as well as genetic markers, e.g. DNA polymorphisms, and describe the methods associated with the statistical analysis of genetic data, such as linkage analysis. They emphasize that "the tools provided by molecular genetics can be used for the detection of specific causes of abnormal psychopathology whether ultimately genetic or nongenetic." The important "Diagnostic Advances in Anatomical and Functional Brain Imaging in Schizophrenia" comprise the next chapter offered by Drs. Pahl, Swayze, and Andreasen of the United States. Structural brain imaging as delineated through x-ray computed tomography and magnetic resonance imaging is reviewed along with the clinical applications of this imaging, e.g. diagnosing psychoses of focal organic etiology. Also discussed is functional brain imaging (assessing in vivo neurochemistry and metabolic function of the brain) utilizing such techniques as cortical probe-flow, photon emission computed tomography, and positron emission tomography along with their potential clinical applications, e.g. determining optimal neuroleptic drug doses. Dr. Goldstein of the United States next discusses "Risk Factors and Prevention in Schizophrenia." In so doing, he considers the vulnerability-stress model and looks at childhood and adolescent precursors of vulnerability in high-risk groups as well as family environmental stressors and how these factors relate to the course of schizophrenia and strategies for intervention with the family (e.g., reducing high expressed emotion). Drs. Mueser, Liberman, and Glynn, also of the United States, discuss their work on "Psychosocial Interventions in Schizophrenia," in particular, the behavioral therapies (social skills training, behavioral family therapy, and token economy) as well as their clinical implementation. Recent advances in social skills training and behavioral therapy have led to the development of the "modular approach" to psychosocial treatment, which targets the full spectrum of necessary living skills for chronic schizophrenics. Moving to the psychopharmacologic area, two papers by United States authors follow. The first, by Dr. Meltzer, "Clozapine:

Mechanism of Action in Relation to its Clinical Advantages," describes the major clinical advantages of this atypical antipsychotic drug in treating both positive and negative symptoms in treatment-resistant schizophrenic patients as well as its minimal extrapyramidal symptoms and lack of producing tardive dyskinesia. The atypical mechanism of action of clozapine in relation to these clinical advantages is also discussed, particularly the drug's influence on the dopaminergic-serotonergic system. The second chapter, by Dr. Kane, "Psychopharmacologic Treatment of Schizophrenia," discusses the general principles of pharmacotherapy for schizophrenia including predictors of response, the management of negative symptoms, maintenance treatment, side effects (especially tardive dyskinesia), and the potential role of a new atypical antipsychotic, clozapine. The chapter also emphasizes new approaches (intermittent and targeted strategies) based on establishing minimum effective dose requirements.

In the final section of the book, "Delivery Systems for Managing Schizophrenic Patients" in various parts of the world are described. Authors from the United States, Canada, Italy, United Kingdom, Africa (Kenya), and China offer, amidst diverse historic and cultural backgrounds, a current spectrum of community experiences in mental health care including: mental health policies; models of delivery services; what is known about outcome measures; and future trends and directions. Dr. Talbott from the United States in "Current Perspectives in the United States on the Chronically Mentally Ill" offers a historical background regarding the reliance on state hospitals prior to the 1960s, the onset of deinstitutionalization and the subsequent problems that occurred (e.g., depopulation rather than deinstitutionalization, a lack of adequacy of community care and care in mental hospitals, inadequate training and limited role of psychiatrists, and lack of assessment of program efficacy) with attempted and proposed solutions. He concludes with a look at the future and describes a few promising and innovative initiatives. Dr. Harnois from Canada discusses "Policy on Chronic Mental Illness in Canada: Current Status and Future Directions," first describing the provincial and federal contributions to health care in Canada; the fact that federal support for psychiatric hospitalization is provided to the general hospital and not the mental hospital leads to a disparity in care offered between these two types of hospitals. Quebec is the only province in Canada with a formal mental health policy. This policy, which has seven priorities for improving the delivery of mental health care, "stresses that the priority of the person's needs, not those of the system should be primary." "Psychiatric Reform in Italy: Implications for the Treatment of Long-Term Schizophrenic Patients" is described by Dr. Tansella. Rather than mass deinstitutionalization, he describes a model of "closing the front door of psychiatic hospitals" and the development of the community priority as illustrated by the South-Verona experience. In a follow-up study, the community-based model was superior to hospital-based services in: treatment of acute and chronic syndromes; prevention of secondary handicaps; and correction of extensive disadvantages such as inadequate social skills and unemployment. Representing the United Kingdom, Drs. Tarrier and Barrowclough discuss "Mental Health Services and New Research in England: Implications for the Community Management of Schizophrenia." They discuss the British National Health Service as a system of comprehensive medical care with specific reference to the Salford District Health Authority and its Family Intervention Project. Relapse rates were significantly lower when stress was reduced within the home environment with important components including the reduction of high expressed emotion in relatives and improvement in the patient's social skills. Dr. Mustafa, addressing "Delivery Systems for Schizophrenic Patients in Africa—Sub-Sahara" outlines the problems in delivering psychiatric services to vast, underdeveloped regions where basic health services, especially mental health services, may be lacking and a reliance on traditional healers may complicate efforts to deliver community-based psychiatric services. Some solutions have included building psychiatric units in general hospitals as well as developing mobile units for rural areas, educating village health workers, and training the general health nurse in recognition, treatment, and referral of mental illnesses. Finally, "Delivery Systems for Research in Schizophrenia in China" are described by Drs. Zhang and Xia who outline the Chinese working diagnostic criteria for schizophrenia. They also detail the various levels of mental health care at municipal, district or county, and grass-roots levels as well as other models for mental health care in general hospitals and community services. Finally, they describe the general conduct of both clinical and laboratory research in China including genetic studies, biochemical investigations, psychopharmacological studies, and research in immunology, endocrinology, neuropathology, and physiology.

The editors' goal for this volume is to provide an integrative perspective on basic and clinical approaches to the understanding and treatment of schizophrenia. Such work is advancing rapidly throughout the world and reflects the global consensus that the time has come to mount an attack on this major public health problem from all fronts: the genetic, the biologic, the pharmacologic, the psychosocial, and the delivery systems for care. The editors hope and wish that this volume will help to increase the momentum of these efforts and to stimulate others around the world to continue their efforts to conquer this devastating illness.

The editors express their deep appreciation to all of the authors for their important and valuable contributions. We also gratefully acknowledge the immeasurable help and skilled assistance of several of our colleagues in completing this book: Drs. Edward Bixler, Rocco Manfredi,

Constantin Soldatos, and Alexandros Vgontzas. Finally, we are indebted to our patients and their families who represent people from every walk of life, from all countries and nationalities who are waiting for the healing that can come only through the concerted effort of researchers and clinicians from around the world working together.

ANTHONY KALES
COSTAS N. STEFANIS
JOHN A. TALBOTT

Contents

Part I.   Conceptualization of Schizophrenia

Part II.   Recent Advances in the Diagnosis and Treatment of Schizophrenia

Part III.   Delivery Systems for Managing
Schizophrenic Patients

Contributors

MARTIN L. ALBERT, M.D., Professor of Neurology and Director, Behavioral Neuroscience and Geriatric Neurology, Boston VA Medical Center, Boston University School of Medicine, Boston, Massachusetts, U.S.A.

NANCY C. ANDREASEN, M.D., PH.D., Professor of Psychiatry and Director, Mental Health Clinical Research Center, University of Iowa, Iowa City, Iowa, U.S.A.

CHRISTINE BARROWCLOUGH, B.A., M.SC., Principal Clinical Psychologist, District Department of Clinical Psychology, Salford District Health Authority, Prestwich Hospital, Manchester, United Kingdom.

ROBERT W. BUCHANAN, M.D., Research Assistant Professor, Maryland Psychiatric Research Center and Department of Psychiatry, University of Maryland School of Medicine, Baltimore, Maryland, U.S.A.

WILLIAM T. CARPENTER, JR., M.D., Professor of Psychiatry and Director, Maryland Psychiatric Research Center, Department of Psychiatry, University of Maryland School of Medicine, Baltimore, Maryland, U.S.A.

JOHN M. CLEGHORN, M.D., Professor of Psychiatry and Coordinator, Brain and Behavior Research Program, McMaster University Faculty of Health Sciences, Hamilton (Ontario), Canada.

TIMOTHY J. CROW, M.D., PH.D., Deputy Director and Head of the Division of Psychiatry, Clinical Research Centre, Northwick Park Hospital, Harrow, United Kingdom.

LYNN E. DELISI, M.D., Associate Professor of Psychiatry and Director, Schizophrenia Research Unit at Kings Park Psychiatric Center, State University of New York at Stony Brook, Stony Brook, New York, U.S.A.

SHIRLEY M. GLYNN, PH.D., Research Psychologist and Clinical Psychologist, UCLA School of Medicine, Brentwood VA Medical Center & NPI/Camarillo Clinical Research Unit, Camarillo State Hospital, Los Angeles, California, U.S.A.

MICHAEL J. GOLDSTEIN, PH.D., Professor of Psychology and Psychiatry and Director of the UCLA Family Project, Department of Psychology, University of California at Los Angeles, Los Angeles, California, U.S.A.

GASTON P. HARNOIS, M.D., Director, Montreal/WHO Collaborating Centre and Associate Professor, McGill University, Montreal (Quebec), Canada.

JOYCE D. KALES, M.D., Professor and Director, Division of Community Psychiatry, Department of Psychiatry and Associate Director, Central Pennsylvania Psychiatric Institute, Pennsylvania State University College of Medicine, Hershey, Pennsylvania, U.S.A.

JOHN M. KANE, M.D., Chairman, Department of Psychiatry, Hillside Hospital Long Island Jewish Medical Center, Glen Oaks, New York and Professor of Psychiatry, The Albert Einstein College of Medicine, Bronx, New York, U.S.A.

BRIAN KIRKPATRICK, M.D., Research Assistant Professor, Maryland Psychiatric Research Center and Department of Psychiatry, University of Maryland School of Medicine, Baltimore, Maryland, U.S.A.

ROBERT P. LIBERMAN, M.D., Professor of Psychiatry, UCLA School of Medicine and Chief, Rehabilitation Medicine Service, Brentwood VA Medical Center, Los Angeles, California, U.S.A.

MICHAEL LOVETT, PH.D., Director, Human Genetics, Genelabs, Redwood City, California, U.S.A.

HERBERT Y. MELTZER, M.D., Douglas D. Bond Professor of Psychiatry and Professor of Pharmacology, Case Western Reserve University School of Medicine, Cleveland, Ohio, U.S.A.

ZHANG MINGDAO, M.D., Professor, Department of Psychiatry, Shanghai Second Medical University and Vice Director, Shanghai Mental Health Center Shanghai, The People's Republic of China.

KIM T. MUESER, PH.D., Assistant Professor of Psychiatry and Coordinator of Schizophrenia Treatment Program, Medical College of Pennsylvania and Eastern Pennsylvania Psychiatric Institute, Philadelphia, Pennsylvania, U.S.A.

GHULAM MUSTAFA, M.D., Chief Psychiatrist and Vice-President, African Psychiatric Association, Ministry of Health, Mathari Hospital, Nairobi, Kenya.

JÖRG J. PAHL, M.D., F.C.P. (S.A.), Associate of Psychiatry, Department of Psychiatry, University of Iowa, Iowa City, Iowa, U.S.A.

JOSEF PARNAS, M.D., Associate Professor of Psychiatry, University of Copenhagen, and Director of research, Psychological Institute, Copenhagen Municipal Hospital, Copenhagen, Denmark.

FINI SCHULSINGER, M.D., Professor of Psychiatry, University of Copenhagen, Denmark and Secretary General, World Psychiatric Association.

VICTOR W. SWAYZE, M.D., Assistant Professor of Psychiatry, Department of Psychiatry, University of Iowa, Iowa City, Iowa U.S.A.

MICHELE TANSELLA, M.D., Professor of Medical Psychology and Director, South-Verona Mental Health Centre, Institute of Psychiatry, University of Verona, Verona, Italy.

NICHOLAS TARRIER, M.SC., PH.D., Top Grade Clinical Psychologist and Head of District Services (Psychology), District Department of Clinical Psychology and Chairman, District Services Management Team, Mental Health Unit, Salford District Health Authority, Prestwich Hospital, Manchester, United Kingdom.

ANTONIO VELA-BUENO, M.D., Professor, Department of Psychiatry, Autonomous University and Director, Massachusetts Institute de España, Madrid, Spain.

XIA ZHENYI, M.D., Professor, Department of Psychiatry, Shanghai Medical University and Honorary Director, Shanghai Mental Health Center, Shanghai, The People's Republic of China.

Part I
Conceptualization
of Schizophrenia

1
Schizophrenia:
Historical Perspectives

ANTHONY KALES, JOYCE D. KALES, AND
ANTONIO VELA-BUENO

[Whereas mental aberrations have been described throughout history, and even inferred in prehistoric times, psychiatry as a distinct medical discipline and the birth of the nosological concepts of schizophrenia are both only about two centuries old.][However, before these relatively recent systematic and scientific efforts to study mental disorders, one can find references and descriptions pertaining to mentally ill individuals that date back to early civilizations.][1-10] [An understanding of diseases of the mind seems to have rested in general on prevailing religious, social, and philosophical views of behavior, reason, and human volition.][Nonetheless, there were numerous efforts to classify descriptively symptoms and syndromes and to propose hypotheses concerning causation that provide interesting historical links to our contemporary systems of classification and theories of etiology.[2]]

[It is probable that in ancient times what we now call schizophrenia was subsumed under the two terms used to describe most mental diseases: mania and melancholia.][11,12] [Mania was in the classical world a term equivalent to madness, and it was defined by the presence of excitement, aggression, rage, and lack of control.][Thus, it is possible that catatonic excitement and acute schizophrenic episodes were included in this definition.][Melancholia served to describe conditions of reduced behavioral activity, hallucinations, paranoia, and even demented states.][Although it is likely that many of these states correspond to what we now call psychotic depression, others correspond to the current definition of schizophrenia.]

The term "schizophrenia" was introduced by Bleuler in his 1911 book, *Dementia Praecox or the Group of Schizophrenias*.[13] He built on concepts that had been developing for more than 100 years.[14] [For a number of centuries before that time persons who we now describe as suffering from schizophrenia were variously considered to be possessed by evil spirits, endowed with special prophetic powers, affected by witchcraft, and much less frequently considered to be mentally ill.][1,5-7] However, a review of ancient medical writings indicates an awareness even in these early times that mental illnesses are diseases, as are other illnesses, and have naturalistic causes.

Our attempts to comprehend the evolving views of mental illness, and especially to define what schizophrenia is, can be better understood as we review attempts to interpret irrational and psychotic phenomena within a historical context. Thus, this chapter provides a historical review of mental illness in general and schizophrenia.

Prehistoric Times

The study of mental illness among prehistoric people can be assessed only indirectly by examining and speculating about the archaeologic evidence of now extinct cultures and by studying certain primitive tribes that currently inhabit remote regions of the earth.[1,6,7] Fieldwork must be done by research teams with diverse skills and knowledge and often must rely on scanty remnants and ruins to reconstruct a complex picture of the culture.[5,15] Thus, it is not surprising that little objective data exist on the nature of and attitudes toward mental illness and the type of care provided among these early people.

There emerges, however, a recurring theme regarding the concept of mental illness as well as physical illness among these early tribes. This common thread is the belief that there exists some external, malignant, and supernatural force that invades the body, creating symptoms and affecting behavior so that the afflicted individual is seen as only a host for the invading spirit.[3,5] Clearly the hallucinations and delusions of the schizophrenic person would seem to represent an external force; this would be particularly true in the case of persecutory or abusive voices. Mental illness often was considered by these tribes to be the gods' spell or punishment for violation of taboos or being neglectful of rituals. Explanations of this sort are believed to be particularly frequent in illnesses featuring extreme behavioral changes.[3,5]

In accordance with these religious beliefs, "possession" of the individual became the focus of rituals that were performed with the hope of removing or exorcizing a malicious spirit or inviting a benevolent spirit to restore the afflicted person's original behavior. Typically, their rituals included chanting, dancing, application or ingestion of herbal medicines, and manipulation of magic objects, all directed at the invading spirit rather than the afflicted person.[5,7] In some instances the shaman, who was thought to possess special powers and was the ritual leader, would arrange for the disease to be transferred to a scapegoat or sacrificial animal or symbolically expelled by dramatically plucking some object such as a stone from his own mouth. The concept of shamanism is one that persists today, providing considerable evidence for informed speculation about preliterate cultures and their view of the mentally ill.[5,7]

The practice of trepanation, whose beginning can be traced to the end of the Paleolithic period, was common during the Neolithic period.[5,16,17] This surgical procedure involved actually boring a hole into the skull and removing bone. Anthropologists postulated that the purpose of this procedure was either to liberate evil spirits or to allow or facilitate entry of healing spirits.[5,17] Support for this theory is provided by the continued use of this procedure over time (Figure 1.1) and even today among some undeveloped cultures for the treatment of epilepsy, retardation, and mental illness.

Dawn of Civilization

Our understanding of the concepts of mental illness among the world's earliest literate cultures comes from writings and other remnants of early Middle Eastern and Eastern civilizations.[1,5,7] Reconstruction of these societies by researchers reveals strong evidence for the intertwining of psychological and religious concepts, blurring the definition needed to identify and study mental illness among these peoples.

The early Egyptian people strived for a balance between what they con-

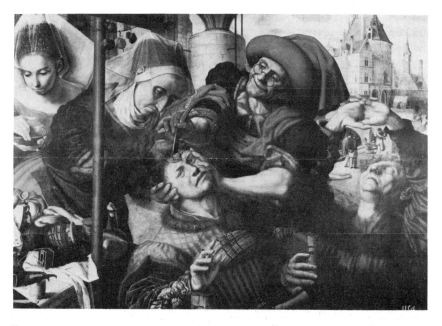

FIGURE 1.1. The Extraction of the "Stone of Madness" by Sanders Hemessen (1500?–1566). Reprinted with permission. Copyright © by Museo del Prado, Madrid.

sidered to be internal and external powers and focused on the cycles of life from birth to death. They were influenced deeply by what they perceived as supernatural events, particularly attempts at communication with the departed spirit. This communication was achieved during sleep in a healing process termed incubation. Integration of body, mind, and spirit through the power of benevolent forces was the focus of treatment for mental illness.[1,5,18]

Among the early Indians there was clear differentiation between the mind and the brain and belief that the soul never dies.[1,5,7,10] Hindu medicine considered the heart to be the site of mental activity. Constitutional imbalance caused by an excess of passion or of darkness was thought to cause mental illnesses. These illnesses, considered as endogenous or exogenous, seem to correspond to what we know today as schizophrenic (hebephrenic, paranoid, and catatonic) and manic-depressive disorder.[5,8,19,20] Magic formulas, chanting, fasting, "divine agents" (sun, water, air), drugs (including rauwolfia), and even sacrifices were brought to bear by the practitioners of Vedic medicine against the offending forces.[5,10]

Chinese culture attributed mental illness to weakness of moral character, and as early as 1,000 BC reference was made to violent behavior, convulsions, insanity, and dementia among the Chinese.[5,21] The prevailing philosophy was that mental activity is not separated from physical function and that the heart plays the role of regulator of the mind. Failure to observe filial piety and loss of face were considered major causes of mental illness. The spirits of the ancestors were appeased through special ceremonies conducted by priests. There is some evidence that nonviolent, afflicted individuals who did not respond to attempts at restoring psychic balance were left to wander the countryside.[5,21]

Abundant evidence of the awareness of mental disorder in the Judaic culture is documented in the Talmud and the Old and New Testaments.[1,5,7,22] Madness, with symptoms such as those associated with schizophrenia and manic-depressive psychosis, and other mental conditions such as epilepsy were attributed to evil spirits and moral turpitude and were not well differentiated. There prevailed a fatalistic attitude that mental illness was punishment for wrongdoing or visited upon one by divine decree.[1,5,7,23] Among the Judaic community views of mental illness varied greatly, ranging from an enlightened attitude to one of prejudice, neglect, and even hostility.[1]

Ancient Times

Our knowledge concerning mental illness in ancient Greek and Roman culture is derived from writings, archaeological investigations, myths handed down over the centuries, and popular folklore.[5,7] As with other early civilizations, many persons afflicted with madness or bizarre behavior were presumed to be possessed by evil spirits emanating from the gods, whereas others were regarded as objects of reverence or sacredness.[1,5,7,24] Because the mentally ill person was viewed as being punished by the gods, he was not held legally responsible for his actions; however, he might be banished from his town or made to undergo a religious purification.[5,7] Because mental illness was believed to have spiritual causes, it is understandable that the ancient priests often made recommendations concerning a humanitarian approach to treatment; about the ninth century BC kindness was recommended as well as physical and recreational activities to assist the ill person with his or her affliction.[3]

Despite these earlier popular, supernaturally held views regarding mental disorder, the Greeks later in about the sixth century BC began to study mental disorder from a naturalistic standpoint. Thus, in Greek medical literature, mental phenomena are separated from religious influences.[6,25] In the fourth century BC, Hippocrates' writings included madness as being caused by excesses of the four bodily humors—blood, yellow bile, black bile, and phlegm. Temperament and personality were regulated through the balance of the humors, and one's emotional responses might be sanguine, choleric, melancholic, or phlegmatic.[1,2,25,26] Hippocrates wrote about mania, melancholia, phrenitis, and also applied the term paranoia. In his writings, the natural origins of mental illness are emphasized and the brain is the seat of the human ability to feel, think, and dream.[3,6] Hippocrates states:

Men ought to know that from nothing else but thence (from the brain) come joys, delights, laughter, and sports; and sorrows, griefs, despondency, and lamentations . . . by the same organ we become mad and delirious, and fears and terrors assail us, some by night and some by day. . . . All these things we endure from the brain when it is not healthy.[5,26]

Aristotle also believed that sensory and affective disturbances were caused by temperature changes of the black bile.[5,7] This widely held theory of vital fluids was later rejected by the Greco-Roman physician Asclepiades who delineated phrenitis (mental excitement with fever), mania (with continuous excitement and without fever), and melancholia.[5,7,27] Asclepiades, as well as the Roman Celsus, suggested a psychotherapeutic approach including use of treatment modalities such as music and intellectual stimulation, as well as working with groups of mentally afflicted persons.[1,5,7,25]

In Greek tragedies madness is often portrayed, and repeatedly there are key protagonists afflicted with madness,[5,24,28] such as Ajax,[29] Heracles,[30] Orestes,[31] and Pentheus.[28] Plato's writings also elaborated on four types of "divine" madness: prophetic, ritual, poetic, and erotic.[5,24,32] Aristotle described emotions such as fear, anger, and joy and recognized the therapeutic function of arousing and releasing repressed feelings; he noted that music and the theater were thus often cathartic of emotions.[1,2,5,25] He defined tragedy as: "an imitation of action which commands serious attention . . . and by means of pity and fear producing the purgation (Katharsis) of such emotions."[33] Accordingly, Aristotle believed that the release of expression of emotions through theater was a way of gaining emotional balance and stability. Besides catharsis through the theatre, he recommended the application of wine, music and aphrodisiacs as effective in treating mental disorder, particularly melancholia.[5]

Under Roman rule, the culture of Greece continued to hold sway and included many of the theories held by the Greeks concerning madness.[5,6] Although the influence of the humors continued to be held to be important, writers such as Celsus placed an emphasis on the passions or emotions as the essential causative factor as well as the essential treatment consideration for the mental patient. In his work, *De Re Medica*, he discussed mental disorders and described the importance of treatment techniques, some of which were harsh or restrictive or used fright to restore a mentally ill person to his senses.[1,6] Seneca, in the first century AD, emphasized the role of reason for correct human behavior and stressed that the passions or emotions per se should be differentiated from mental diseases.[5]

The great physician Galen, also writing in the first century AD, was strongly influenced by Hippocratic writings and espoused the doctrine of the four humors. In cases of melancholia, the excess of bile needed to be released through phlebotomy or the use of cathartics.[2,5] Additionally, Galen elaborated on types of melancholia such as paranoia, resulting from false sensory impressions, and dysthymia, including fear and despair. Galen also suggested the therapeutic effect of sexual activity on hysterical symptoms which he thought were caused by sexual abstinence.[5,34]

While the common attitude toward the mentally ill continued to be neglect, there were notable exceptions. Among these was Soranus at the beginning of the second century AD who applied humanitarian treatment to the management of the mentally disturbed.[1,5,25] A milieu was provided in which disturbing stimuli were eliminated. Those caring for patients were taught to be kind and sympathetic, and, when possible, those with mental illness were encouraged to participate in reading and group meetings in a type of experience that seemed to be a forerunner of psychodrama, using tragedy for mania and comedy for depression. In his admonitions to these attendants, Soranus also cautioned them, "The room should be perfectly quiet, unadorned by paintings, not lighted by low windows, and on the ground floor rather than on the upper stories, for victims of mania have often jumped out of windows."[35]

When dynamic psychiatry appeared in the twentieth century, there was great interest in reviewing the therapeutic methods used by the ancients including the interpretation of dreams, incubation techniques, and therapy with words or psychotherapy based on a relationship with the healing person.[1,36,37] Plato's writings stressed the beneficial effect of harmony between body, psyche, and soul.[5] Thus, the importance placed by the ancients on the necessary conditions for health, which would include the spiritual condition, the physical condition, and the psychological condition,[25] would seem to be instructive to the present state of our understanding of the approach to schizophrenia. This approach requires an integration of these most important components, to gain an understanding of the biological as well as of the psychosocial environment of the schizophrenic patient.

Medieval Times

An accurate account of the approach to and treatment of schizophrenia in medieval times is complicated by the fragmentary nature of references, which are primarily religious and superstitious in scope.[1,5,7] In addition, with Christianity established as the official religion of the Roman Empire by Constantine in approximately 300 AD, the study of Plato, Aristotle, and pagan philosphers and physicians was forbidden. Furthermore, with the short life span due to plagues and epidemics as well as chronic illnesses and extremely high infant mortality, medicine had little to offer aside from prognosis. Christians could only hope for paradise after death, and sought the salvation of their souls which only the church could provide.[38]

The understanding and treatment of the mentally ill was thus a spiritual matter and influenced by the superstitions and preoccupation concerning the devil that was part of the times.[6] The writings of St. Augustine in the fourth century detailed his life of excess and his conversion. In his *Confessions,* he emphasized psychological introspection and self-analysis.[1,2,39] However, most other theological works stressed the role of the devil and his legions having the ability to enter into men or women and execute their evil powers.[38] Because there was no scientific understanding of mental or physical illness or natural disasters, and no effective remedies, it is understandable that witchcraft offered a plausible explanation and solution. Certainly persons who were mentally ill exhibited symptoms suggestive of witchcraft or demonic possession, which then led to the death sentence. The usual punishment was to be burned alive in public.[38] Symptoms of delusions and hallucinations, bizarre postures and speech, written and artistic productions, as well as imagining being possesed were all supportive of accusations of witchcraft.

Several writers, however, caution against stereotypic thinking that the middle ages were uniformly characterized by beliefs that mental illness was caused by sin.[40-43] There is evidence in medieval sources to indicate an awareness that mental illness could be due to humoral imbalance, diet and alcohol intake, excessive work, or grief due to loss. The practical view then, as now, included everyday experiences in the understanding of mental disorder.[41,44] A notable example of humane treatment was the colony of Gheel, established toward the end of the sixth century and still located in presentday Belgium.[5,7,45] Here, mental patients came to pray at the shrine of St. Dymphna to be relieved of the spirit of evil. When healing was not immediately achieved and as more pilgrims came awaiting a miracle, the compassionate population of Gheel began to provide lodging and shelter in their homes and thus established a form of family treatment.

In Arab countries as well as those with Arabic influence, for example, Spain, physicians were free to build upon the ideas of the Greek and the Roman classical writers as well as absorb certain Christian influences.[1] The study of medicine continued in the tradition of Hippocrates, Aristotle, and Galen. Although there is scant specific knowledge about the Arabs' understanding of mental illness, according to the Prophet, the insane person, rather than being possessed by evil, was beloved of God and thus selected to tell the truth. Among the Arabs, asylums for the benevolent care of the mentally ill were founded between the eighth and thirteenth centuries in Bagdad, Damascus, Aleppo, Cairo, Fez, and Kalaoma.[1,5]

Renaissance

The early Renaissance period beginning in the thirteenth century ushered in a revival of teaching from classical times, and great universities were established in England, Spain, France, Italy, and elsewhere.[1,5,7] Notable teachers of scholastic philosophy included Albert the Great and his pupil St. Thomas Aquinas who both incorporated the writings of Hippocrates and Galen, as well as the Arabic physicians, into Christian teaching.[1] They rejected the idea that the soul or spirit could become sick, thus, insanity was regarded as a somatic disease.[5] Mental illness occurred because of a deficiency in the use of logic which could be caused by an excess of powerful emotions or because of alteration of the physical state such as through dreams or intoxication. A number of psychotic symptoms, including hallucinations as well as loss of memory and epilepsy, were described by Aquinas. From a legal standpoint, persons with mental illness were unable to distinguish right from wrong. Thus, their responsibility for crimes was absolved. Humane procedures such as baths and sleep were recommended.

However, by the middle of the thirteenth century, the Inquisition was established to eliminate heresy leading to an interference with independent thought.[7] There appeared to be a preoccupation with sexuality as a particular manifestation of the influence of demons, in that it was believed that demons could enter into sexual relationship with those possessed.[6,7] Thus, a man or woman who had an erotic dream could believe that a demon, the devil himself, or a witch had come during the night and had sexual intercourse with him or her. Apparently exorcism was widely practiced as a form of treatment.

The most well-known treatise on witchcraft was *Malleus Maleficarum (The Witch's Hammer)* by two Dominican monks, Sprenger and Kramer, appearing in 1486. The book, which became the authoritative text for the Inquisition, included lewd sexual details, and, because the majority of witches proved to be women, was also grossly antifemale.[7] It was a reaction to the growing social and political instability of Christian Western Europe and was the official textbook approved by the church authorities for proof of existence, description, and legal persecution of witches.[7] The authors recognized the existence of mental illness, but they regarded it as only of supernatural origin; that is, phenomena such as auditory and visual hallucinations were due to the devil's possession.[46] Zilboorg suggests that many people burned at the stake represented cases of schizophrenia, senility, syphilitic insanity, and involutional melancholia.[5,7]

Several individuals who held more humanistic and enlightened views both concerning the status of women and those with mental disorders stand out in opposition of the generally held beliefs in witchcraft. Paracelsus, writing in 1520 on the *Diseases Which Lead to a Loss of Reason,* maintained that mental disturbances are natural diseases and not due to possession by demons.[2,46] Paracelsus also was among the first to note a hereditary tendency in mental disorder.[2,46,47] Vives advocated the education of women, and subsequently wrote a treatise on more humanistic views toward the poor suggesting that particular care be given to those who were sick from mental illness and recommended the building of special hospitals to treat compassionately "so great a disaster to the health of the human mind."[2,5,46] Johann Wyer, writing in 1563, also opposed the beliefs of supernatural possession by demons describing them as "absurd" and explained mental disorders from a psychological standpoint.[48] Considered by many to be the first psychiatrist, his clinical experience permitted him to outline the symptoms of psychoses, epilepsy, nightmares, delusions, paranoia, and depression. Wyer's ability to study mental phenomena with an open mind, free from the prejudice of his day, placed him ahead of his time.[42]

Despite the popular beliefs and practices concerning witchcraft and demons, several institutions were established for the humane care of mental patients in a number of places throughout Europe: in Metz in 1100, Uppsala in 1305, Bergamo in 1325, Florence in 1385, and Valencia in 1409.[5,45,49] It is unknown whether patients in mental hospitals uniformly received adequate care, because these patients were commonly placed on exhibition at places like Bethlehem Hospital in London up until the nineteenth century.[7]

The physician Paolo Zacchia in 1650 advocated that a physician rather than priests or lawyers should evaluate disturbed patients and assess their responsibility for their behavior.[2] Undoubtedly, numerous individuals with schizophrenia were judged as devil possessed and burned at the stake, condemned to jail, or kept chained at home.[9] The term "lunatic," relating aberrant behavior to the moon's influence, gained general use by the fifteenth century.[42] The neuroanatomist Thomas Willis, who described the circle of Willis, appears to have described mentally ill young adults with dementia praecox, who from a childhood status of intelligence and attractiveness became dull and physically ungraceful in young adulthood.[50] Nonetheless, Willis also adhered to a belief in possession by the devil and the use of harsh treatments for those with mental disorders that included threats, chains, and physical abuse as a part of the medical treatment to induce the mind to give up irrational ideas.[6]

Era of Enlightenment

The Eighteenth Century

By the seventeenth and eighteenth centuries, the Copernican Revolution brought a changing concept of the world with a decline in astrological beliefs and superstition. The work of scientists, such as Harvey with circulation and Galvani with physiology, and philosophers, such as Descartes in psychology and philosophy, led to a more rational and scientific approach to diseases and the study of the mind. Thus, the empiricism and rationalism that dominated the picture during the seventeenth century had a strong impact on the eighteenth century zeitgeist.[1] The beginning of scientific psychiatry can be dated to this period. The study of mental disorders reflected the two main trends in medical thinking; first, the concept of an organic etiology of disease and second, in parallel with advances in the natural sciences, the development of taxonomy in medicine.

The origin of the concept of an organic etiology in medicine can be traced back to the work of the Italian pathologist Giovanni Battista Morgagni.[51] He maintained that diseases have an organic basis, a conviction that dominated the field of clinical medicine in this epoch. Thus, many physicians interested in understanding the origin of mental disease began a persistent but unsuccessful search for brain lesions underlying mental disease. For example, outstanding psychiatrists, such as the Frenchman, Philippe Pinel, believed that the basis of mental derangement might be a lesion in the central nervous system.[52]

The rapid accumulation of data and observations throughout this period made systematization and classification of mental disorders necessary. William Cullen was the author of a comprehensive attempt at classification of mental disorders, in which he was the first to use the term "neurosis" to refer to diseases without fever or localized pathology. He thought "neurosis" was due to a decay either of the intellect or of the voluntary or involuntary nervous system. He subdivided neurosis into comata (conditions such as stroke), adynamiae (alterations of the involuntary or autonomic nervous system), spasmi (disturbances of voluntary muscles such as convulsions), and vesaniae (intellectual impairment).[1]

During the second part of the eighteenth century, description and classification of mental disorders according to their symptoms was attempted. Noteworthy are Pinel's descriptions of the alterations of different psychological functions (such as memory, attention, judgment, and thought).[52,53] His system was simple and practical, and divided psychotic illnesses into melancholias, manias without delirium, manias with delirium, and dementia (ie, intellectual deterioration and idiocy).[52]

Other scientists attempted to classify mental disorders according to their origin. William Battie, an English author, classified them into those that were due to an "internal disorder" (we would call them today endogenous), and those that were due to extrinsic or exogenous factors. Although he recognized that the exogenous illnesses resulted from brain damage, he did not consider that some mental illness might derive from life experiences.[54] At variance with Battie's view, Pinel thought that in addition to hereditary vulnerability, deficiencies in education or different passions could lead to mental derangement. Thus, he was convinced that mental illness resulted from a combination of both heredity and life experiences.[52]

Besides his clinical contributions, Pinel became known for his efforts to reform the generally inhumane outlook in the treatment of mental patients. Along with other psychiatrists, both in Europe and America, Pinel transformed the madhouses into hospitals, where he advocated moral treatment. For example, he reformed two important mental hospitals in France at the time of the French Revolution: Bicetre in 1793 and 2 years later the Salpetrière. In both hospitals, patients were released from their chains, treated kindly, and fed appropriately.[1,7]

In summary, throughout this period the care of mental patients developed in a way that can be considered both more scientific and compassionate. There was a break from the magic and inhumane practices of previous periods.

The Nineteenth Century

During the nineteenth century, psychiatry was consolidated as a medical specialty. Advances made in the previous century planted the seeds for the development of the concept of schizophrenia as well as other mental disorders as clinical entities. Three factors had a decisive influence in the description, identification, and classification of the diagnostic categories as we know them today: development of the clinicoanatomical view, evolution of a psychological definition of behavior, and changes that occurred in taxonomy.[55]

During the first half of the century, the nosographic trend initiated by Pinel was continued by his students, most notably Jean Etienne Dominique Esquirol. He made outstanding contributions to clinical psychiatry with precise descriptions of symptoms and syndromes. He introduced the term hallucinations, differentiated them from illusions, and also proposed a classification of mental illnesses based on affective monomania or disturbance in a particular aspect of behavior.[56]

Esquirol's students continued this tradition, and two of them, Jean Pierre Falret[57] and Jules Baillarger,[58] labelled what later was to be classified as manic-depressive psychosis, with the terms "folie circulaire" and "folie a double forme," respectively. Another clinician of this school, Etienne Georget, described with great precision a severe form of psychosis that might correspond to what later became known as hebephrenia.[1]

In general, it can be said that the descriptive work accomplished by the school initiated by Pinel and continued by Esquirol laid the foundation for the nosology of the second half of the century, as developed by several German psychiatrists.[59] Pinel and his students, in addition to their nosological contributions, implemented hospital reform and contributed to the development of forensic psychiatry.[1,7]

Description of symptoms, patterns of behavior, and syndromes was eclectic, and there was no attempt to correlate them with disorders of personality. With the beginning of the nineteenth century and the many movements toward social reform, a new trend in psychiatry emerged as part of the general romantic and idealistic reaction against the rationalism of the previous period.[1] Certain psychiatrists of the romantic period emphasized the subjective aspects of mental processes. This resulted, from a descriptive standpoint, in an important contribution; it added a new dimension to the study of overt behavior.[55]

An outstanding representative of this school of psychiatry was Jacques-Joseph Moreau de Tours.[60] A student of Esquirol, he proposed a more dynamic approach to psychopathology by attempting to understand clinical manifestations as expressions of malfunctioning of personality. He stressed the importance of introspection and also gave paramount importance to dreams in the understanding of disordered mental functions. Finally, he suggested a similarity between dreams and psychotic manifestations such as delirium.

Moreau de Tours had a number of German counterparts. One of them Johann Christian Reil, a brain anatomist, published the first book on psychotherapy in 1803.[1,7] He clearly described the interaction between psychological and physiological phenomena. Similarly, the psychiatrist Johann Christian Heinroth advanced ideas analogous to those found years later in Freud's work.[61] He also was the first to use the term "psychosomatic."

However, all of the ideas and other psychodynamic postulates that began to emerge in the first part of the nineteenth century were obscured by the observations and ideas of the "new wave" of organicists and clinical psychiatrists of the second half of the century. Scientific medicine was profoundly influenced by major advances in several fields. For example, advances in microbiology by Pasteur, the formulation of the tissue theory of disease by Bichat, and the cell theory of pathology by Virchow, all had a major impact in the second half of the century. In this context, there was an emphasis on relating mental disease with brain lesions and dysfunctions. This was the beginning of the era of neuropsychiatry.[1]

Wilhelm Griesinger is often considered the most outstanding neuropsychiatrist.[62] His major claim was that all mental diseases should be regarded as brain diseases. However, at this time, only in individuals with syphilitic general paralysis was there any evidence of brain lesion; that is, in 1822 Bayle described chronic arachnoiditis in paretic patients.[63] Thus, Griesinger was representative of a clinical movement that minimized the value of psychological concepts in the understanding of mental diseases and considered them the result of abnormal brain states.[62]

Brilliant neurologists and psychiatrists such as Karl Westphal, Theodore Meynert, and Karl Wernicke continued Griesinger's endeavors of finding brain structural lesions or dysfunctions in different clinical syndromes.[7] Important discoveries included those of Wernicke, who, for example, found amnesia for recent events in organic brain syndrome patients.

Three groups of clinical entities maintained the hope of finding an organic basis for all mental diseases by psychiatrists from the organic school. These clinical disorders were the toxic psychoses, especially the alcoholic, the infections such as syphilis, and the dementing states. However, due to the lack of diagnostic technologies, the organic basis would continue to be limited to these three types of disorders for many years. Thus, physicians turned their attention to the natural history of diseases by observing their clinical courses over time.

At this time, neurologists were involved in developing a neurologic taxonomy based on clinicopathological correlations.[1] Under the influence of their neurological colleagues, neuropsychiatrists using the same model attempted to develop a psychiatric nosology based on the existing descriptions of previous years. Whereas taxonomy during the eighteenth century was inspired by the principles of natural sciences, such as botany, the classifications of the nineteenth century were based on empirical methods. These included symptom comparison, analysis of frequency distributions, and etiological speculations. In this way, natural history also was incorporated.[55]

In the middle of the century the idea of the unitary psychosis was maintained by distinguished psychiatrists such as Griesinger, whose professor, Albert Zeller was the first to formulate this theory in a clear way.[64] He maintained that there is only one fundamental process: madness. Melancholia, mania, delusional insanity, and vesanic dementia were successive stages of the same process. This idea of an unitary psychosis can be explained, at least in part, as a reaction of some psychiatrists to the limited usefulness of the complex classifications of the time.[55]

During the nineteenth century it became clear that three groups of mental functions (intellectual, emotional, and volitional) could be disturbed separately. The "intellectual insanities" were the primordial forms of schizophrenia and paranoia.[55]

The Beginning of the Concept of Schizophrenia

In the decade of 1850, Benedict Augustin Morel described what he called "demence précoce," a progressive deterioration evolving quickly in young persons. He did not suggest that it was a distinct nosologic entity, but he thought the condition was the result of a progressive degeneration in the family, with successive generations showing gradually more severe impairment until the family became extinct.[65]

In 1863 Karl Ludwig Kahlbaum in his work, *Grouping of Psychic Diseases*, attempted to move beyond a description of "symptom complexes" and arrived at more precise diagnoses based on onset, course, and outcome.[66] He initially described a clinical entity he called hebetic paraphrenia, characterized by an insidious onset in young individuals, that after a protracted clinical course led to alienation. Some years later he added a related disorder, characterized by the predominance of disturbed muscle tone, stupor, and a tendency to adopt bizarre postures and attitudes. He called the disorder "catatonia" and considered its motor manifestations as a direct result of brain dysfunction.[67]

In 1871, Ewald Hecker, a student of Kahlbaum, wrote what is considered a masterful description of hebephrenia. The disorder, starting in puberty, evolved rapidly through successive episodes of melancholia, mania, and confusion, ultimately resulting in a state of psychological weakness and mental deficiency.[68] Years later, Christian described the same disease with a rapid evolution to dementia.[69] In 1880, Fink described some cases that presented with both catatonic and hebephrenic symptoms, which until then were considered as manifestations of two different syndromes.[70] The term hebephrenia survived controversies and polemics, and one can find it as a clinical form in contemporary classifications.

In 1885, Kahlbaum described heboidophrenias, a group of syndromes similar to hebephrenia but with certain unique characteristics. They appeared in subjects slightly older than those suffering from hebephrenia and were characterized by moral perversity, distorted behavior, and psychological failure, with little tendency to progressive worsening. Hereditary factors were considered to be crucial in the etiology.[64]

Emil Kraepelin took from Kahlbaum the ideas about catatonia and used the term dementia praecox, taken from Morel, to define quite precisely Hecker's description of hebephrenia.[64] Kraepelin was the one to unify several states in which catatonia, apathy, and various types of delusions were present in variable proportions in one disease.[64] He initially thought the disease was a hereditary condition and later that it was related to a metabolic derangement and more specifically to an "autotoxin."[64]

In 1883, the first edition of Kraepelin's *Kompendium der Psychiatrie* appeared.[71] In its sixth edition (1899), Kraepelin devoted a chapter to dementia praecox and included three clinical varieties: hebephrenic, catatonic, and paranoid (including paranoid dementia and paranoia).[69] The three clinical forms could occur in the same patient. The clinical picture was characterized by thought blocking, negativism, impaired judgment, a decrease in psychological productivity, motor impairment, loss of energy, and affective worsening.

After receiving numerous criticisms, especially from French psychiatrists, for including paranoia among the clinical types of dementia praecox, Kraepelin created a new term to define the clinical presentations mimicking paranoia. He called them paraphrenias, with two main varieties: the systematic (ie, well-organized delusions) and the nonsystematic (i.e., expansive, confabulatory, and fantastic).[69]

Also, Kraepelin differentiated dementia praecox from other organic psychoses and from those considered to be functional, that is, the manic-depressives. The main differentiating feature between manic-depressive disorder and dementia praecox was the evolution of the latter to a demented state. He placed the disease in the realm of the endogenous disorders, a concept he took from Moebius.[72]

Eugen Bleuler,[13] introduced the term schizophrenia and made important contributions to the knowledge of this disease. He challenged many of the Kraepelinian notions; Bleuler not only changed the name of dementia praecox to schizophrenia, but also the general approach to this clinical entity. Bleuler put the main emphasis on content and less on etiology, clinical presentation, or outcome.[13]

Although he always supported the notion that schizophrenia had an organic etiology, Bleuler insisted that the psychological aspect of this illness should be studied.[73] He worked together with C. G. Jung and tried to determine the psychodynamic dimensions of the schizophrenic.[74] Under the influence of psychoanalytic thinking he paid more attention to the unconscious symbolic aspects of thought; he described these primitive processes as "autistic thinking." He claimed these processes were similar to dreaming, were archaic, and did not follow the laws of logic. They were characterized by wishful symbolic thinking that was not influenced by reality.[73]

Bleuler proposed that there is more than one type of schizophrenia. All these types have a common psychopathology, that is, an affective–intellectual split. In schizophrenia (literally means split mind) some psychological processes are abnormal, whereas other remain intact even many years after the onset of the disease.[13] Bleuler suggests that as a consequence of the split in the psychological functions of these patients, there would be an interiorization of psychic life and a loss of contact with the social environment. He called this autism.[13] Also, these patients have in common ambivalence and depersonalization. He pointed out that the life experiences of the patient had a strong influence both on symptomatology and evolution of the disorder. Bleuler also believed that the name dementia praecox was misleading. The age of onset was not always precocious, and the disorder did not necessarily result in dementia.[75]

Bleuler divided the symptoms of schizophrenia according to their origin, that is, as primary or secondary.[13] Primary symptoms were direct manifestations of brain dysfunction and secondary symptoms were consequences of the affective–intellectual split. Based on the frequency of the symptoms, he further classified them into fundamental and accessory.[13] The former symptoms were loose associations, affective disturbance, ambivalence, and autism. The latter ones were, among others, hallucinations and delusions. Bleuler also added two more clinical types of schizophrenia to those described by Kraepelin;[75] the so-called simple and the latent.

In this historical overview (Table 1.1), we have been able to observe a pendulum-like oscillation of trends over time regarding mental disorder and particularly schizophrenia. Various schools of thought including reli-

TABLE 1.1. Historical perspectives on mental illness/schizophrenia.

Historical period	Predominant concept/contribution
Prehistoric times	Some malignant, supernatural force invades the body and creates symptoms
Dawn of civilization	Intertwining of psychological and religious concepts
Ancient times	Separation of mental phenomena from religious influences
Hippocrates	Madness caused by excesses of bodily humors
Aristotle	Described emotions (anger, fear, and joy, etc) and the therapeutic function of releasing feelings
Galen	Espoused the doctrine of four humors
Medieval times	Religious and superstitious beliefs leading to persecution of mentally ill
St. Augustine	Emphasized psychological introspection
Renaissance	Demonology and witchhunting *vs* mental illness due to natural causes; first psychiatric hospitals in Europe
Paracelsus	Mental disturbances are natural diseases
Wyer	Explained mental disorders psychologically
Era of enlightment	Mental disorders become a focus of medicine
Pinel	Described psychological functions, classified mental illness, introduced moral treatment
Esquirol	Differentiated hallucinations from illusions and developed a classification for mental illness
Moreau de Tours	Emphasized introspection and dreams in the understanding of mental disorders
Griesinger	Espoused an organic reductionistic approach
Development of concept of schizophrenia	Disorder of schizophrenia becomes a distinct entity
Kahlbaum	Diagnosis based on onset, course, and outcome
Hecker	Described hebephrenia
Kraepelin	Introduced the term "dementia praecox" and included three clinical types of schizophrenia: hebephrenic, catatonic, and paranoia
Bleuler	Introduced the term schizophrenia—four main symptoms described: loose associations, autism, ambivalence, and affective disturbance

gious, medical, psychological, and philosophical provided significant and often useful perspectives over the centuries. Even the "dark" ages were illuminated by strands of thought that were harbingers of future enlightenment. Generally, the level of understanding reflected the overall cultural and scientific spirit of the times. With the emergence of the biopsychosocial model introduced in 1977 by Engel,[76] strict reductionism has given way to a more comprehensive integration of the models of understanding of schizophrenia. In this spirit, the International Perspectives Series on Recent Advances in Schizophrenia encompasses an integration of the latest and most important biological and psychosocial advances from around the world.

Summary

Before the development of the concept of schizophrenia in the last two centuries, there were many efforts to describe and classify mental disorders and attempts to understand their causation. In prehistoric times, the general belief about mental aberrations was that they were a result of supernatural forces. As civilization emerged in early Middle Eastern and Eastern cultures, strong religious beliefs toward mental illness were maintained but intertwined with psychological considerations of mental dysfunction as evidenced by efforts to restore the balance of an individual through such healing processes as incubation, fasting, chanting, and the casting out of evil spirits.

Early in ancient times there were contrasting views of schizophrenia; as in earlier civilizations, persons affected with madness were presumed to be possessed by evil forces, whereas others were regarded as sacred. Later, Greek physicians recognized the naturalistic causes of mental illness, separating mental phenomena from religious influences. Hippocrates emphasized the role of bodily humors in the regulation of temperament and personality and of the brain as the seat of thinking, dreaming, and feeling. Also, early classification of mental illness was formulated, and therapeutic approaches were developed.

In medieval times, disasters and epidemics led to an emphasis on the immortality of the soul and the attainment of paradise, as opposed to a reliance on medicine. Superstitions concerning the devil and his works, dominated the perception of mental illness. Many deranged people were burned at the stake because of their delusions, hallucinations, and other bizarre behavior. Nevertheless, some awareness existed that mental illness might derive from naturalistic causes.

The Renaissance ushered in a resurgence of classical ideas, the establishment of great centers of learning, and humane approaches for the care of the mentally ill. However, the Inquisition established in the thirteenth century to eliminate heresy exacerbated preoccupation with witchcraft. The treatise, *Malleus Maleficarum,* became the basis upon which persecution of witches was legalized. The physicians Paracelsus, Vives, and Wyer stand out as exceptions to beliefs in witchcraft.

[The beginning of scientific psychiatry arose in the eighteenth century with emphasis on empiricism and rationalism. The study of mental disorders was based on a premise of organic etiology; Pinel believed that mental illness was caused by lesions of the central nervous system. Also, through reforms, maltreatment was replaced by a movement toward moral treatment.]

The concept of schizophrenia evolved from Morel's description of "demence precoce." Kahlbaum further elaborated on related clinical entities such as catatonia, and Hecker described hebephrenia. Kraepelin brought together a variety of conditions (hebephrenic, catatonic, and paranoid) with the term, dementia praecox. The term schizophrenia was first introduced by Bleuler. In addressing both the organic and the psychological aspects of the disorder, his work serves as a forerunner to our presentday awareness of the need to address both brain dysfunction and the psychosocial aspects of schizophrenia.

References

1. Alexander FG, Selesnick ST: *The History of Psychiatry: an Evaluation of Psychiatric Thought and Practice from Prehistoric Times to the Present.* New York, Harper & Row, 1966.
2. Kaplan HI, Sadock BJ: History of psychiatry, in Kaplan HI, Sadock BJ (eds): *Synopsis of Psychiatry,* ed 5. Baltimore, MD, Williams & Wilkins, 1988, pp 1–17.
3. Kolb LC, Brodie HKH: The beginnings of psychiatry, in Kolb LC, Brodie HKH (eds): *Modern Clinical Psychiatry,* ed 10. Philadelphia, WB Saunders, 1982, pp 1–7.
4. Kolb LC, Brodie HKH: Development of modern psychiatry, in Kolb LC, Brodie HKH (eds): *Modern Clinical Psychiatry,* ed 10. Philadelphia, WB Saunders, 1982, pp 8–26.
5. Mora G: Historical and theoretical trends in psychiatry, in Freedman AM, Kaplan HI, Sadock BJ (eds): *Comprehensive Textbook of Psychiatry,* ed 2. Baltimore, MD, Williams & Wilkins, 1975, vol 1, pp 1–75.
6. Zegans LS, Victor BS: Conceptual issues in the history of psychiatry, in Goldman HH (ed): *Review of General Psychiatry,* ed 2. Norwalk, CT, Appleton & Lange, 1984, pp 5–19.
7. Zilboorg G, Henry GW: *A History of Medical Psychology.* New York, WW Norton, 1941.
8. Bark NM: On the history of schizophrenia. Evidence of its existence before 1800. *NYS J Med* 1988;July:374–383.
9. Chandrasena RD: Phenomenology and nosology of schizophrenia: historical review. *Rev de Psychiatrie de l' Univ d'Ottawa* 1983;8(2):17–24.
10. Haldipur CV: Madness in ancient India: concept of insanity in *Charkara Samhita* (1st century AD). *Compr Psychiatry* 1984;25:335–344.
11. Simon B: Models of the mind and mental illness in ancient Greece: II. The Platonic model. *J Hist Behav Sci* 1972;8:389–404.

12. Diethelm O: Mania. A clinical study of dissertations before 1750. *Confina Psychiatrica* 1970;13:26–49.
13. Bleuler E: *Dementia Praecox or the Group of Schizophrenias*. New York, International Universities Press, 1950.
14. Kraepelin E: *One Hundred Years of Psychiatry*. New York, Citadel Press, 1962.
15. Ackerknecht EH: Psychopathology, primitive medicine, and primitive culture. *Bul Hist Med* 1942;14:30–67.
16. Margetts EL: Trepanation of the skull by the medicine-men of primitive cultures, in Brothwell D, Sandison AT (eds): *Diseases in Antiquity*. Springfield, IL, Charles C Thomas, 1967, pp 673–701
17. Lisowski FP. Prehistoric and early historic trepanation, in Brothwell D, Sanderson AT (eds). *Diseases in Antiquity* Springfield Il; Charles C Thomas 1967, pp 651–672.
18. Laver AB: Precursors of psychology in ancient Egypt. *J Hist Behav Sci* 1972;8:181–195.
19. Dube KC: Nosology and therapy of mental illness in Ayurveda. *Comparative Medicine East and West* 1978;6:209–228.
20. Rao AV: India, in Howells JG (ed): *World History of Psychiatry*. New York, Brunner Mazel, 1975, pp 624–649.
21. Veith I: Psychiatric thought in Chinese medicine. *J Hist Med* 1955;10:261–268.
22. Gold H: Psychiatry and the Talmud, *Jewish Heritage,* 1957;1:9–12.
23. Deuteronomy 28:28, in *The Bible*. Michigan, Zondervan Corp, 1985, p 150.
24. Robbins RA: Contributions to the history of psychology: XLVIII. ancient Greek roots of the assumptions of modern clinical psychology. *Percept Mot Skills* 1988;66:903–921.
25. Drabkin IE: Remarks on ancient psychopathology. *Isis* 1955;46:223–234.
26. Hippocrates: *The Medical Works of Hippocrates*. Oxford, Blackwell, 1950.
27. Parkin A: Neurosis and schizophrenia: I. historical review. *Psychiatr Q* 1966;40:203–216.
28. Perry R: Madness in Euripides, Shakespeare, and Kafka. *Psychoanalytic Rev* 1978;65:253–279.
29. Sophocles: Ajax, in Oates WJ, O'Neill E (eds): *The Complete Greek Drama*. New York, Random House, 1938,1:315–360.
30. Euripides: Heracles, in Oates WJ, O'Neill, (eds): *The Complete Greek Drama*. New York, Random House, 1938;1:1017–1053.
31. Aeschylus A: The choreophori, the eumenides, in Oates WJ, O'Neill E, (eds): *The Complete Greek Drama*. New York, Random House, 1938;1:167–307.
32. Dodds ER: *The Greeks and the Irrational*. Berkeley, CA, University of California Press, 1951.
33. Long AA: Aristotle, in Easterlins PE and Knox BMW (eds) *The Cambridge History of Classical Literature, I Greek literature,* 1985, Cambridge University Press, Cambridge, pp. 527–540.
34. Galen: *On the Passions and Errors of the Soul*. Columbus, Ohio State University Press, 1963.
35. Veith I: Psychiatric nosology: from Hippocrates to Kraepelin. *Am J Psychiatry* 1957;114:385–391.
36. Openheim AL: The interpretation of dreams in the ancient Near East. *Trans Am Philos Soc* 1956;46:179–373.

37. Edelstein L, Edelstein E: *Aesculapius,* vol II. Baltimore, Johns Hopkins Press, 1945.
38. Hemphill RE: Historical witchcraft and psychiatric illness in western Europe. *Proc R Soc Med* 1966;59:891–902.
39. St. Augustine: *Confessions,* Pusey EB (trans). New York, Modern Library, 1949, pp 166–167.
40. Jackson SW: Unusual mental states in medieval Europe. I. Medical syndromes of mental disorder: 400–1100 AD. *J Hist Med* 1972;27:262–297.
41. Kroll J, Bachrach B: Sin and mental illness in the Middle Ages. *Psychol Med* 1984;14:507–514.
42. Neugebauer R: Medieval and early modern theories of mental illness. *Arch Gen Psychiatry* 1979;36:477–483.
43. Schoeneman TJ: Criticisms of the psychopathological interpretation of witch hunts: a review. *Am J Psychiatry* 1982;139:1028–1032.
44. Wright E: Medieval attitudes toward mental illness. *Bull Hist Med* 1939;VII:352–356.
45. Rumbaut RD: The first psychiatric hospital of the western world. *Am J Psychiatry* 1972;128:1305–1309.
46. Evans JL: Witchcraft, demonology and Renaissance psychiatry. *Med J Aust* 1966;11:34–39.
47. Mora G: Paracelsus' psychiatry: on the occasion of the 400th anniversary of his book *"Diseases that Deprive Man of His Reason"* (1567). *Am J Psychiatry* 1967;124:803–814.
48. Mora G: On the 400th anniversary of Johann Weyer's *"De Praestigiis Daemonum"*—its significance for today's psychiatry. *Am J Psychiatry* 1963;120:417–428.
49. Chatel J, Joe B: Psychiatry in Spain: past and present. *Am J Psychiatry* 1975;132:1182–1186.
50. d'Estrube P: Diagnostic labels in the history of schizophrenia. *Can Psych Assoc J* 1966;11;356–357.
51. Lopez Piñero JM: Clinica y Patologia de la Ilustracion. Italia, in Lain Entralgo P (ed): *Historia Universal de la Medicina,* Barcelona, Salvat, 1973, vol 5. pp 79–83.
52. Pinel P: *Traite Medico-Philosophique sur L'aliénation Mentale,* ed 2. Paris, Richard, Caille et Ravier, 1801.
53. Pinel P: *Nosographie Philosophique ou la Methode de l'Analyse Appliqueé à la Medicine,* ed 6. Brosson, Paris, 1818, 2 vols.
54. Battie W: *A Treatise on Madness.* London, J Whiston and B White, 1785.
55. Berrios GE: Depressive and manic states during the nineteenth century, in Georgotas A, Cancro R, (eds): *Depression and Mania.* New York, Elsevier, 1988, pp 13–25.
56. Esquirol JED: *Mental Maladies* New York, Hafner Press 1965.
57. Falret JP: Memoire sur la folie circulaire. *Bulletin de l'Academia de Medicine* 1854;19:382–415.
58. Baillarger JGF: De la folie a double-forme. *Annales Medico Psychologiques* 1854;6:367–391.
59. Gracia D, Espino JA: Desarrollo histórico de la Psiquiatría, in Gonzalez de Rivera GJL, Vela Bueno A, Arana J, (eds): *Manual de Psiquiatria.* Madrid, Karpos, 1980, pp 3–37.

60. Bollotte G: Moreau de Tours (1804–1884). *Confrontations Psychiatriques* 1973;11:9–26.
61. Heinroth JC: *Lehrbuch der Storungen des Seelenlebens* (original version 1818), Schmorak J (trans). Baltimore, Johns Hopkins Press, 1975.
62. Griesinger W: Mental Pathology and Therapeutics New York, Hafner Press, 1965.
63. Bayle AL: *Description of General Paralysis*. Paris, Didot le Jeune, 1822.
64. Colodrón A: *Las Esquizofrenias*. Madrid, Siglo Veintiuno de España Editores S.A. 1983.
65. Morel BA: *Traite de Dégénérescenses Physiques, Intellectuelles et Morales de L'espèce Humaine*. Paris, Bailliere, 1857.
66. Kahlbaum K: *Gruppierung der Psychischen Krankheiten*. Danzig, Kafemann 1863.
67. Kahlbaum DL: *Die Katatonie oder das Spannungsirresein*. Berlin, Hirschwald, 1874.
68. Hecker E: Die Hebephrenie. *Arch Pathol Ant Physiol Klin Med* 1871;52:394–429.
69. Guiraud P: E. Kraepelin. *Confrontations Psychiatriquez* 1973;11:83–101.
70. Fink E: Beitrag zur Kenntnis des Jugendirresins. *Allg Z Psychiat* 1880:37:490–520
71. Kraepelin E: *Kompendium der Psychiatrie*, Leipzig, Abel, 1883.
72. Mobius PJ: *Abriss der Lebre von Nervenkrankheiten*. Leipzig, Abel, 1893.
73. Bleuler E. Jung CG Komplexe and Krankheitsursachen bein Dementia praecox. *Zb. Nervenheilk Psychiat* 1908;31:220–227
74. Jung CG: *The Psychology of Dementia Praecox*, Monogr 3. New York, Nervous and Mental Diseases Publishing Co., 1936.
75. Bleuler E: Die prognose der dementia praecox (Schizophrenie gruppe). *Allg Z Psychiat* 1908;65:436–464.
76. Engel GL: The need for a new medical model: a challenge for biomedicine. *Science* 1977;196:129–136.

2
On the Concept of Schizophrenia

Costas N. Stefanis

[Schizophrenia is much more than just the most prominent word in psychiatry. Psychiatry, both as a medical discipline and as a profession, was born out of the condition that is currently known as schizophrenia.]In many respects, the development of the theory and practice of psychiatry has been determined by its effectiveness in reliably diagnosing schizophrenia, formulating plausible explanations of the symptoms, understanding its nature, and discovering effective modes of treatment. It is, therefore, worth reviewing the evolution of the concept of schizophrenia over time and relating its present state with current advances in neurosciences and clinical research.

The Concept over the Ages

The medical definition and history of schizophrenia are relatively new. It was only about 150 years ago that schizophrenia formally drew the attention of medicine.[1,2] Nonetheless, what currently is considered as schizophrenia was in existence from antiquity. It is generally assumed that melancholia in Hippocrates' time corresponds to what we now call psychotic melancholia.[3] However, many of the descriptions of melancholia referred to by Hippocrates are probably schizophrenia or mania, as we define them today, rather than psychotic depression.

The Hippocratic approach to schizophrenic and other psychotic patients was in essence a medical one as was to some extent the approach of his successors up to the time of Aretaeus the Cappadocian.[4] During the Middle Ages a purely magical, that is, nonmedical, approach to mental patients, especially those who were psychotic, was followed. Over time, changes occurred in the concept of schizophrenia with the resurgence of medical thinking about mental illness in the eighteenth century.

Pinel and Esquirol, who laid the foundation of French psychiatry, followed a purely descriptive approach to the various mental conditions and produced a detailed listing of symptoms upon which decision for hospitalization was based.[5,6] By focusing on the cross-sectional clinical picture of the patient, they were the formal initiators of the syndromal approach to mental disorders, producing a naturalistic representation of insanity (folie) and avoiding speculation on causative factors and pathogenetic mechanisms. Pinel and Esquirol allocated their mental patients into four main categories (mania, melancholia, dementia, and imbecility), drawing mostly from the taxonomic system of Boissiere de Sauvage[7] in which two of the seven major categories (delusions or errors of judgement and transient delusions) are relevant to the concept of schizophrenia. Esquirol added a separate category, the monomanias, which in contradistinction with the manias, refers to individuals who retain the integrity of their cognitive functions (folies partielles).

The historical landmark in the evolution of the illness concept of insanity was Bayle's presentation of his doctoral thesis in Paris in 1822 with the telling title "Research on Mental Illnesses."[8] He actually introduced the first genuine medical model for mental illnesses, by presenting evidence that in a number of mental patients the clinical symptomatology is associated with pathological lesions in the central nervous system and with a clinical course that develops in stages.[8] This model established the notion of patienthood for individuals with mental disorders, a model contemporary psychiatry is striving for by applying it at least in the major mental illnesses such as schizophrenia. The criteria for identification of patients with general paralysis were purely medical: symptomatology causally related to organic lesions, as well as a predictable clinical course.

During this early period in the development of psychiatric nosology no clear concept of an illness entity close to what we currently know as schizophrenia had been formulated. The rudiments of such a concept can be traced in the description of the well-known case of "demence précoce" by Morel and in the frame of his general theory of degeneration.[1] Behavioral manifestations of mental disorders within the broader theory of Morel came to be considered stigmata rather than symptoms of an illness. Morel would have provided a conceptual frame about schizophrenia much earlier than Kraepelin[9] and Bleuler,[10,11] if he had limited his theorizing only to what he considered to be the prerequisites for a particular type of mental disorder (predisposition, provoking agent to activate this predisposition and evolutionary course) and had not extended it to a Darwinian-type theory of general biological degeneration.

Morel's observations[1] were subsequently enriched by eminent French clinicians like Magnan, Lasengue, and Fahiret, who identified particular types of insanity very close to certain subtypes of schizophrenia or schizophrenia-like conditions, such as the chronic systematic delusional states and the boufée délirante.[7] Viewed from an historical perspective, the contribution of the French school of psychiatry would be considered as a fermentation process that led to the formulation of the clinical concept of schizophrenia.

The German-speaking clinicians were privileged to make use of this fermentation process and to give birth to the clinical entity of schizophrenia, as we currently conceive this condition. Kraepelin and Bleuler were the dominant figures in this task and their work continues to be used up to this day as a frame of reference, as a measure of validity, and as a starting point for new hypotheses and new theories.[9-11]

The building blocks of the synthetic concepts on schizophrenia by Kraepelin and Bleuler had been laid by several earlier German clinicians; most distinguished were Kahlbaum, who described catatonia and his assistant Hecker, who described hebephrenia[12,13] They did not limit themselves to listing symptoms, but used symptoms and behavioral manifestations to identify separate clinical entities based on their respective clinical course. Other names who preceded Kraepelin are mentioned because of the relevance of their work and theory to the current divergent views on the validity of the clinical concept of schizophrenia. Heinroth advanced the notion that there are many separate mental illnesses (he listed 48 of them) on the basis of ill-defined and confusing criteria[14] while Henrich Neumann maintained that there is only one mental illness, insanity.[15]

Griesinger actually introduced neuropsychiatry to the academic medical field.[16] Through his perceptive clinical mind not only did he advance considerably and substantially the knowledge of psychiatric disorders, but he worked out elaborate hypotheses on the origin and nature of these disorders. He advocated the unitary theory of psychosis (Einheitspsychose) and with his textbook (*Pathologie und Therapie der Psychischen Krankheiten*) lent heavy support to the concept of the organicity of psychiatric disorders and considered them as brain diseases.[16] He believed in hereditary predisposition to these illnesses, yet he viewed the psychiatric symptomatology in the context of the cultural background of the individual. He even went as far as to consider participation of psychological mechanisms and motives of which the patient was unaware in the pathogenesis of mental illness. In dealing with Griesinger's "Functional Psychoses," all schools of psychiatry today could easily find parts of his work that would fit their paradigm. He was among the first eclectics in psychiatry but nevertheless did not produce an integrative theory that would have secured a long historical survival of his contribution.

The entrance of Emil Kraepelin onto the scene of psychiatric nosology marked a turning point in clinical psychiatry.[2,9,17] It took him 30 years to elaborate his diagnostic concepts. From the first (1883) to the last (1927) edition of his "Compendium der Psychiatrie" and up to this day, Kraepelin's work has had a profound impact on the shaping of our ideas and our concepts about schizophrenia. He introduced the term "dementia praecox," defining it by three main characteristics: early onset, progressive and chronic course, and termination in dementia. On the grounds of these criteria he excluded psychotic conditions with intermittent course and with affective symptoms prevailing in the clinical picture. Thus, he introduced the concept of manic-depressive psychosis as being a separate disease entity from dementia praecox.

Kraepelin was a keen, clinical observer, not a theorist. He adhered to and advanced the medical concept of mental illnesses. He viewed them as separate from other clinical entities, primarily on the grounds of the differential course and outcome. Although delusional, hallucinatory, and catatonic symptoms were described as the outstanding features of his dementia praecox, he was quite ambivalent in proposing them as criteria with predictive value.

Emil Kraepelin is undoubtedly the father of psychiatric classification. However, when one refers to Kraepelinian concepts of diagnosis and classification, one has to be aware that his clinical concepts went through several developmental stages. The early Kraepelin firmly viewed the unremitting course and outcome as the descriptor of illness identification, while later he reported that 13% of his dementia praecox patients did not deteriorate and thus separated the paraphrenias from the main track of dementia praecox and became more lenient to the syndromal approach of mental illness. The early Kraepelin also linked schizophrenia with organic brain dysfunction and although he maintained this view, he later also considered symptomatology in the context of the patient's cultural background.

Neo-Kraepelinians is the name that has been given to those groups in the USA who developed strict diagnostic criteria for identifying mental illness mainly on the basis of presenting symptoms.[18] However, it would be more fitting to call them Neo-classics because to consider somebody as Kraepelinian—or Neo-Kraepelinian for that matter—with regard to schizophrenia, one has to conceptualize schizophrenia as an illness entity and only secondarily to adopt symptom-based criteria.

With Eugen Bleuler a new period in the conceptualization of schizophrenia began.[10,11,19] By coining in 1911 the term schizophrenia, which withstood the test of time, he focused on presenting symptoms and more specifically on those related to thought processes. He deviated substantially from the single illness entity concept of Kraepelin and in a way revived the Esquirol symptomatic and syndromal approach to understanding and diagnosing schizophrenia.

Even by the title of his monograph, "Dementia Praecox oder die Gruppen der Schizophrenien," Bleuler indicated that clinically we may deal with more than one schizophrenia of unknown but still variant origin. He pointed out that not necessarily all of them follow a deteriorating course but all of them share a common characteristic, a constellation of basic symptoms which he differentiated into primary and secondary ones. Among the basic symptoms that he considered to be rather specific and permanent, he included four groups. The first was derived from dissociation of thinking (incoherence, condensation of ideas, tendency to stereotypic thinking, poverty of ideas and other thinking disorders); the second group was derived from inappropriate affect (absence of or blunted affect, paraphrenia and paramania); the third was derived from ambivalence (in sentiments, volition, and cognition); the fourth group comprised all the descriptive features of autism. Among the accompanying and the complimentary symptoms, he listed the delusional experiences, the hallucinations and the psychomotor disturbances, because he viewed them as unspecific and not rarely encountered in other psychopathological conditions.

Thus, Bleuler produced a plausible diagnostic system for schizophrenia with criteria based solely on presenting symptoms; he did not include criteria of course and outcome nor did he include exclusion criteria. Being influenced to some extent by Freudian psychodynamic concepts, he viewed symptoms as manifestations of underlying psychological mechanisms, but he avoided binding himself to any causation theory.

Bleuler's diagnostic concepts and particularly his main or basic criteria for the diagnosis of schizophrenia were honored by clinicians all over the world but particularly by psychiatrists in the USA who expanded them by including the capacity for establishing effective interpersonal relationships. However, they were not valued as much by clinical researchers of schizophrenia, not because they were considered irrelevant but because they scored very low in reliability studies. This is reflected in the construction of the DSM-III[20] which, although basically syndromal (Bleulerian) in its approach, includes among the presenting symptoms of diagnostic significance only one of Bleuler's basic symptoms and even this is dependent on certain conditions.

Bleuler's approach to schizophrenia was further advanced by other German speaking investigators, the most eminent among them being Kurt Schneider.[21] Although Bleulerian in his approach, Schneider was not satisfied with the basic symptoms Bleuler had proposed as pathognomonic for schizophrenia. Out of his vast clinical experience and not in the context of any theoretical model, he proposed eleven symptoms of his own as pathognomonic (first rank) and a few others as complimentary (second rank) for the diagnosis of schizophrenia. According to his view the incontestable and unequivocal presence of even a single first rank symptom was an adequate criterion for identifying schizophrenia, while he did not exclude its diagnosis even in the absence of all first rank symptoms. Four of the first rank symptoms refer to disordered perceptions and sensations (audible thoughts, voices heard conversing, voices making comments on one's actions and experiences of somatic passivity). The subsequent three refer to thought disorders (stealing away one's thoughts, imposition and interference with one's thoughts and divergence of thought). The following one (delusional experiences) reserves a place in itself and the final three refer to disordered instincts, affects and volition (imposed feelings, impulses and volition).

In rating symptoms by their frequency of occurrence, ranking them in a hierarchical order and distinguishing the basic from the complimentary ones, Schneider produced a basically Bleulerian diagnostic system in which, however, symptoms described by Kraepelin for dementia praecox were preferred. The atheoretical empirical description of schizophrenic symptoms by Schneider, although challenged frequently regarding its discriminating and predictive value,[22] had a profound influence on the formulation of inclusion criteria for schizophrenia in several recently developed diagnostic systems including the ICD-9 and the DSM-III.

Among the classics who have contributed to the conceptualization of schizophrenia are Kleist [23] and Leonhard[24] of the German school. Kleist advanced the illness concept of schizophrenia in conjunction with his localization theory, viewing it as an organic brain disease due to pathological (degenerative) lesions in well-circumscribed areas of the brain. He also narrowed its nosological terrain by separating the typical schizophrenias from other schizophrenia-like conditions. His pupil Leonhard, in 1936, replaced the concept of typical schizophrenia with the concept of systematic schizophrenias including three major types (systematic hebephrenias, systematic catatonias and systematic paraphrenias) which he subdivided into a total of sixteen subtypes.

Following Kleist's inception of cycloid psychosis (Cykloide Psychosen) and based on his clinical observations and family studies, Leonhard provided empirical evidence that cycloid psychosis is a clinical entity separate from both schizophrenia and manic depressive psychosis. There are current investigators who defend its nosological validity.[25,26] However, cycloid psychosis is not included in any of the new classification systems, and it is usually conceptualized as being interchangeable with the schizoaffective disorders.

Last to be mentioned among the classics is Langfeldt[27] whose concepts about schizophrenia still exert a degree of influence on Scandinavian psychiatry and in the nomenclature of both the ICD-9[28] and DSM-III.[20] Langfeldt's approach to schizophrenia was basically Kraepelinian; he relied heavily on the course and outcome criterion for diagnosing schizophrenia. However, he introduced the notion of two types of schizophrenia: one that is equivalent to Kraepelinian dementia praecox and another that he called schizophreniform or reactive psychosis. The latter, although in terms of its symptomatology was similar to process schizophrenia, had a non-deteriorating course ending after a certain period in full recovery and often was the result of a discernible psychologically traumatic event.

Two additional features in Langfeldt's notion of schizophrenia are worth mentioning: one relates to symptomatology, in which he added "massive derealization and depersonalization" as one of the main symptoms; and the other relates to the prognostic criteria by emphasizing the dimension of personality structure. Non-schizoid, (non-schizotypal as we would have said), well-adjusted pre-morbid personality types were more likely to have a benign course (reactive psychosis) than those with process schizophrenia.

With Langfeldt, the pantheon of great clinicians who laid the foundations for the descriptive empirical approach to the schizophrenia riddle can be considered as completed. Intercepted among them, though, there are other mainly German-speaking eminent figures in European psychiatry who exerted a great influence on subsequent developments of our approaches and theories on schizophrenia. Jaspers,[29] Biswanger,[30] and Minkowski[31] founded the Central European phenomenological-existential school, and their work gave rise to the empathic understanding of the schizophrenic patient. Their theoretical proposition was to de-emphasize the formal aspects of schizophrenic symptomatology. The mainstay of their proposition was to understand and even share the patients' life experiences and to accept unquestionably these experiences in their own right without any reference to etiological factors or pathogenetic mechanisms.

Freud was a contemporary of all the classics in Europe. His views on schizophrenia fell within the framework of psychoanalytic theory that embraced all psychopathology.[32] Out of his specific references to this condition we might extract the following basic propositions. Schizophrenia is a profound deep-lying disturbance in object relations ("narcissistic psychosis"). The symptoms of schizophrenia, as those of any other psychopathological condition, are the result of the interaction of psychological defense mechanisms against anxiety resulting from unconscious conflicts deeply rooted in the person's early life experiences. The phenomenological aspects of the symptoms are important for identifying the condition, but it is mainly the content of the symptoms that carries the personal meaning of the underlying psychological processes. The developmental-regression hypothesis put forward by Melanie Klein[33] further elaborated and enriched the Freudian-psychoanalytic tenets about the pathogenesis of schizophrenia.

A great part of the psychoanalytic and psychodynamic theory was incorporated into Adolf Meyer's conceptualization of schizophrenia.[34] In the frame of his psychobiological theory, Adolf Meyer brought the individualization notion of schizophrenia to its extreme. He viewed it as a highly idiosyncratic experiential state, comprehensible only in the context of the uniqueness and the totality of each person's life. His ideas in conjunction with environmentalistic and psychosocially oriented views of several of the new Freudians, had a profound impact on the conceptualization of schizophrenia by American psychiatrists before the advent of psychopharmacology and the resurgence of interest in diagnosis and classification of mental disorders.

Current Developments in Classification

It is a capricious turn of history that all work regarding diagnostic criteria began and flourished in the USA, the country in which a rather unitary mental illness approach had prevailed for many years and where issues of diagnosis and classification were neglected and often scorned. Several factors have contributed to this change of attitude and paved the way to current developments in American and, by extension, world psychiatry.

Resurgence of Interest in Diagnosis and Classification

An important factor for the change in psychiatrists' attitudes was the advent of psychopharmacology. The new compounds were found to be differentially effective in treating various diagnotic groups of mental disorders. Thus, the therapist had to determine the appropriate diagnostic class in order to provide the patient with rational drug treatment. From this arose the issue of poor reliability of psychiatric diagnosis evidenced by a series of studies, the most notorious being the comparison of diagnostic practices in the U.K. and the USA showing that in the latter the diagnosis of schizophrenia was fourfold higher than in the former.[35]

Two other developments greatly contributed to the resurgence of interest in diagnosis and classification. One factor was the challenge to psychiatry by the anti-psychiatric movement, and another factor was the rapid progress of neurosciences providing new insights and reviving the vision of a new scientific psychiatry. In conjunction with this progress, the explosive advancement in computer technology made it possible for a huge amount of clinical data to be stored, processed, and analyzed through the use of newly developed and sophisticated statistics.

Further, social factors were involved, most notable among them the growing involvement of social care systems or third party payers with the profession of psychiatry. Not only institutions and psychiatric hospitals but private psychiatrists as well have had to be increasingly accountable. Another social factor of particular significance was the increased public concern about medical ethics and particularly those pertaining to psychiatric practice including patient commitment or enforced treatment in accordance with newly reformed laws. All this occurred in the midst of the rising movement for patients' rights and community care. Finally, there has been the need of clinical investigators to obtain homogeneous diagnostic groups of patients for research purposes.

The metric approach to psychological phenomena dates back to Galton in Great Britain in 1905.[36] In France, Binet and Simon applied successfully the principles of quantification[37,38] and actually initiated the era of psychometrics. Rating scales for psychopathology, in which scoring was derived from a selected list of symptoms, were published and used for several major mental disorders including schizophrenia.[39] These may be considered as antecedents to: the formulation of diagnostic criteria; the construction of the current classification systems for diagnosis; and the development of standardized instruments for psychiatric diagnosis such as the PSE (Present State Examination) of Wing,[40] the DIS (Diagnostic Interview Schedule) of Robins and co-workers,[41] the AMDP (Arbeitsgemeinschaft fur Methodik und Dokumentation in der Psychiatrie),[42] the SCID-R (Structured Clinical Interview for DSM-III-R),[43] and the CIDI (Composite International Diagnostic Interview).[44]

In 1972, the St. Louis group published an article titled Diagnostic Criteria for Use in Psychiatric Research. This work served to initiate the recent trend to systematize the practice of psychiatric diagnosis by introducing specific diagnostic criteria which facilitated a clear definition and subsequently, were demonstrated to have an increased reliability for the corresponding diagnostic category.[45]

The main principles for the diagnostic criteria proposed by the St. Louis group may be summarized as follows. They are agnostic or atheoretical regarding etiology and pathogenetic factors. However, the illness concept predominates; selection of symptoms have to be clinically understood and empirically validated as well as clustered in a way that leads to the formation of distinct categories with a predictive value. Moreover, the selected symptoms must maintain their distinguishing features for the category to which they belong during the entire clinical course of the condition. All these features speak for phenomenological aspects of a condition, which like physical illness is characterized by a distinct clinical picture, and imply specific, although as yet unknown, etiology and pathogenesis.

The originality and novelty of the St. Louis approach to mental disorders lies not in conceptual issues but in the systematization of the empirical clinical knowledge and subsequent formulation of diagnostic rules. These rules secure clinical homogeneity of patients as a means of conducting scientific research in psychiatry and advancing validation of clinical judgement. Thus, following further elaboration, they appeared as the Research Diagnostic Criteria (RDC).[46]

The St. Louis criteria for schizophrenia best exemplify the diagnostic rules in which in addition to the presenting symptomatology, course, family history, pertinent demographic data and implicit prognosis are included. With their further elaboration by the New York group,[46,47] the St. Louis operational criteria have laid the foundation for the DSM-III.[20]

Concurrent with the RDC criteria, the New Haven Schizophrenic Index (NHSI) developed by Astrakhan and co-workers has appeared.[48] It also derived from the need to increase diagnostic reliability among American psychiatrists by formulating criteria based on symptoms listed in the DSM-III which are generally referred to by clinicians in making the diagnosis of schizophrenia. The NHSI derives from a complex calculation of a long list of symptoms and signs rated according to their significance. It relies heavily on the presenting symptomatology and does not include duration criteria.

The so-called flexible system for the diagnosis of schizophrenia of Carpenter et al had the same motivational origin as the NHSI, that is, to improve the descriptive criteria of the DSM-II for the diagnosis of schizophrenia and provide an instrument that would more reliably distinguish schizophrenia from affective disorders.[49] It is in fact a checklist of symptoms and signs originating from the PSE.[40] These symptoms were found to be discriminant for the diagnosis of schizophrenia during the application of the PSE in the International Pilot Study on Schizophrenia by the WHO.[40,50] Thus, the symptoms may be considered as being empirical and internationally applicable.

In subsequent years, Taylor and Abrahams on the basis of a comparative study of their own criteria and those of the RDC have proposed two modifications of the initial list.[51,52] These changes may be considered as an attempt to narrow even further the diagnosis of schizophrenia as their initial proposals in 1972 on comparative studies were found to rank very low in terms of reliability.[53]

Lastly, mention should also be made of the criteria used by Rosenthal, Kety and their co-workers for the well-known Danish-American study of population groups in Denmark at high risk for schizophrenia.[54] Out of these genetic studies the concept of schizophrenia spectrum disorders has emerged and the strict or discriminant diagnostic criteria proposed by the RDC, the NHSI and the CSB could be challenged as being under-inclusive for the diagnosis of schizophrenia.

All the aforementioned proposals share a common characteristic: they attempt to formulate operational criteria for the diagnosis of schizophrenia in the conceptual frame of empiricism. Moreover, they have contributed significantly to the formulation of diagnostic criteria and the classificatory principles on which the DSM-III is based.

Current Diagnostic and Classification Systems (DSM-III, DSM-III-R, ICD-9-CM and ICD-10)

The DSM-III was published in 1980 and stirred worldwide attention reflected in its rapid translation into several languages and in publications unprecedented in number. Regardless of praise or criticism, the DSM-III and its revised form published in 1987, testified to the fact that through a national diagnostic and classificatory system the conceptual framework of world psychiatry has changed radically.[20,55]

What is novel and important in DSM-III and its revised form, DSM-III-R? How does it compare with other national systems and the ICD-9[28] and the forthcoming ICD-10?[56] What is its impact on current and future research of schizophrenia? For schizophrenia, as for other mental disorders, the DSM-III has adopted an agnostic, atheoretic stand regarding pathogenetic mechanisms and etiological factors. This is due to the fact that in schizophrenia, as well as in the other non-organic mental disorders, inference to pathogenetic mechanisms and etiological factors is still hypothetical, contradictory and potentially confusing.

Based on the provisions of DSM-III and DSM-III-R, the clinical symptomatology on which diagnosis must be made is determined by inclusion and exclusion criteria. Although these clinical features are proposed as being operational criteria, in fact they are just rules on which there is consensus by professionals, at least by those who participated in their formulation. Thus, inclusion criteria have been established based on symptoms that are characterized by high frequency and long duration, as well as by manifest features that are recognizable and easy to assess clinically. Most of these symptoms are not different from the first rank symptoms of Schneider, however, none by itself is considered obligatory or sufficient (pathognomonic) for the diagnosis. In DSM-III and DSM-III-R the notion of the threshold is introduced because the presence of at least a minimum number of the symptoms is required for the diagnosis. Thus, the approach regarding presenting symptoms is polythetic.

The requirement of a six-months duration of the syndrome, including the prodromal and the residual symptoms in the revised DSM-III is obligatory. It implies chronicity which at least partly endorses the Kraepelinian concept of the disorder. Outcome and treatment response are not included as diagnostic criteria. Instead, impairment of functioning during the course of the disorder acquires diagnostic significance. Schizoaffective disorder and mood disorder with psychotic features constitute exclusion criteria, unless they are present in the active phase and have brief duration compared to the total duration of the schizophrenic syndrome. Course is classified in five types, the last one being remission, the differentiation of which from no mental disorder depends on clinical judgement rather than specific criteria. Schizophrenia itself is divided into five types (catatonic, disorganized, paranoid, undifferentiated and residual) exclusively on the grounds of the prevailing cross-sectional symptomatology.

With the exception of the 6-month duration of the illness, antecedents are not included among the diagnostic criteria. Pre-morbid personality of any type, including the schizoid or the schizotypal and borderline personality disorders if noted, are placed in a separate axis, axis II. In order to avoid etiological inferences and violation of the principle of atheoreticism, family history and possible genetic predisposition are not listed among the criteria. If patients meet the criteria for diagnosis of schizophrenia but their disorder lasts for less than six months, their condition is categorized as psychotic disorder not elsewhere classified with the specific rubric of schizophreniform disorder. Whenever a patient who is suffering from schizophreniform disorder continues to present symptoms for more than 6 months, he or she is rediagnosed as suffering from schizophrenia. Delusional (paranoid) disorder is classified separately as being characterized by persistent non-bizarre delusions which are not due to any other mental disorder such as schizophrenia, schizophreniform disorder or a mood disorder.

The multi-axial evaluation system consisting of five axes (axes I and II for diagnosing mental disorders and axis III physical disorders, axis IV for the description of the severity of psychosocial stressors and axis V for the global assessment of functioning) is applied in the diagnosis of schizophrenia as is the case for all mental disorders in the DSM-III. The multi-axial system aims at providing a biopsychosocial approach to assessment. With regard to compatibility with ICD-9-CM, all DSM-III diagnoses are legitimate in relation to their corresponding ICD-9-CM codes. However, legitimacy does not imply correspondence in assessment criteria or in nomenclature and typing of the disorders across the two systems.

In my view, the current concept of schizophrenia has not been changed by the DSM-III and DSM-III-R. Nonetheless, with the wide acceptance of their diagnostic rules, these classifications provide a common frame of reference to which research findings can be related. In conjunction with the instruments for standardized psychiatric interviews developed specifically to fit their diagnostic criteria (the DIS, the SCID and the SCID-R), DSM-III and DSM-III-R undoubtedly maximize diagnostic reliability of schizophrenia and pave the way for a more factual and accurate clinical understanding of this disorder.

The empirical–atheoretical approach to schizophrenia and schizophrenic disorders is based on the assumption that inferences to mechanisms and etiological factors have been excluded. Although this approach is quite acceptable considering the present state of our knowledge, the question arises as to how atheoretical a diagnostic system can be. No system based on explicit diagnostic criteria can be entirely atheoretical and purely empirical. Extraction of criteria implies judgement, which is not necessarily based on observable, quantifiable and predictable manifestations of a scientifically validated mechanism and/or causal factor.

A number of examples can be cited to illustrate that atheoreticism and pure empiricism have not been practiced absolutely in the DSM-III formulation of schizophrenia. More importantly, some of the theoretical inferences are in fact conflicting.

The notion of patienthood, which prevails in the description of schizophrenia, speaks in itself for a theoretical bias that favors the disease concept (i.e., medical) as opposed to other concepts (e.g., social). Moreover, the adoption of a multiaxial system with personality traits, life events and social functioning each providing separately an axis status equal to that of the clinical syndrome, implies a concept promoting the biopsychosocial model of the disorder.

It is also within the context of a theoretical approach to infer etiological factors, such as family history (genetic loading) when differentiating between schizophrenia and delusional paranoid disorder. It is even more theoretical to label a disorder as "reactive psychosis" implying a distinct relationship between this disorder and life experiences.

There is an underlying theoretical concept in preferring content rather than form, when distinguishing among the various diagnostic groups. Some might argue that symptom form rather than symptom content characterizes a patient's condition, whereas symptom content is part of the individual's past experience. Further, how atheoretical could it be to ascribe to personality traits and disorders an axis status equal to clinical symptomatology? Many clinicians would welcome such a close relationship as being consistent with their theory of psychological determinism which links personality development and psychopathological processes. Others, adhering strictly to the disease model, would rigorously object to any intrinsic association between personality development and psychopathology. Both sides, however, would be somewhat puzzled seeing that a part of axis II is incorporated into symptomatology and another is ascribed to a separate section, that of personality disorders.

In spite of these theoretical contaminations, the strategy of the DSM-III, particularly in the area of schizophrenia, is undoubtedly an empirical one, more empirical than that of any other previous system. It is this strategy, however, that invites criticism from those who would have preferred a more flexible approach to understanding mental disorders.[57] Thus, it is claimed that subordinating an individual to strict diagnostic criteria derived from standardized instruments and ascribing the patient to a taxonomic group, results in an impoverishment of the information, diminishes the role of the subject and renders the patient a sheer symptom-emitting object by finally enclaving him or her into a determinism sustained both psychologically and socially by a diagnostic label.

Not all of those who advocate theoretical approaches as a means to generate progress in understanding mental disorders are so critical of the need for empirical criteria in psychiatric diagnosis. As Michels has noted in a discussion regarding diagnostic strategies and theoretical concepts, "scientific strategy is to have some theoretical bias or assumption or model or attitude which will inform one's first guesses about the concepts or operations or measurements and try to reach a reasonable level of reliability in those areas and then to have a kind of reciprocal back and forth relationship between improving reliability, searching for external validators, coming back to them and modifying the criteria to again improve reliability, recognizing the importance of theory from the very first formulation of the criteria."[58]

There are other debatable issues regarding conceptual and organizational aspects of DSM-III in terms of the diagnostic criteria for schizophrenia. Despite its merits the multi-axial system runs the risk of being misused or abused in clinical practice and even in research by endless addition of information to axes III, IV, and V, the clinical relevance of which lies entirely in the judgement of the interviewer. Thus, the main features may be obscured by irrelevant information and diagnostic clarity may be substituted by a hodge-podge of elements embracing physical health and experiences in life. In contrast, family history and response to treatment in schizophrenia have not been given an axis value neither were they included as information worth mentioning for the diagnosis of schizophrenia in DSM-III. This is despite the fact that the presently available knowledge on these two areas is sufficient to be integrated into our diagnostic considerations.

Another issue worth commenting on is the adding, removing and renaming of syndromes in the schizophrenia spectrum, such as "schizophrenia," "delusional paranoid disorder," "psychotic disorders not elsewhere classified," etc. This issue brings forth the question how comprehensive and applicable these terms are in various settings around the world as well as to what extent schizophrenia and related disorders in DSM-III and DSM-III-R correlate with the corresponding disorders in the ICD-9 and the forthcoming ICD-10 and in other national classification systems. There is abundant literature on this issue and particular reference should be made to two books: *International Perspectives on DSM-III* and the *International Classification of Psychiatry: Unity and Diversity*.[59,60]

Undoubtedly schizophrenia in the DSM-III is a diagnostic concept much narrower than in the DSM-II and also much narrower than in the ICD-9 and ICD-10. This is due to the symptoms selected (the majority observable and objectively assessed) and to the restrictive criterion of the six-months duration. By applying seven different diagnostic formulations among 200 first admissions for functional psychosis Berner and his co-workers[61] have found in a descending order of strictness of the diagnosis of schizophrenia the following: 121 patients with at least one first rank symptom of Schneider; 91 with at least one basic symptom of Bleuler; 80 with DSM-III diagnosis of schizophrenic or schizophreniform disorder; 53 with at least two As of Bleuler's basic symptoms; 49 with only the diagnosis of a schizophrenic disorder; 36 with a diagnosis of endogenomorphic schizophrenic syndrome; and 22 with at least three As of Bleuler's basic symptoms.

The orientation towards narrowing the diagnosis of schizophrenia is also manifested in DSM-III by considering separately at the same hierarchical level "schizophrenia," "delusional (paranoid) disorder" and "psychotic disorder not elsewhere classified" whereas brief reactive psychosis, schizophreniform disorder, schizoaffective disorder, induced psychotic disorder and psychotic disorder not otherwise specified (atypical psychosis) were included as subgroups under "psychotic disorders not elsewhere classified." Conversely, in the forthcoming ICD-10 schizophrenia is housed under a group of disorders named "schizophrenic, schizotypal and delusional disorders."

The strict diagnostic criteria in DSM-III are substituted by diagnostic guidelines in the ICD-10. Schizophrenia proper is subdivided into five types in DSM-III and in nine subtypes in ICD-10 by retaining simple schizophrenia and adding post-schizophrenic depression, other schizophrenias and unspecified schizophrenias. Validation of the pluses and minuses between the two systems remains to be shown. Simple schizophrenia is assimilated into the schizotypal personality disorder in DSM-III and it is a type of schizophrenia in ICD-9 and ICD-10. A group from our department failed to validate this entity with phase, descriptive, and predictive validation criteria.[62] During a follow-up period averaging ten years, they noted that patients in whom the initial diagnosis of simple schizophrenia was made had a variable course ranging from complete remission associated with normal social functioning to a continuously deteriorating course compatible with the diagnosis of process or continuous schizophrenia. These results could hardly justify assimilation of simple schizophrenia to schizotypal personality disorders neither could they support the traditional and ICD taxonomic autonomy.

Related to the issue of the diagnostic validity of simple schizophrenia is the introduction of the notion of positive and negative schizophrenia by Andreasen.[63,64] This notion is based on Jackson's neurophysiological theory according to which functional deficiencies arise directly from cortical lesions while the positive symptoms are secondary manifestations resulting from disinhibition of subcortical functions.[65] The negative symptoms described by Andreasen correspond roughly to the Bleulerian primary (pathognomonic) symptoms that for several years were neglected due to low interrater reliability. Although satisfactory reliability is claimed with the use of developed instruments, the predictive validity of the proposed three types of schizophrenia (positive, negative and mixed) in terms of treatment response, course and associated structural brain deficit has to be confirmed by additional studies. If confirmed, particularly in longitudinal studies, which has not been the case thus far, this notion could legitimately claim a place in the structure of the forthcoming diagnostic systems for schizophrenia.

Naming is a useful and necessary exercise to the degree that newly accumulated knowledge leads to restructuring of our concepts regarding a certain entity and a new name is required to reflect more accurately this restructuring. This, however, is not the case in many of the DSM-III renaming practices. Substituting the time-honored and so familiar term of hebephrenia with the term "disorganized type of schizophrenia" is indicative of such a trend, that is, compensation for the lack of knowledge by cosmetic innovations and renaming. This is a trend that results in confusion and hardly contributes to the promotion of a common language for psychiatry the world over.

Other National Classification Systems

It is interesting to see to what extent certain peculiarities that exist in some national diagnostic systems relate to DSM-III concepts.

The peculiarity of the French system is mainly characterized by the inclusion of two entities which are considered separate from schizophrenia proper.[66,67] One is that of acute delusional episode (bouffée délirante) and the other is the chronic hallucinatory psychosis. Both terms are widely used in diagnostic practice in France. The boufée délirante is used practically as a diagnostic term for every first delusional and/or hallucinatory condition with sudden onset and also for every new episode recurring following an interval free of psychopathology. The schizophreniform disorder of the DSM-III introduces in American psychiatry for the first time a category that is very close to the French concept of boufée délirante. Also, chronic hallucinatory psychosis, which is included under the category of chronic delusional states as a separate type in the official classification by INSERM and is considered to be separate from schizophrenia now comes very close to the DSM-III-R delusional (paranoid) disorder.[67]

In a recent study, data for the French concept of boufée délirante and chronic hallucinatory psychosis were reviewed and compared with the correspondent DSM-III concepts.[68] The results indicated that both of these syndromes on reclassification correspond to various DSM-III categories among which DSM-III schizophrenia is dominant. On a five-year follow-up study most of the patients initially diagnosed with acute delusional episode and/or chronic hallucinatory psychosis were assigned to the schizophrenia syndrome according to the DSM-III criteria.

Comparison of the Soviet diagnostic system with DSM-III, ICD and other national classificatory systems is difficult to make, because empirical comparative studies are lacking. The prevailing diagnostic system in the Soviet Union is the one developed by Snezhnevsky.[69] It follows the traditional Russian clinical approach, but is overwhelmingly influenced by the classical Central European schools of psychiatry.

The mode of onset and the initial symptomatology, according to the Soviet view, is a valid predictor of the course and the outcome of psychosis. According to Nadzharov and Sternberg,[70] clusters of symptoms can be recognized and proven to have distinctive diagnostic value for four age groups (children, adolescents, adults and the elderly). Schizophrenia is subtyped into three categories based on course and outcome: continuously progressive, attack-type progressive and recurrent. A theoretical frame of "psychopathological structure of the psychosis as a developmental dynamic whole"[71] is understood in connection with genetic factors and earlier pre-morbid attributes of personality.

It is apparent from the above that it is mainly our limited knowledge of pathogenetic mechanisms and etiological factors of schizophrenia and schizophrenia-related disorders that justifies the time and effort to formulate descriptive and operational criteria for diagnosis and subsquently for our research plans and our treatment choices. Limitations of this approach in both reliability and validity measures are quite obvious and a search for external validating criteria is more than imperative. Diagnostic reliability not only has a heuristic value and serves the sheer purpose of science, but has also profound pragmatic (therapeutic, legal and moral) consequences, both for the individual and the society.[72] Obtaining a high interrater reliability, however, does not necessarily imply increased validity, particularly when based on rules that originate from consensus and are an integral part of the definition process.

Universality of the Concept

The universality of the concept of schizophrenia has been a longstanding and vigorously debated issue; opposing views have been defended either on purely theoretical grounds or on the basis of scanty empirical findings obtained from studies flawed with methodological deficiencies. The issue, however, is of paramount importance because it is linked closely with any attempt to conceptualize schizophrenia and understand its nature.

For several years, the main constraining factor in resolving this debate was a lack of explicit and strict criteria for defining and diagnosing schizophrenia, a condition in which symptomatology is expected to be heavily influenced by culture-bound beliefs and attitudes. Kraepelin himself, after visiting Java, indicated the potential interference of sociocultual factors in certain symptoms of mental disorders including dementia praecox, that is, schizophrenia.[73] He indicated that only if the same investigator undertook a cross-cultural study might it be possible to discern and define the contribution of these factors to the clinical picture of mental disorders.

In the past, several authors, mainly deriving from sociology and anthropology, contended that the prevalence of schizophrenia is much higher in the western industrial societies, very low in non-westernized developing countries and hardly present in illiterate tribal societies.[74,75] Psychiatrists, on the other hand, did not endorse this contention based on limited empirical findings. The debate went on. Due to the scarcity of systematic transcultural research for mental disorders that would satisfy basic methodological requirements, a series of studies by the World Health Organization (WHO) which started in the late sixties acquires particular significance and may be viewed as a landmark in this area of research on schizophrenia.[76–80]

There were several merits in the WHO studies. They were based on a large sample of patients from carefully selected centers in 17 countries, ranging from the most developed to the least developed, with pronounced cultural and ethnic differences. Assessment was made on a clinical basis by experienced psychiatrists in each particular center and intercenter reliability of diagnosis was one of the study aims. Moreover, in order to increase the reliability and degree of comparability, a standardized semi-structured instrument was developed and used in equivalent versions of the local language of the various centers. Additional advantage of the WHO series of studies was the multiple followup assessments taking place at intervals of one, two and five years.

In the WHO series,[50,76–80] the first study[50] is the well known international pilot study of schizophrenia (IPSS), the second[77] is the study on the assessment and reduction of psychiatric disability and the third very recent study[78] deals with the determinants of the outcome of severe mental disorders.

The main findings of all these studies relate to the question of universality of schizophrenia and to potential factors related to possible differences in phenomenology, course and outcome across various cultures and countries.[76–80] The outstanding finding that emerged is that schizophrenia is indeed found to be present in all cultures and countries covered by the WHO investigations and surprisingly the clinical picture presented was not substantially different from one cultural setting to another.

The clinical diagnosis matched sufficiently well with the results of the statistical analysis of data (through the CATEGO system) derived from the standardized examination by the instrument employed (PSE) and the subsequent classification according to the ICD-9 criteria[78,40] In fact, the investigators of the IPSS identified a number of symptoms composing two groups, the "nuclear syndrome" and the "auditory hallucination syndrome" which in conjuction were found to be of high discriminative value for schizophrenia. Further, one of these symptoms, that is, voices speaking to the patient (non-emotional and out of cultural context) emerged as an almost exclusive symptom for schizophrenia.

Apart from the basic symptoms, the WHO investigators have noted differences in the clinical picture of patients between developed and developing countries. The latter displayed fewer affective symptoms such as depression, less delusional mood and thought insertion and more auditory and visual hallucinations. These clinical features, however, could not be clustered together in a way to establish a separate syndrome and were considered as variations of the basic clinical syndrome rather than a cultural-specific entity.

Variations in both frequency and content of delusional and hallucinatory experiences may occur even in two or more regions of the same country with different sociocultural norms and traditions, as shown also by Mantonakis in our department in a comparative study of the symptomatology of schizophrenia in patients from the islands of Crete and Corfu.[81]

Incidence rates for the schizophrenic syndrome measured by the annual rate of first-in-lifetime contacts with any type of service was found to vary by only a factor of three between study areas of high incidence and areas of low incidence. Once the strict criteria for defining schizophrenia according to the CATEGO CLASS S+ were employed, the interarea variation of the incidence rates was further reduced and led to the conclusion that the nuclear schizophrenic syndrome is distributed almost evenly across the study areas despite their gross sociocultural differences.

Whereas the overall clinical symptomatology at first contact was strikingly similar among the centers, the followup studies [79] showed a differential course and outcome between patients from developing and developed countries. An excellent example is offered by the finding that 58% of the study patients in Nigeria and only 6% in Denmark had a remission as defined by the study criteria. It was, thus, concluded that patients from developing countries do considerably better than patients in developed industrialized countries, both in terms of duration of illness as well as in functional capacity.

In critically reviewing the results of the WHO studies[50,76–80] the following remarks can be made. Schizophrenia is not a culturally preferred condition in so far as its core nuclear symptoms are concerned. Contrary to the aphorism by Devereux that schizophrenia is the typical ethnic psychosis of complex civilized societies,[74] it was identified clinically among areas in the world with profound variances in cultural, ethnic and socioeconomic characteristics.

This finding has had a profound impact on our concepts and our approaches to this disorder. Some of the observed differences in phenomenology as well as the significant dissimilarity in course and outcome of patients with schizophrenia from developed and developing countries may require further comments. Regarding differences in phenomenology, it would be rather surprising if they were not found. The lay concept of the illness differs greatly across cultures and exerts a profound influence on illness behaviour patterns. In a great number of cultures of the Western World, distinction between mind and body is not conceived. What in Western cultures is considered to be a symptom, in many other cultures is part of living myth and belief systems. In some cultural settings there is not even a word to denote certain feelings such as depression. Undoubtedly, these culture-bound elements impinge upon the presenting symptoms of schizophrenia and for that matter of any illness, be it mental or physical.

Regarding the differences in course and outcome between patients from developing and developed countries, two sets of arguments are offered. One pertains to confounding factors in methodology as well as in the criteria for classification of the disorders. A version of the PSE[40] was used which included basically Schneiderian first rank symptoms, and it is, thus, conceivable that for certain study areas the PSE was under-inclusive for schizophrenia while for others it was over-inclusive. Further, the diagnosis of schizophrenic syndrome was based on the presenting symptoms and because duration and outcome, particularly social functioning, were not used as diagnostic criteria, an uneven distribution of schizophreniform states, such as reactive psychosis, bouféé délirante and paranoid states, according to various classificatory systems, is likely to have occurred across centers.

The second set of critical arguments relates to the role of sociocultural factors. It is expected that, as mentioned, such factors may not only play a pathoplastic role in the phenomenology of the disorder but they also may exert an influence on its course and outcome. This would not be a unique phenomenon in nosology exclusive for schizophrenia. Any disorder may result not only from biological and/or psychosocial stress, but it may act as a stress factor itself capable of inducing symptoms causally unrelated to the primary disease process.

Quite often, with mental patients it is difficult to draw the line between stressors resulting in and originating from the morbid condition. Stressors are experienced by the individual in the context of the cultural tradition and social setting. Similarly stress-coping mechanisms vary considerably among individuals from different cultures and their effectiveness to a large extent is dependent upon the available psychosocial support systems or inversely on societal demands. Sociocultural settings that exert great pressure upon the individual for compliance to demanding social norms are less likely to provide the kind of beneficial care for course and outcome, compared to cultures that are more lenient, less demanding and provide for increased institutional and family support to individuals with behavioral derangements.

Last is the issue of incidence. The WHO study was based on data from patients who were seeking help either in health care facilities or other help-providing agencies. The ideal of course would be to conduct field surveys in order to increase representativeness. It is to be noted, however, that patients with severe mental illness, schizophrenics in their overwhelming majority, do contact such agencies provided that appropriate services exist. This was shown in our recent field survey studies in which the prevalence of mental disorders in the community as well as the utilization of services by the patients were investigated.[82]

Although the issue of universality of schizophrenia seems to have been resolved by the WHO studies, the issue of differential prevalence has not been dealt with adequately. Also the factors influencing the variability, not only in prevalence but also in symptomatology across countries and cultures, have not been researched appropriately. Such factors, if identified, could provide a clue to the pathophysiology and possibly to the etiology of schizophrenia. Populations of either high or low prevalence of schizophrenic or schizophrenic-like disorders should be thoroughly scrutinized to extricate relevant genetic and environmental (physical and sociocultural) factors.

We might conclude that the available data provide sufficient evidence that the schizophrenic syndrome is a universal phenomenon manifested, at least in the onset and early phase of its development, by a cluster of symptoms of distinctive value that permit diagnosis across various cultures, countries and ethnic groups. Furthermore, it is a condition, which in terms of symptom content, course and outcome, varies considerably from individual to individual and from culture to culture. Such variation, however, does not challenge its basic diagnostic identity as it does not for a large number of worldwide-spread organic illnesses with even greater variations in their clinical presentation.

Other Issues Related to the Concept

A major problem in the ascertainment of the diagnosis of schizophrenia is the lack of external validating criteria or diagnostic indices, especially on the biological level. In spite of a scarcity of such diagnostic indices in psychiatry, a wealth of data related to a number of biological and other factors in the etiology of psychiatric conditions, including schizophrenia, has been accumulated over the years. Thus, it is worth discussing briefly the relative value of these data in the context of their eventual usefulness for the development of diagnostic indices.

A number of studies have shown that first-degree relatives of schizophrenic patients run a risk of having schizophrenia 5 to 15 times higher than would be expected in the general population.[83–87] However, this so-called consanguinity method of providing support to the notion of a genetic etiology of schizophrenia has its limitations, the main one being that the family environment itself could have played a role in the high prevalence of this disease in the families of schizophrenics.

More substantive support to the genetic hypothesis in the etiology of schizophrenia came from studies demonstrating differences in concordance rates for schizophrenia between monozygotic and dizygotic twins; the concordance rates for monozygotic twins was found to range from 35% to 55%, whereas the concordance for the dizygotic twins was not substantially higher than that which would have been expected for any siblings of schizophrenic patients.[88–94] These studies have made clear that there is a definite genetic liability for schizophrenia. However, because half or more of the monozygotic twins are not afflicted by the illness, the interaction of genetic and environmental factors needs to be considered.

The joint American–Danish study of the genetic contribution to schizophrenia showed that children adopted away from biological parents suffering from schizophrenia were afflicted by this disease in rates higher than those children adopted away from biological parents free of schizophrenic illness.[54,95] Furthermore, it was demonstrated that being reared by schizophrenic parents was, at least in this study, not found to be a substantial factor contributing to the development of schizophrenic illness.

Fischer, in a twin study, showed that many factors play an important role in the development of schizophrenia.[89] In that study, it was pointed out that there is no way to identify the specific nature of the pathogenic environmental factors, because there were several intra-pair differences among the group of concordant pairs of monozygotic twins that were inconsistent from pair to pair. The study also scrutinized the hypothesis of a dominance-submissiveness relationship being a factor contributing to the development of schizophrenia among the group of discordant monozygotic twins. However, one of the major findings of Fischer's study was that in both members of discordant monozygotic twin pairs there was the same prevalence of schizophrenia in their offspring regardless of whether or not their parent was the one who was afflicted by the illness.

As a whole all classical genetic studies (that is, consanguinity, adoptive and twin studies) have failed to identify the mode of genetic transmission as well as exactly what is transmitted. There were several hypotheses presented in review papers and the prevailing hypothesis was that what is inherited is the combination of several different genes, that is, a polygenic hypothesis.[96,97]

Currently, the advent of improved technology in molecular genetics (recombinant DNA techniques) offers promising perspectives for the unravelling of the mysteries of schizophrenia.[98] With the research design that was used in identifying the approximate locus of the abnormal gene in Huntington's disease (restriction fragment length polymorphisms), the road is open to link schizophrenia to high density pedigrees.[99] Thus far, in the field of psychiatry, this work is limited mainly to the area of affective disorders, more particularly of bipolar illness. The well-known Amish study[100] together with other investigations for gene location in pedigrees of patients with bipolar illness[101,102] indicate that the genetic loci for this illness may be different in different genetic pools or in different pedigrees. The Amish study assumed that the gene responsible for bipolar illness is autosomally linked although the two other studies have shown the loci to be situated on the X chromosome. There are some investigations, however, that failed to find any loci in other pedigrees.[103] All of these studies suggest that there might be several genetic sub-types leading to the same clinical entity. If this is true for bipolar affective disorder, it should be more so for schizophrenia.

The work in schizophrenia employing the new tools of molecular genetics has just been initiated by Basset who reported that a schizophrenic proband and his affected maternal uncle have a trisomy of the long arm of chromosome 5 while his non-affected mother has a balanced abnormality on the same chromosome.[104] Lately there are unpublished reports presented in meetings by the Middlesex group, which based on the study of three large pedigrees of schizophrenic patients indicate that a gene location for schizophrenia is the short arm of chromosome 5.

It is too early to draw definitive conclusions regarding the genetic loading in schizophrenia families. Whatever results may emerge from this research, one has to consider that genetic traits associated with one or several types of schizophrenia may be necessary but not sufficient for the development of the illness, that is, environmental factors, either biological or psychosocial, interact with the genetic trait to produce manifest symptoms of schizophrenia. This is quite understandable for schizophrenia, which is such a complicated illness that affects all levels of human affective, cognitive and behavioral functions in a most troubling and unpredictable way. If this holds true for the manifestations at the onset of the illness, it is even more true for the formation of clinical symptoms, the course and the varying outcome of this disorder.

One also needs to consider the extremely complicated interaction of genes particularly those with low penetrance. Equal significance is attached to the protective as well as to the pathogenic genes. Another consideration is that exposure to environmental factors as well as response-sensitivity to environmental stimuli also might be genetically determined.[105]

A number of studies have suggested a possible involvement of the immune system in the pathogenesis of schizophrenia.[106-110] Some have been carried out using the Human Leukocyte Antigen (HLA) System, others the number and morphology of T and B lymphocytes as well as their in vitro cultures. Inconsistent and diverse findings from such studies could be attributed to variances in patient material and methods employed. The results of our own studies indicate that there is indeed a degree of defect in the immune system of schizophrenics.[111] This deficiency is not related to medication, duration of illness, or to other variables that have been implicated in previous studies. The observed skin anergy in the majority of our schizophrenics, in the absence of any immunosuppressive treatment, indicates the existence of a serious defect in cellular immunity in these patients.

A detailed study of peripheral lymphocytes demonstrated the presence of a significantly greater percentage of transformed cells in schizophrenics.[111] Beta-lymphocytes were found to be significantly higher and T-lymphocytes significantly lower in schizophenic patients compared with controls. Blastic transformation index and cumulative transformation index in the presence of phytohemagglutinin (PHA) were found to be significantly diminished in schizophrenic patients compared with those of the controls. These findings strongly suggest the existence of defective cellular immunity in schizophrenics. Finally, migration indices of mononuclear cells from the peripheral blood of schizophrenics in the presence of PHA were definitely abnormal. The autoimmune hypothesis would best explain these findings. This hypothesis would not be in conflict with either genetic susceptibility or a host of potential epigenetic factors, among which viral infection requires special mention in view of the recent findings.

The assumption that an exogenous agent, more specifically a virus, might be associated with the etiology of schizophrenia was initially advanced on the basis of observations that encephalitis lethargica, which followed the large influenza epidemic of 1918, in many respects resembled schizophrenia and occasionally presented with schizophrenia-like symptoms.[112-113] This assumption was revived in the past few years by various authors who proposed that schizophrenia either is a reaction to one of the known-viruses or is caused by an as yet unknown neurotropic virus. One of the arguments in favor of this hypothesis is the observation that there are geographical pockets with increased prevalence of schizophrenia.[114] As an extention of this hypothesis, there even were claims that physical proximity rather than genetics might account for the high prevalence rate of schizophrenia among monozygotic twins.

Further support of the viral hypothesis derived from the observation of some seasonal variations in births of schizophrenic patients.[97] The speculation was that children born during the winter months are more susceptible to infections of viral origin. In addition, Crow, by analyzing the age of onset in pairs of siblings with schizophrenia, has shown that horizontal or contagious transmission probably does not occur at the time of onset of the illness or at any time in post-natal life.[115] Based on laterality differences between the two hemispheres and other empirical observations, he advanced the hypothesis that schizophrenia might be due to a retrovirus or transposon which becomes integrated in the human genome.[116] He proposed that the psychosis-responsible gene is acquired by the schizophrenic individual either from an affected or predisposed parent or by an integration-transposition event occurring during pregnancy.

Recently Mednick and co-workers reported findings consistent with an affliction of the individual possibly by a viral infection particularly during the second trimester of gestation.[117] This conclusion was based on the finding of a high incidence of schizophrenia among cohorts exposed in utero to influenza A-II virus in 1957.

There are several other hypotheses regarding the etiology of schizophrenia which may eventually provide a useful tool for the diagnosis of this condition: the most prominent among them is the biogenic amine hypothesis, more specifically the dopamine hypothesis, a biochemical theory formulated following the observation that neuroleptics found to be effective in treating schizophrenic patients block the D2 receptors.[118]

Other etiological and pathogenetic mechanisms have been traced following findings supporting the existence of structural and functional alterations in the brain of schizophrenics. Johnstone and associates have described structural changes that seem to be pronounced features particularly of chronic schizophrenic patients.[119] They concluded that the changes are more likely a developmental defect than secondary atrophy. A number of studies have indicated that changes of the left hemisphere are important in schizophrenia.[120–122] Pertinent to this view are the results from psychophysiological studies of electrodermal parameters in schizophrenic patients and controls by Rabavilas and colleagues in our department that support a functional abnormality lateralized in the left hemisphere.[123]

The above examples indicate the difficulty that exists in integrating findings from various investigations. Biological findings including positron emission tomography (PET) data do not seem to be consistent; one study showed an increase of D2 receptors in the brain of schizophrenics[124] while another failed to do so.[125] Even the metabolic underactivity of the frontal lobe, the so-called hypofrontality, is confirmed by some groups and not by others.[126-133] Further, the gradient between cortical and subcortical activity is disputed.[132,133]

Despite all these inconsistencies regarding schizophrenia, it seems that we are dealing with a condition that has several dimensions. Definitely there is a genetic dimension, clearly there are biological aberrations, but there is also a variety of psychosocial factors which may contribute to its pathogenesis and definitely contribute to its course. All these factors have to be taken into account together. Thus, an integrative approach is essential in order to deal with the many dimensions of schizophrenia.

Summary

Various concepts of schizophrenia can be retrospectively traced back to the early descriptions of melancholia by Hippocrates. In the 19th century Morel provided the rudiments of a description of schizophrenia by describing a case of "demence précoce." Since the 18th century there have been three prevailing concepts regarding schizophrenia: the syndromal, the nosological and the theoretical. The syndromal concept is based on clusters of symptoms and behaviors with no particular consideration attached to etiology, pathogenesis and clinical course. The nosological concept proposes schizophrenia as a medical disease, a clinical phenomenon with a predictable onset, course and outcome. The theoretical concept attempts to explain or hypothesize underlying etiologic and pathogenic mechanisms and the course of the disease.

The French school (Pinel and Esquirol) initiated the syndromal approach to the diagnosis of mental disorders. Kraepelin advanced the nosological concept and was the founder of systematic classification systems. In contrast, Bleuler emphasized the primacy of the presenting symptoms for the diagnosis of schizophrenia; underlying mechanisms, however, were not ignored. In Europe, the syndromal approach was further advanced by Schneider who introduced his list of first rank symptoms for the diagnosis of schizophrenia. After World War II, the psychodynamic concept emerged. Since the mid-1950s with the development of neuroleptic drugs, and subsequent social shifts toward patient rights, accountability as well as technologic advances in data acquisition and processing, the biologic and nosologic points of view have become preeminent.

All of these concepts are reflected in the categories for schizophrenia in the current ICD-9 and -10 and in the DSM-III and DSM-III-R. These concepts reflect the state-of-the-art in the area of diagnosis and classification. Although the claim is made that the DSM-III and DSM-III-R descriptions are atheoretical, this is not actually the case. DSM-III and DSM-III-R do not change the concept of schizophrenia. They include criteria that are much narrower than those in ICD-9 and ICD-10; whereas DSM-III applies strict diagnostic criteria, ICD-10 uses diagnostic guidelines. It needs to be noted that obtaining a high interrater reliability does not necessarily imply increased validity especially when the criteria originate from consensus and are also an integral part of the definition process. Because external validating criteria are not as yet adequate, we must still rely on clinical assessment in which presenting symptoms, the duration of symptoms, pattern of symptoms and outcome must all be considered.

A series of landmark studies on schizophrenia have been conducted by the WHO. The concept of schizophrenia was shown to be a universal one with schizophrenia found to be present in all countries and cultures studied. Incidence rates for the schizophrenic syndrome measured by the annual rate of first-in-lifetime contacts with any type of service were found to vary by only a factor of three between study areas of high incidence and areas of low incidence. While the overall presenting clinical picture did not differ substantially from one cultural setting to another, patients in developing countries displayed fewer affective symptoms and more auditory and visual hallucinations than schizophrenic patients in developed countries. A differential course and outcome was found; patients in developing countries did considerably better than patients in developed industrialized countries, both in terms of duration of illness as well as in functional capacity.

Other issues that bear on the concept of schizophrenia are related to the search for biological indices that will provide data to support the current concepts of schizophrenia based on inclusion and exclusion criteria. These indices include data based on: genetic studies; studies of the immune system; the search for a viral causation; biochemical/metabolic data; and structural brain abnormalities. Thus, the current concept of schizophrenia represents a multifaceted condition with definite contributions from genetic, biochemical and psychosocial factors affecting the symptomatology and course and possibly pathogenesis as well, thus requiring an integrative approach to its understanding.

References

1. Morel BA: *Traite de Dégénérescenses Physiques, Intellectuelles et Morales de l'Espèce Humaine.* Paris, Bailliere, 1857.
2. Kraepelin E: *One Hundred Years of Psychiatry.* New York, Citadel Press, 1962.
3. Hippocrates: *The Medical Works of Hippocrates.* Oxford, Blackwell, 1950.
4. Kotsopoulos S: Aretaeus the Cappadocian on mental illness. *Compr Psychiatry* 1986;27:171–179.

5. Pinel P: *Nosographie Philosophique ou la Methode de l'Analyse Appliquée à la Medicine*. Paris, Brosson, 1818.
6. Esquirol JED: *Mental Maladies*. New York, Hafner Press, 1965.
7. Zilboorg G, Henry GW: *A History of Medical Psychology*. New York, WW Norton, 1941.
8. Bayle AL: *Description of General Paralysis*, Paris, Didot le Jeune, 1822.
9. Kraepelin E: *Dementia Praecox and Paraphrenia*. Edinburgh, Livingston, 1919.
10. Bleuler E, Jung CG: Komplexe and krankheitsursachen bei dementia praecox. *Zb. Nervenheilk Psychiat* 1908;31:220–227.
11. Bleuler E: *Dementia Praecox Oder die Gruppe der Schizophrenien*. Leipzig, Deuticke, 1911.
12. Kahlbaum K: *Die Gruppierung der Psychischen Krankheiten und die Einteilung der Seelenstoerungen*. Danzig, Kafemann, 1863.
13. Hecker E: Die Hebephrenie. *Arch Pathol Ant Physiol Klin Med* 1871;52:394–429.
14. Heinroth JC: *Lehrbuch der Storungen des Seelenlebens* (orig. 1818, translated by Schmorak J) Baltimore, Johns Hopkins Press, 1975.
15. Neumann H: *Blodsinnigkeitserklarung*. Erlangen, 1860.
16. Griesinger W: *Mental Pathology and Therapeutics*. New York, Hafner Press, 1965.
17. Kraepelin E: *Psychiatrie*, 8th edit. Leipzig, JA Barth, 1915.
18. Klerman GL: The significance of DSM-III in American psychiatry, in Spitzer RL, Williams JBW, Skodol AE (eds). *International Perspectives on DSM-III*. Washington, DC, American Psychiatric Press, 1983.
19. Bleuler E: Die prognose der dementia precox (Schizophreniegruppe). *Allg Z Psychiat* 1908;65:436–464.
20. American Psychiatric Association: *Diagnostic and Statistical Manual of Mental Disorders*, third edit. Washington, DC, American Psychiatric Association, 1980.
21. Schneider K: Primare und sekundare Symptome bei Schizophrenie. *Fortschr Neurol Psychiatr* 1957;25:487.
22. Carpenter WT, Strauss JS: Cross-cultural evaluation of Schneider's first rank symptoms of schizophrenia: a report from the international pilot study of schizophrenia. *Am J Psychiatry* 1974;131:682–687.
23. Kleist K: Uber zycloide, paranoide und epileptoide Psychosen und uber die Frage der Degenerationpsychosen. *Schweiz Arch Neurol Psychiatry* 1928;23:3–37.
24. Leonhard K: *Die Defekt Schizophrenen Krankheits Bilder*. Leipzig, Thieme, 1936.
25. Clayton RJ, Rodin L, Winokur G: Family history studies: schizoaffective disorder, clinical and genetic factors. *Compr Psychiatry* 1968;9:31–49.
26. Perris C: A study of cycloid psychoses. *Acta Psychiatr Scand* 1974;*Suppl*, 253.
27. Langfeldt G: *The Schizophreniform States*. Copenhagen, Munksgaard, 1939.
28. World Health Organization: ICD-9-CM: International Classification of Diseases, 9th revision, Clinical Modification. Ann Arbor, Commission on Professional and Hospital Activities, 1980.
29. Jaspers K: *General Psychopathology*. Chicago, University of Chicago Press, 1963.

30. Binswanger L: *Being-in-the-world*, in Needleman J (ed). New York, Basic Books, 1963.
31. Minkowski E: *La Schziophrenie, ed. 2*. Paris, Desclee de Brouwer, 1953.
32. Freud S: *The Origin of Psychoanalysis*. New York, Basic Books, 1954.
33. Klein M: Notes on some schizoid mechanisms. in Klein M, Heimann P, Isaacs S, Riviere J (eds). *Developments in Psychoanalysis*. London, Hogarth Press, 1952, p. 292.
34. Meyer A: Fundamental conceptions of dementia praecox, in *Collected Papers of Adolf Meyer, Vol. 2*. Baltimore, Johns Hopkins Press, 1950: 432.
35. Kendell RE, Cooper J, Gourley A, Copeland J: Diagnostic criteria of American and British psychiatrists. *Arch Gen Psychiatry* 1971;25:123–130.
36. Pearson K: *Life, Letters and Labours of Francis Galton II*, 1924.
37. Binet A, Henri V: La psychologie individuelle. *Année Psychol* 1896;2:411–465.
38. Binet A, Simon T: Methodes nouvelles pour le diagnostic du niveau intellectuel des anormaux. *Année Psychol* 1905;11:191–336.
39. Overall JE, Gorham DR: The Brief Psychiatric Rating Scale. *Psychol Rep* 1962;10:799–812.
40. Wing JK, Cooper JE, Sartorius N: *The Description and Classification of Psychiatric Symptoms: An Instruction Manual for the PSE and Catego System*. London, Cambridge University Press, 1974.
41. Robins LN, Helzer JE, Croughan J, Ratcliff KS: National Institute of Mental Health diagnostic interview schedule: its history, characteristics and validity. *Arch Gen Psychiatry* 1981;38:381–389.
42. Helmchen H: *Das AMDP-System Manual zur Dokumentation Psychiatrischer Befunde*. Berlin, Springer-Verlag, 1979.
43. Spitzer RL, Williams JBW, Gibbon M, First MB: *Instruction Manual for the Structured Clinical Interview for DSM-III-R (SCID, 1988 Revision)*. New York, New York State Psychiatric Institute, 1988.
44. Helzer JE, Robins LN: The diagnostic interview schedule: its development, evolution and use. *Soc Psychiatry Psychiatr Epidemiol* 1988;23:6–16.
45. Feighner JP, Robins E, Guze SB, et al: Diagnostic criteria for use in psychiatric research. *Arch Gen Psychiatry* 1972;26:57–63.
46. Spitzer RL, Endicott J, Robins E: Research Diagnostic Criteria: rationale and reliability. *Arch Gen Psychiatry* 1978;35:773–782.
47. Spitzer RL, Endicott J: *Schedule for Affective Disorders and Schizophrenia (SADS), 2nd ed*. New York, New York State Psychiatric Institute, Biometrics Research, 1975.
48. Astrachan BM, Harrow M, Adler D, et al: A checklist for the diagnosis of schizophrenia. *Br J Psyhiatry* 1972;121:529–539.
49. Carpenter WT, Strauss JS, Bartko JJ: Flexible system for diagnosis of schizophrenia. Report from the WHO international pilot study of schizophrenia. *Science* 1973;182:1275–1278.
50. WHO: *Report of the International Pilot Study of Schizophrenia. Vol. I*. Geneva, World Health Organization, 1973.
51. Taylor MA, Abrams R: A critique of the St. Louis psychiatric research criteria for schizophrenia. *Am J Psychiatry* 1975;132:1276–1280.
52. Taylor MA, Abrams R: The prevalence of schizophrenia: a reassessment using modern diagnostic criteria. *Am J Psychiatry* 1978;135:945–948.

53. Kendell RE: The uses and abuses of diagnosis, in Dongier M, Wittkower E (eds). *Controversial Issues in Psychiatry*. New York, Harper & Row, 1979.
54. Rosenthal D, Kety SS, eds: *The Transmission of Schizophrenia*. Oxford, Pergamon 1968, pp. 345–362.
55. American Psychiatric Association: *Diagnostic and Statistical Manual of Mental Disorders (Third Edition-Revised)*. Washington, DC, American Psychiatric Association, 1987.
56. International Classification of Diseases, 10th Revision (ICD-10): *1986 Draft of Chapter V: Mental, Behavioral and Developmental Disorders*. Geneva, World Health Organization, Division of Mental Health, 1987.
57. Klerman GL, Vaillant GE, Spitzer RL, Michels R: A debate on DSM-III. *Am J Psychiatry* 1984;141:539–553.
58. Michels R: Discussion, in Freedman AM, Brotman R, Silverman I, Hutson D (eds). *Issues in Psychiatric Classification*. New York, Human Sciences Press. 1986, pp. 111–115.
59. Spitzer RL, Williams JBW, Skodel AE, eds: *International perspectives on DSM-III*. Washington DC, American Psychiatric Press, 1983.
60. Mezzich JE, von Cranach M (eds): *International classification of Psychiatry: Unity and Diversity*. New York, Cambridge University Press, 1989.
61. Berner P, Katschnig H, Lenz G: The polydiagnostic approach in research on schizophrenia, in Freedman AM, Brotman R, Silverman I, Hutson D (eds). *Issues in Psychiatric Classification*. New York, Human Sciences Press, 1986;70–91.
62. Kontaxakis V, Markidis M, Verveniotis S: The validity of the diagnosis of schizophrenia simplex. *Encephalos* 1984;21:143–150.
63. Andreasen NC: Negative symptoms in schizophrenia. Definition and reliability. *Arch Gen Psychiatry* 1982;39:784–788.
64. Andreasen NC, Olsen S: Negative v positive schizophrenia. Definition and validation. *Arch Gen Psychiatry* 1982;39:789–794.
65. Hughlings-Jackson J: *Selected Writings*. Taylor J (ed). London, Hoder & Stoughton, 1931.
66. Pull CB, Pull MC, Pichot P: Des criterières empiriques francais pour les psychoses. I. Position du probleme et methodologie. *Encephale* 1984;10:119–123.
67. Pichot P: *DSM-III et Psychiatrie Francaise*. Paris, Masson, 1984.
68. Lazaratou H: *The Taxonomic Approach of Schizophrenic Psychoses in the French and American Nosologies* (Doctoral Thesis). Athens, University of Athens, 1987.
69. Snezhnevsky AV: On the nosologic specification of the psycho-pathological syndromes. *Zh Nevropatol Psikhiatr* 1960;1:91–107.
70. Nadzharov RA, Sternberg EY: Die Bedeutung der Berucksichtigung des Altersfaktors fur die psychopathologishe, klinische und nosologische Forschung in der Psychiatrie. *Schweiz Arch Neurol Neurosurg Psychiatr* 1970;106:159.
71. Yosiphovich KI: In search of a common language. *Biol Psychiatry* 1987;22:525–528.
72. Freedman AM, Silverman I, Brotman R, Hutson D: The range of issues in psychiatric classification, in Freedman AM, Brotman R, Silverman I, Hutson D (eds). *Issues in Psychiatric Classification*. New York, Human Sciences Press, 1986.

73. Kraepelin E: Vergleichende psychiatrie. *Centralblatt fur Nervenheilkunde und Psychiatrie.* 1904;27:433–437.
74. Devereaux: *Essais d'Ethnopsychiatrie Generale.* Paris, Gaillimard, 1970.
75. Murphy HBM: *Comparative Psychiatry: The International and Intercultural Distribution of Mental Illness.* Berlin, Springer-Verlag, 1982.
76. WHO: *Schizophrenia. An International Follow-Up Study.* Chichester, Wiley, 1979.
77. Jablensky A, Schwarz R, Tomov T: WHO collaborative study on impairments and disabilities associated with schizophrenic disorders. *Acta Psychiatr Scand* 1980;62,Suppl 285:152–163.
78. Sartorius N, Jablensky A, Korten A, et al: Early manifestations and first-contact incidence of schizophrenia in different cultures. *Psychol Med* 1986;16:909–928.
79. Jablensky A, Sartorius N: Is schizophrenia universal? in Jansson B, Perris C (eds). *Berzelius Symposium XI: Transcultural Psychiatry in Stockholm, Sweden, April 8–10, 1987. Acta Psychiatr Scand* 1988;78,Suppl 344:65–70.
80. Sartorius N, Jablensky A, Shapiro R: Cross-cultural differences in the short-term prognosis of schizophrenic psychoses. *Schizophr Bull* 1978;4:102–113.
81. Mantonakis J: *The Religious Aspects in the Psychopathology of Schizophrenics from the Island of Crete, A Comparative study. (Postdoctoral Thesis).* Athens, University of Athens, 1982.
82. Madianos M, Stefanis C, Madianou D: Prevalence of mental disorders and utilization of mental health service in two areas of Greater Athens, in Cooper B (ed). *Psychiatric Epidemiology. Progress and Prospects.* London, Groom Helm 1987, pp. 372–382.
83. Tsuang MT, Winokur G, Crowe RR: Morbidity risks of schizophrenia and affective disorders among first degree relatives of patients with schizophrenia, mania, depression, and surgical conditions. *Br J Psychiatry* 1980; 137:497–504.
84. Mendlewicz J, Linkowski P, Wilmotte J: Relationship between schizoaffective illness and affective disorder in schizophrenia: morbidity risk and genetic transmission. *J Affective Disord* 1980;2:289–302.
85. Guze SB, Cloninger CR, Martin RL, Clayton PJ: A follow-up and family study of schizophrenia. *Arch Gen Psychiatry* 1983;40:1273–1276.
86. Kendler KS, Gruenberg AM, Tsuang MT: Psychiatric illness in first-degree relatives of schizophrenic and surgical control patients. *Arch Gen Psychiatry* 1985;42:770–779.
87. Gershon ES, DeLisi LE, Maxwell ME, et al: A controlled family study of psychosis. *Arch Gen Psychiatry* 1988;45:328–337.
88. Gottesman II, Shields J: *Schizophrenia and Genetics: A Twin Study Vantage Point.* Orlando, FL, Academic Press, 1972.
89. Fischer M: Genetic and environmental factors in schizophrenia. *Acta Psychiatr Scand* 1973;238(Suppl):1–158.
90. Gottesman II, Shields J: *Schizophrenia: The Epigenetic Puzzle.* New York, Cambridge University Press, 1982.
91. Kendler KS: Overview: a current perspective on twin studies of schizophrenia. *Am J Psychiatry* 1983;140:1413–1425.
92. McGuffin P, Farmer AE, Gottesman II, Murray RM, Reveley AM: Twin concordance for operationally defined schizophrenia: confirmation of familiarity and heritability. *Arch Gen Psychiatry* 1984;41:541–545.

93. Bertelsen A: Controversies and consistencies in psychiatric genetics. *Acta Psychiatr Scand* 1985;71(*Suppl* 319):61–75.
94. Farmer A, McGuffin P, Gottesman I: Twin concordance in DSM-III schizophrenia. *Arch Gen Psychiatry* 1987;44:634–641.
95. Rosenthal D, Wender PH, Kety SS, et al: The adopted away offspring of schizophrenics. *Am J Psychiatry* 1971;128:397–411.
96. Gottesman II, McGuffin P, Farmer A: Clinical genetics as clues to the "real" genetics of schizophrenia. *Schizophr Bull* 1987;13:23–47.
97. Wyatt RJ, Alexander RC, Egan MF, Kirch OG: Schizophrenia, just the facts. What do we know, how well do we know it? *Schizophr Res* 1988;1:3–18.
98. Gershon ES, Merrill CR, Goldin IR, et al: The role of molecular genetics in psychiatry. Biol Psychiatry 1987;22:1388–1405.
99. Gusella JF, Wexler NS, Conneally PM, et al: A polymorphic DNA marker genetically linked to Hungtinton's disease. *Nature* 1983;306:234–238.
100. Egeland JR, Gerrhard DS, Pauls DL, et al: Bipolar affective disorders linked to DNA markers on chromosome 11. *Nature* 1987;325:783–787.
101. Baron M, Rainer JD: Molecular genetics and human disease: implications for modern psychiatric research and practice. *Br J Psychiatry* 1988;152:741–753.
102. Mendlewicz J, Sevy S, Brocas H, et al: Polymorphic DNA marker on X chromosome and manic depression. *Lancet* 1987;i:1230–1232.
103. Detera-Wadleigh S, Berretlini WH, Goldin LR, et al: Close linkage of c-Harvey-ras-1 and the insulin gene to affective disorder is ruled out in three North American pedigrees. *Nature* 1987;325:806–808.
104. Bassett AS, McGillivray BC, Jones BD, Pantzar JT: Partial trisomy chromosome 5 cosegregating with schizophrenia. *Lancet* 1988;i:799–801.
105. Kendler KS, Lindon JE: Models for the joint effect of genotype and environment on lability to psychiatric illness. *Am J Psychiatry 1986;143:279–289.*
106. Vartanian ME, Kolyaskina GI, Lozovsky DV: Aspects of humoral and cellular immunity in schizophrenia, in Bergsma D, Goldstein AL, (eds). *Neurochemical and Immunologic Components in Schizophrenia.* New York, Alan R. Liss, 1978.
107. Liedeman RR, Prilipko LI: The behavior of T lymphocytes in schizophrenia, in Bergsma D, Goldstein AL (eds). *Neurochemical and Immunologic Components in Schizophrenia.* New York, Alan R. Liss, 1978.
108. Coffey CE, Sullivan JL, Rice JR: T lymphocytes in schizophrenia. *Biol Psychiatry* 1983;18:113–119.
109. Ivanyi P, Droes J, Schreuder GM, et al: A search for association of HLA antigens with paranoid schizophrenia: A_9 appears as a possible marker. *Tissue Antigens* 1983;22:186–193.
110. Miyanaga K, Machiyama T, Juji T: Schizophrenic disorders and HLA-DR antigens. *Biol Psychiatry* 1984;19:121–129.
111. Theodoropoulou-Vaidaki S, Alexopoulos C, Stefanis CN: A study of the immunological state of schizophrenic patients, in Stefanis CN, Rabavilas AD (eds). *Schizophrenia. Recent Biosocial Developments.* New York, Human Sciences Press, 1988, pp. 69–85.
112. Torrey EF, Petersen MR: The viral hypothesis of schizophrenia. *Schizophr Bull* 1976;2:136–146.
113. Crow TJ: A reevaluation of the viral hypothesis: is psychosis the result of

retroviral integration at a site close to the cerebral dominance gene? *Br J Psychiatry* 1984;145:243–253.

114. Torrey EF, McGuire M, O'Hara A, et al: Endemic psychosis in Western Ireland. *Am J Psychiatry* 1984;141:966–969.

115. Crow TJ, Done DJ: Age of onset of schizophrenia in siblings: a test of the contagion hypothesis. *Psychiatry Res* 1986;18:107–117.

116. Crow TJ: Genes and viruses in schizophrenia. The retrovirus/transposon hypothesis, in Stefanis CN, Rabavilas AD, (eds). *Schizophrenia. Recent Biosocial Developments*. New York, Human Sciences Press, 1988, pp. 54–68.

117. Mednick SA, Machon RA, Huttunen MO, Bonet D: Adult schizophrenia following prenatal exposure to an influenza epidemic. *Arch Gen Psychiatry* 1988;45:189–192.

118. Meltzer HY, Stahl SM: The dopamine hypothesis of schizophrenia: a review. *Schizophr Bull* 1976;2:19–76.

119. Johnstone EC, Crow TJ, Frith CD, et al: Cerebral ventricular size and cognitive impairment in chronic schizophrenia. *Lancet* 1976;ii:924–926.

120. Newlin DB, Carpender B, Golden CJ: Hemispheric asymetries in schizophrenia. *Biol Psychiatry* 1981;16:561–582.

121. Wyatt RJ, Cutler NR, DeLisi LE, et al: Biochemical and morphological factors in the etiology of the schizophrenia disorders, in Grinspoon L (ed). *Psychiatry, 1982 Annual Review*. Washington DC, American Psychiatric Press, 1982.

122. Reveley MA, Reveley AM, Daldy R: Left hemisphere hypodensity in discordant schizophrenic twins. *Arch Gen Psychiatry* 1987;44:625–633.

123. Rabavilas AD, Liappas JA, Stefanis CN: Electrodermal laterality indices in paranoid schizophrenics, in Stefanis CN, Rabavilas AD, (eds). *Schizophrenia. Recent Biosocial Developments*. New York, Human Sciences Press, 1988:122–134.

124. Wong DF, Wagner HN, Tune LE, et al: Positron emission tomography reveals elevated D2 dopamine receptors in drug-naive schizophrenics. *Science* 1986;234:1558–1563.

125. Farde L, Hall H, Ehrin E, Sedvall G: Quantitative analysis of D2 dopamine receptor binding in the living human brain by PET. *Science* 1986;231:258–261.

126. Ingvar DH, Franzen G: Abnormalities of cerebral blood flow distribution in patients with chronic schizophrenia. *Acta Psychiatr Scand* 1974;50:425–462.

127. Buchsbaum MS, Ingvar DH, Kessler R, et al: Cerebral glucography with positron tomography. Use in normal subjects and in patients with schizophrenia. *Arch Gen Psychiatry* 1982;39:251–259.

128. Sheppard G, Gruzelier J, Manchanda R, et al: O-positron emission tomographic scanning in predominantly never-treated acute schizophrenic patients. *Lancet* 1983;ii:1448–1452.

129. Widen L, Blomquist G, Greitz T, et al: PET studies of glucose metabolism in patients with schizophrenia. *Am J Neurol* 1983;4:550–552.

130. Williamson P: Hypofrontality in schizophrenia: a review of the evidence. *Can J Psychiatry* 1987;32:399–404.

131. Bushbaum MS, Haier RJ: Functional and anatomical brain imaging: impact on schizophrenia research. *Schizophr Bull* 1987;13:115–132.

132. Gur RE, Resnick SM, Alavi A, et al: Regional brain function in schizophre-

nia, I. A positron emission tomography study. *Arch Gen Psychiatry* 1987;44:119–125.
133. Gur RE, Resnick SM, Gur RC, et al: Regional brain function in schizophrenia, II. Repeated evaluation with positron emission tomography. *Arch Gen Psychiatry* 1987;44:126–129.

3
Modular Disjunction in Schizophrenia: A Framework for a Pathological Psychophysiology

JOHN M. CLEGHORN AND MARTIN L. ALBERT

This chapter is an attempt to synthesize contemporary research data from neurobiology, neuropsychology, and cognitive science for the purpose of understanding schizophrenic psychosis. Our principal conclusions constitute a framework for a pathological psychophysiology of schizophrenia. Because we consider variability or a lack of neurocognitive modulation to be a fundamental characteristic of schizophrenic behaviour, our framework focuses on explanations of this variability. We suggest that although individual modules of cognitive and emotional function may be intact in schizophrenia, messages are inappropriately sent to parts of the brain not specialized for the required information. Neural networks that form the substrate for cognitive or emotional modules are activated or inactivated in a disorganized or inappropriate temporal sequence, and, thus, desynchronization ("modular disjunction") of widely distributed neural systems develops, causing the signs and symptoms of schizophrenic psychosis.

This chapter is organized in the following manner. First, we consider the notion of "modularity" in cognition and demonstrate ways in which desynchronization of modular function (modular disjunction) may underlie psychotic symptoms. We then move from phenomenology to neuropsychological mechanisms, analyzing the relations among information processing, perseveration, and modularity. Next we discuss neurophysiological, neuropharmacological, and neuroanatomical systems that serve as the biological substrate for those neuropsychological mechanisms that we theorize may underlie modular disjunction. We conclude by synthesizing the data and summarizing our new conceptual framework whereby modular disjunction leads to signs and symptoms of schizophrenic psychosis.

By way of introduction we wish to comment on those clinical features of schizophrenia that seem to be relevant for our analysis. First, a large proportion of schizophrenic patients demonstrate persistent neurocognitive impairment, and we assume that this neurocognitive impairment is a central component of the psychopathology, which can neither be explained by the negative symptoms nor relegated to a secondary role as part of a residual deficit state.[1]

Clinical examination of most schizophrenics, in episode and to a lesser extent in remission, reveals one or more of the following: conscious awareness of dysfunction is reduced and attentiveness is impaired; the registration and recall of verbal and/or spatial information is less complete than in normal controls; and anticipation and planning and goal-directed behaviour are restricted. In fact, conscious monitoring of behaviour is ineffective,[2] and lacking is the sense that certain actions are intended.[3,4] Emotional colouring of experience is muted. The awareness of self, self–other distinctions, self-cohesion, and continuity in time may be impaired. It is therefore hardly surprising that communication is incoherent, as the neuropsychological background is fragmented.

These observations indicate a lack of modulation of communication systems in the brain. Further evidence for a lack of modulation can be detected in the variability in many functions measured repeatedly over time. The variability can be observed in symptomatic behaviour,[5,6] neuropsychological test performance,[7-9] neuroendocrine responses to drug challenges,[10,11] symptomatic responses to neuroleptic treatment,[12] and in measures of neurotransmitter metabolites in cerebrospinal fluid.[13] These studies have all demonstrated greater variability in patients than in controls when the measures are repeated at different times.

Because there is an enormous gulf between psychopathology and dysfunctional units of the brain, the bridging concept of cognitive module is being proposed to permit a reinterpretation of existing data.*

Cognitive Modules

Contemporary cognitive science recognizes a partition between brain data and behavioural data in general, and proposes the bridging concept of cognitive modules.[14-17] A cognitive module is one kind of functional unit of the brain. The concept of cognitive module has emerged from numerous observations that certain cognitive functions can be specifically disturbed by local brain lesions.

The term cognitive module has been given added meaning recently as a computational unit, a nonanatomic concept derived from computer science.[14] Brain anatomy and chemistry provide fixed structures and widely distributed circuits that are essential to the production of language, memory, attention, emotion, and so on. However, the actual manifestation of coherent language, memory for the emotional significance of perceived phenomena, and the critical differentiation of real and false (all disordered

---

*Cleghorn JM, Albert ML: A neurobiological model of schizophrenic psychosis: modular disjunction in widely distributed systems in the brain. In preparation, 1989.

in schizophrenia) must involve computational processes we do not yet understand.

Certain fundamental, elementary operations can be localized in the brain[18]; for example, engaging attention in space. However, the concept of module cannot be reduced to specific brain regions. There is a large gulf between cognitive module, a functional concept, and its neurobiological basis. Isomorphism cannot be assumed.

The heuristic value of the modularity concept for schizophrenia is that it invites us to explore the contributions of cognitive and neural sciences together. Such a multidisciplinary approach may be needed, because the efforts of the separate sciences have been frustrated.

For example, fundamental neurological functions have been found to be largely intact in schizophrenia. Simple tests of attention, language, and motor function reveal minor abnormalities, if any. Therefore, brain mechanisms subserving these functions must be largely intact. Abnormalities emerge when a patient is required to integrate these fundamental functions with affective expression and meaning.

The separation of functions may be analogous to the phenomena observed in split-brain patients. In such patients when a right hemisphere function is activated, the verbal left hemisphere offers a verbal explanation, often fanciful but in a way that makes sense and resolves dissonance.[19] The interhemispheric communication required for this transfer of information may well be disturbed in schizophrenia.[20,21] This is one kind of proximate mechanism proposed to underlie the psychopathology of schizophrenia, one kind of disjunction of cognitive modules.

We now will apply the concept of modular disjunction to the psychopathology of schizophrenia to provide a provisional framework for organizing possible ways of thinking. Because data are lacking to define fully the content and interactions of modules, and because knowledge of the chemical and anatomical nature of modules is unknown, it must be acknowledged that our model may be oversimplified and wrong in some details. However, our proposal may suggest promising lines of experimentation that will generate data requiring that the model be modified, a process that may help guide some future research directions.

Psychotic Symptoms and Modular Disjunction

We now examine several of the symptoms of schizophrenia to describe the kinds of processes that might underlie the dissociations that gave rise to the name of the disorder. In so doing we begin to propose processes of modular disjunction.

When a patient expresses himself or herself incoherently, there is evidently nothing wrong with his or her ability to process or express language.[22] However, there is evidence for poor discourse planning.[23] A disjunction between processes involved in the preparation of an utterance and its expression may have occurred. This is reflected most obviously in the timing of communication with other people. Responses seem too rapid or interminably delayed. Gaze is abbreviated or avoided. Facial expression and tone of voice do not change much or are poorly modulated.[24] There is either a failure to plan or to activate a plan or failure in the timing of expression.

Furthermore, the decoding of incoming information may be impaired, for example, facial expression.[25] Patients are often not "in tune" with those they are with.[26] They do not share a focus of attention.[27] They may, in addition, fail to interpret the message correctly and therefore respond in a socially inappropriate way.

In addition to errors in timing, the patient and some relatives are unable to screen out as much distracting information as normal people.[28] When two such family members are given a task to discuss, their communication is characterized by misperceptions, vagueness, and lack of focus. An inability to comprehend the social context of communication[24] contributes to this communication failure.

The text of conversation of schizophrenic patients shares features with jargon aphasia,[29] although it is not identical. Inappropriate significance is given to some semantic and phonological features. Sentences may be influenced by previously uttered words rather than the topic of conversation and there are fewer cohesive ties than in other patients or normal people.[30] Thus, there is a disjunction of processes underlying both the expression and reception of social communication.

In some patients, communication is impaired by incongruity of thought and affect. This is particularly evident in the hebephrenic patient who giggles in a fashion that seems silly. When asked what the examiner said that was funny, or what funny thought the patient had, he cannot say, any more than Gazzaniga's split-brain patients[19] can explain their responses to nonverbal stimuli. Similarly, a patient with frontal lobe damage may laugh or cry easily,[19] even though complaining that this behaviour does not reflect the appropriate affect. Such behaviour is observed in some schizophrenic patients during the psychotic state. Thus, one bit of communication perseverates while a new item appears, as though modules that generate verbal and nonverbal communication are operating independently.

The concept of modular disjunction also may serve as a basis for understanding the development of some delusions. Early in the psychosis, a delusional perception (primary delusion or idea of reference) occurs. There is a sudden insight that a perception or event has special significance for the person. This is a mismatch of the sense of significance of an event which has not been correctly checked with an expectancy based on personal memory. The loss of boundaries with other persons also may involve a mismatch of internal emotional state and the inappropriate attribution of personal significance to the acts of another person. The patient fails to make a match between a perception and that which is "not part of me."

When a patient experiences thought withdrawal or insertion, part of himself is experienced as alien, there is disjunction of the sense of ownership or familiarity and the thought ("someone else is putting thoughts in my head, or taking them away"). In this experience the patient attributes part of self to nonself, in contrast to the above described merger of self and nonself. In addition his conscious attention may be stuck on a prior event. Thus, the thought is accompanied by a sense that it is unintended and is controlled by an agent outside himself. There is a double disjunction here, that is, of modules subserving the sense of familiarity and the sense of intention.

Auditory hallucinations may represent similar mechanisms in the language systems of the brain. Subvocal speech accompanies auditory hallucinations.[31,32] They are unintended and alien, automatic and repetitive, that is, perseverative. The lack of intention may reflect the absence of a plan for discourse,[3] or if a plan exists it is not connected with language expression. Possibly, the missing link is the absence of conscious awareness of intent.[33] The hallucination, in any event, is experienced as alien, not self. In addition, it is usually located outside the head. Thus, speech articulation and spatial perception are disconnected.

Thought blocking may represent modular disjunction of a speech plan and its articulation or expression. The speech plan may have been transmitted to a nonverbal module, or, alternatively, attention to the train of thought may have been disengaged.

Poverty of thought and spontaneous speech, apathy, and avolition can be conceptualized as perseveration of a state in which both initiative and intentionality are lacking, if not part of a permanent frontal lobe abulia.

The term "ambivalence" arises from the observation that two different emotional responses, or two intentions or thoughts, are given equal weight. The patient vacillates at great length between one and the other. This may represent simultaneous activation of the two components or a failure to inactivate one.

Patients complain of a palpable loss of positive feelings (anhedonia). A much loved friend or relative is still recognized, but with neutral feelings. Fear and anger are still felt, however, and form a rationale for the sense of persecution. An incidental event is associated with negative emotion and creates a sense of suspicion. Thus, the development of paranoia may begin with a loss of the ability to generate positive feelings toward images of familiar people and other stimuli.

The persistence of auditory hallucinations may reflect recurrent or continuous perseveration within a modular system that involves subvocal speech, middle ear activity, and hearing. Compulsions, stereotypies, mannerisms such as grimacing, and rhythmic rocking and tapping may also represent continuous perseveration in complex motor behaviour.[34]

Perseveration also may explain the persistence of delusions. The development of a delusional interpretation is simply the construction of a theory that attempts to make sense of the peculiar experience, as Gazzaniga[19] suggested occurs in split-brain patients. It is a system of belief that often persists when other symptoms respond to neuroleptic treatment. The persistence of a delusion, its impermeability to contrary information and persuasion, is congruent with the concept of cognitive module as a computational unit containing an overlearned program.

In conclusion, much of the behaviour and experience of schizophrenic patients is congruent with the notion that cognitive modules, although functionally intact, are not properly integrated with each other. We propose that modular disjunction is normally prevented by processes that underlie conscious monitoring, intentionality, goal-initiated behaviour,[4] and emotional colouring of meaning. These processes are disrupted by errors in the timing of information processing and in the execution of acts.

Systematic studies of information processing in schizophrenia are examined next. They add specificity and quantification to the clinical observations.

Information Processing, Perseveration, and Modularity

Dysfunctional Information Processing

Six forms of dysfunctional information processing and their significance for disjunctive processes in schizophrenia are described below.

Slow Initial Evoked Responses

Whereas the initial reception of stimuli within the first hundred milliseconds is often normal in schizophrenic patients,[35] the input threshold is elevated in some patients as it is in brain damaged patients.[36] When patients are given stimuli at relatively long intervals (1 second) they do not stay focused on the correct channel, particularly if they have a poor premorbid history.[37,38] These two measures may reflect the failure to register new information often observed.

Attenuated Responses

The response to stimuli during the 200 to 500 milliseconds after they have been presented is attenuated.[35,36,39] The P300 response is delayed over left frontal and temporal regions.[40] Because the hippocampus is a source of the P300 and is involved in giving significance to events, the delay may underlie mismatching of subjective state and perception of events.

Episodic Interruptions Underlie Deficits in Performance

Increased incidence of extraneous eye movements in smooth pursuit eye tracking[41] and attentional lapses that contribute to high error rates on complex tasks such as the Wisconsin Card Sort Test[42] are examples of such deficits. The maintenance of attention and the sequential flow of meaning in communication may be thus disrupted.

Failure in Selective Attention

Failure in selective attention is observed in patients who are acutely psychotic, those in remission, and those at risk for schizophrenia on the basis of family history.[43–45] Numerous studies reviewed by Nuechterlein and Dawson[46] indicate that tasks with a high momentary processing load elicit deficits in selective attention. When two members of the same family are found to be poor attenders they demonstrate deviant and incoherent communication when talking together.[28]

Slow Channel Switching

Schizophrenic patients are slow to make a change from one channel to another, for example, auditory to visual when a reaction time task requires such a shift in attention.[47–49] A delay in communication between perceptual modules may reside in dysfunction of these brain regions. Rapid switching between modalities is required for normal human communication.

Slow and Repetitive Motor Responses

Slow information processing and channel switching are also reflected by slow and repetitive motor responses. Perseveration, the repetitive production of the same response to different stimuli or commands, is frequently observed on examination.[50] Sandson and Albert[34] call this *stuck-in-set* perseveration. Patients respond to a new stimulus as though it were the previous one.[39] The P300 electroencephalogram (EEG) response fails to occur, as though there were no new stimuli of significance. When the response is planned, an expectancy wave or contingent negative variation (CNV) is observed. This is normally resolved when the response is executed. Schizophrenic subjects often fail to resolve the CNV after performing a task,[51] possibly indicating that feedback has not been received. The fact that a response has been made is not registered. Perhaps this is one reason behaviours are repeated.

Several anomalies of the timing of information processes may reflect failures of conscious processing. The channel capacity is usually low and it fails to remain tuned, varying at different times to over- or underuse input. It further fails to match stimuli with memories and is slow to change modalities. The capacity is so limited, the context of sensory information is not used. Access to expectancies based on experience is therefore restricted. Furthermore, connections required to give a correct response are missing. In contrast, according to an interpretation by Calloway and Naghdi,[52] automatic processes that operate unconsciously and in parallel are normal or superior in schizophrenia. Thus, fundamental processes are intact, as stated earlier, but parallel processing of an integrative nature is defective.

To proceed we require a more sophisticated understanding of normal modular function. Such an understanding is being developed by Posner et al.[53,18] They have defined a computational component in which exact times to engage, disengage, or move attention can be calculated. These are called modules of attention. Furthermore, the anatomic location of regions involved in these functions is being determined. Evidence has been gathered to support the existence of separate brain systems for visual and auditory attention, and a connected but separate system for the location of sounds and sights in space, and a separate system for the location of language in space.

The regional activation of cerebral blood flow by module-specific stimuli provides strong support for the localization of elementary operations of visual, phonological, and semantic codes and for an anterior attention system that selects for action.[53] All the modules exist within a generalized attentional system, the anatomical basis of which is probably widely distributed.

Posner's system of computational modules of attention and their anatomical referents offers a very promising approach to the study of modular disjunction in schizophrenia. Preliminary studies of regional brain metabolism are encouraging. The parietal lobes and strong frontoparietal connections comprise part of a generalized attentional system.[54,55] Evidence for hypometabolism of the parietal lobes recently has been presented in patients suffering an acute psychotic episode[56] and in chronic patients.[57–59] Furthermore, there was a reciprocal relationship between the rate of metabolism in the parietal and prefrontal regions in both patients and controls. In psychotic patients, however, the frontal region was hypermetabolic and the parietal region hypometabolic relative to that of controls. Correct performance of tests of attention requires intact function of frontal or parietal regions or both. Parietal lesions lead to slow disengagement,[60] a conspicuous feature of the studies of modality switching quoted earlier. Perhaps parietal hypometabolism relative to frontal hypermetabolism is also associated with slow switching of sensory modalities.

In the future, it will be possible to present stimuli that call on the capacity of each of the above-mentioned modules and to locate the regional brain metabolic response to such cognitive challenges. Correlations between these brain regions can be computed; for example, those involved in engagement and visual aspects of attention. These computations can test the hypothesis that brain regions subserving different modules of attention are disconnected in schizophrenia.

Neurophysiology of Program Selection and Activation and Brain Imaging

If cognitive modules are disconnected then brain systems must be inappropriately coordinated in schizophrenic psychoses. We next examine brain imaging data that are congruent with that hypothesis. Then we examine mechanisms that normally control neural programs, their selection, activation, and switching. These mechanisms have not yet been examined directly in schizophrenia.

In chronic schizophrenic patients, frontal activation often fails to occur. Most studies have shown them to be "hypofrontal." When presented with the Wisconsin Card Sort test, Weinberger et al[60] found that schizophrenic patients failed to activate the dorsolateral frontal cerebral blood flow, whereas normals do so. It is implied that neuronal traffic is held up or directed to the wrong place. Evidence recently has emerged that a structural abnormality may be at fault, because poor performance on the Card Sort test is related to enlarged lateral ventricles.[61] Thus, a test that provokes perseveration in schizophrenic patients has been shown to fail to activate the dorsolateral frontal cortex.

Next, we tentatively suggest that parts of the brain used for specialized tasks are different in schizophrenics than in normals. One study by Gur et al[62] showed increased right frontal blood flow in response to a verbal task in schizophrenic patients, the opposite of that found in normals. Furthermore, glucose metabolism measured by positron-emission tomography (PET) was found to be inversely related to errors on a spatial task in left frontal and parietal regions in schizophrenic patients and on the right in normal control subjects (Cleghorn, 1988, unpublished data). Thus, two studies support our suggestion that schizophrenics use different parts of the brain for some tasks than do normal people.

The functional relationships between regions must be different in schizophrenia than in normals if the theory of modular disjunction is to be supported. Cognitive challenges that activate regions known to be required for successful performance in normals might activate fewer and different areas in schizophrenia. As a result, correlations between disparate regions would be different and less numerous in schizophrenics than in normals.

Two preliminary studies suggest that activation of different parts of the brain are less highly correlated in schizophrenics than in normal controls. Holcomb et al[63] studied glucose uptake by PET and divided the brain slices into six segments. In schizophrenic patients the correlations between these areas were significantly lower than in normal controls. Somatosensory evoked potentials were measured simultaneously, and their relationship with regional glucose uptake was examined. There were sevenfold fewer significant correlations between these measures in patients than in normal subjects. When measures of glucose metabolism in frontal regions were correlated with each other, 7 of 10 regions were positively and significantly correlated in normals, and only 2 of 10 in patients. In the patients, the significant correlations were negative.[64] Volkow et al[65] also have reported fewer significant correlations between regions in schizophrenics than in normals.

If further data corroborate the hypothesis that brain regions inappropriate to tasks are used in schizophrenia and that brain regions are not coordinated as in normals, then a search for defective mechanisms of regional activation and switching should be undertaken. The following candidates could be examined:

1. The command interneuron defined by Kennedy,[66] ". . . single cells which at modest discharge frequencies, release coordinated behaviour involving a number of output channels." Thus, there is a neuron that could be said to have the properties of a multichannel switch that can activate complex patterns of response in temporal sequence. Complex circuits have been demonstrated in animals to generate varied and specific temporal patterns. Mountcastle et al[67] have described populations of neurons in mammalian parietal association cortex that may play a role in transmitting sensory information into motor commands through projections to the caudate nuclei and could include selector and command interneurons.

2. The striatum may be involved in regulating attention as well as movement. Nauta[68] has considered the possibility that reciprocal links of the striatum with cerebral cortex and limbic system may constitute a common substrate for movement and thought. McKenzie et al[69] review evidence suggesting that dorsal and ventral striatal regions relate to different aspects of motor and cognitive behaviour, respectively. The neostriatum appears to control changes in the direction of attention and motor programs. Involvement of the basal ganglia in complex cognitive processes existing between sensory input and motor execution is generally supported by the evidence.

Data on schizophrenics provided by Manshreck et al[70] also support this integrated view of striatum. An inability to produce synchronous motor (tapping) responses was found to be related to the severity of disturbance in thinking. Disordered functioning of both dorsal and ventral striatum are implicated here.

Swerdlow and Koob[71] have made a most interesting proposal that a mechanism for selecting foci of attention, initiating, and switching programs may be located in a matrix of spiny gamma-aminobutyric acid (GABA) cells in the nucleus accumbens (part of ventral striatum). They propose that excess dopaminergic (DA) inhibition of the firing of these cells could lead to a disruption of selective attention and the execution of responses through connections in ventral pallidum and in turn to ventromedial thalamic nuclei, limbic system, and frontal cortex.

3. The possible role of the thalamus should also be considered.[72]

Among its many functions, the thalamus has two modes of operation and shifts between them. Its transfer mode relays internally stored information and matches it with the neurons activated by perception of external stimuli. The thalamus thus has a role in vigilance and attention. Its other role is quite different. It is a neuronal oscillator, responsible for generating the rhythmic activity of the cortex observed in EEG recordings. It is tempting to suggest that the thalamus may shift from its attention transfer mode to its disengaged oscillatory mode in schizophrenics at those times when patients inappropriately disengage cortical activity required for conscious monitoring and intentional activity. The thalamus may indeed be important as it is one of very few brain regions markedly influenced by neuroleptic drugs in schizophrenia.[57]

In summary, the neurophysiology of selecting and switching motor programs may apply equally to cognitive programs. We propose that abnormal neuronal connections in the ventral striatum, the thalamus, and in cortical association areas be investigated as they may underlie abnormalities in regional brain activation and in the functional relationships between brain regions.

In the final sections of this chapter neurochemical and anatomical data relevant to this proposal are considered.

Neuropharmacology of Tuning and Switching

We now examine the possible neurochemical basis of tuning and switching neural programs and how they might be disrupted to produce modular disjunction.

Pharmacological studies of animal behaviour have examined some of the very same processes that go awry in schizophrenia. The mechanisms of alertness, of timing and direction of impulse transmission, and execution of response are regulated by norepinephrine (NE), dopamine (DA), or both. Hornykiewicz[73] proposed that NE may be as important in schizophrenia as DA appears to be. Iversen and Iversen[74] review evidence that NE and DA neurons interact in the manner proposed by Antelman and Caggiula,[75] that NE pathways are involved in attention and DA pathways in motor execution.

Oades[76] has documented the role of NE in "tuning" or altering the signal-to-noise ratio. He further reviews evidence that DA activity may promote switching between inputs and outputs of information to specific brain regions. He concludes that the tuning principle in NE systems is particularly important for the formation of associations and neural plasticity (interference control) and that "the switching principle of dopaminergic systems modulates the timing, time sharing and initiation of responses (program control)." Oades suggests that perseveration in schizophrenic patients might be associated with DA up regulation and thought intrusions with down regulation of DA and NE activation. Selective destruction of

NE neurons and activation of DA neurons can lead to perseveration. Norepinephrine stimulation modifies the perseverative tendency by influencing exploration or habituation.[77]

Amphetamine, a DA and NE agonist, fixes attention in animals and produces behavioural stereotypy and perseveration.[76,78] (Amphetamines can also produce psychosis.) The behavioural repertoire is reduced and a few elements repeated continuously. Disjunctive postures develop as though body parts operate autonomously.[79]

Although amphetamine-induced abnormalities do not simulate all features of schizophrenic psychosis,[80,81] the attentional and perseverative processes warrant cross-species study.[82] For example, Szechtman et al[83] described complex behavioural changes over time in response to the DA agonist, apomorphine. Initially, the scope of attention extended to distant objects but later shrank and focused on body parts. This experiment provides a model for progressive change in the development of psychotic behaviour. Furthermore, such experiments simulate the variability in cognitive process we propose to be a salient feature of schizophrenia. The transition from scanning to narrow focus may be analogous to the development of a new and less versatile pattern of organization postulated by Ciompi[84] to characterize the psychosis. A similar sequence is seen in the development of amphetamine psychoses in humans.[85]

It is a major challenge to define human psychotic behaviour in terms homologous to abnormalities of animal behaviour. However, the data briefly reviewed here suggest that it is plausible to compare Oades' concept of tuning with the adaptation of attention systems to handle information of varying complexity; and to compare the concept of switching with selective attention, the activation of the correct sensory modality and the correct nonperseverative response.

The dominant hypothesis of schizophrenia, the dopamine (DA) hypothesis, can now be examined in terms of dynamic changes that occur over time. A current form of the DA hypothesis is that there is dysregulation of DA neuronal systems.[86] Van Kammen et al[13] have demonstrated time-dependent changes in DA sensitivity. Patients at different stages of illness may improve or worsen in response to amphetamine. Homovanillic acid (HVA) and methylhydroxyphenolglycol (MHPG) in cerebrospinal fluid vary greatly over time in schizophrenic patients. There is greater variability in DA-regulated growth hormone secretion over time.[10,11,87] Raese et al[88] have observed rapid and slow cyclic changes in retinal oscillatory potentials in schizophrenics and advanced a theory of rapid up and down regulation of DA synthesis.

A reciprocal relationship exists between frontal mesocortical and subcortical dopamine systems. These systems could interact to produce the variability observed above. Frontal lobe lesions in animals increase locomotor activity and behaviour induced by dopamine agonists.[89–92] Temporolimbic and subcortical activity might be released by damage to frontal lobe dopaminergic systems leading to the release of positive symptoms from temporolimbic structures that respond to DA antagonists. Temporal lobe glucose metabolism measured by PET in acutely ill, drug-free schizophrenics is, in fact, significantly greater than in normal controls.[93]

Fluctuations in positive and negative symptoms and cognitive processes could reflect the dynamic reciprocal relationship of mesocortical, mesolimbic, and subcortical dopaminergic systems. These relations can be examined in the living brains of patients by PET. Activation of DA systems with agonist drugs may well have remote postsynaptic effects that are reflected in metabolic changes in several regions of the brain.

To put these proposals to test, it is predicted that DA agonist challenge, known to exacerbate positive symptoms, will also activate temporal lobe metabolic activity. Relatively little activation of frontal cortex would be expected. In addition, it is predicted that DA activation will reduce correlations within frontal regions and between frontal and temporal regions. Such a finding would be consistent with the proposal that crucial brain regions may not be activated appropriately, that there is disjunction between them, and that a hyperdopaminergic state is one neurochemical mechanism.

Localized and Distributed Neuroanatomical Systems

Each of the functions that are disordered in schizophrenia must involve complex interactions of large numbers of neurons distributed in many different brain areas. There are many levels of organization: localized circuits, columns, laminal, and topographic maps. The specific representation of behaviours in these systems is largely unknown. It is therefore premature to propose an exact anatomical model.

Several alternative neuroanatomical proposals have been presented in detail (Cleghorn and Albert, in preparation) and summarized elsewhere.[1] Only our conclusions about neuroanatomical regions possibly involved in schizophrenia can be presented here.

The striking variety of pathological behaviors in schizophrenia implicates many brain regions. Modern pathological studies of schizophrenic patients give support to the notion that many brain regions are involved: (1) dorsolateral prefrontal cortex[94,95]; (2) cingulate gyrus[96]; (3) dominant temporal lobe[97,98]; (4) ventral tegmental area, dopamine neurons in the mesocortical and mesolimbic dopamine systems[99–102]; (5) hippocampus,[103] amygdala, and internal globus pallidum[104]; (6) medial dorsal nucleus of thalamus[105]; (7) corpus callosum[106]; and (8) cerebellar vermis.[107]

Studies of brain metabolism and blood flow to date implicate frontal,[108,58] temporal,[109] parietal,[56,58] and globus pallidum[104] abnormalities. Frontal abnormalities have long been suspected because of the similarity between the negative symptoms and some frontal lobe syndromes.[100,101,110,111] Likewise, temporal lobe abnormalities have long been suspected because of the similarity between positive symptoms and some temporal lobe epilepsies. Possible contributions of striatal and thalamic inputs were presented in the section on the Neurophysiology of Program Selection and Activation and Brain Imaging. The role of the parietal lobes was discussed in the section on Information Processing, Perseveration, and Modularity. We conclude that widely distributed neuroanatomical systems are disrupted in schizophrenia and that a lesion in one location could interfere with the functioning of distant regions.[112,113]

Developmental Considerations

Permanent and stable deficits antedate the illness: the inability to process as large an amount of information as is normal;[46,114,115] EEG evidence of hyperarousal;[116] and social isolation and poor peer relationships.[115,117] These features may be preceded by neurodevelopmental abnormalities[118] and by failure in the development of attachment behavior in infancy.[119] Some of these features characterize 40 to 60% of offspring of schizophrenics, many of whom proceed to develop disorders other than schizophrenia. Nevertheless, such deficits are antecedents of many cases of schizophrenia.

Certain clinical features, that is, the permanent stable deficits such as impaired memory and neurological signs, cannot be conceptualized as modular disjunction. The theory of modular disjunction does not, of course, intend to explain these features. They reflect brain damage which produces both permanent deficits in some functions and disjunctions of others. Their perinatal or prenatal origin is not known. However, new knowledge of prenatal cortical development may give us some clues.

Most cortical neurons are generated during the middle of gestation in primates. A massive migration of cortical neurons occurs during the middle third of the period of gestation. Rakic[120] has proposed that the ependymal layer of cells of the embryonic cerebral ventricle consists of proliferative units that provide a protomap of prospective cytoarchitectonic areas of cortex. The cells migrate along shafts of glial cells to their destination in the cortex. Rakic states that each step in this process can be separately affected by genetic or extrinsic factors.

Because there may be errors in the development of cortical organization in schizophrenia, embryological studies should be pursued. Such a strategy is encouraged by the observation of Mednick et al[121] that a putative viral infection in the middle trimester of pregnancy was associated with an increase in hospital admissions for schizophrenia when the offspring reached their mid-20s.

With the advent of adolescence and the psychotic episode, new developmental changes in the brain need to be considered.

Several processes may be relevant to adolescent onset: (1) the myelinization of the frontal lobes which continues in adult life, and (2) synaptic pruning, or the normal developmental regression of excess neuronal connections in childhood and early adolescence. Both these processes may be associated with specialization of frontal functioning. The onset of illness could be attributed to a failure in the development of specialized dopaminergic afferents to frontal cortex, which is then unable to modulate limbic system activity and unable to cope with stress.[122] Alternatively, developmental changes could bring "on-line" frontal parts well known to be defective before illness onset. (3) Still another alternative has been suggested: developmental delay in certain glutamate receptors in the hippocampus as they assume an adult form postpuberty.[123]

Finally, the psychotic episode is followed, in most cases, by a drop in social and work performance. Neurocognitive assessment may reveal a drop in test scores. Neuroleptic treatment improves performance, but there is usually a net drop in performance from before to after the episode. It is possible that a neurotoxic process occurs during the psychotic episode and is responsible for the disjunctions observed during the episode and for the addition of new deficits after the psychotic episode.

Summary

It has been proposed that many symptoms of schizophrenia and demonstrable perseveration and failures of attention reflect variability in the control of certain neural circuits in the brain. Conscious control and intentionality are intermittent. Messages are sent to parts of the brain not specialized for the required function; other parts are inactivated or activated inappropriately. Thus, desynchronization of widely distributed neurocognitive systems develops.

Psychotic symptoms reflect asynchronous activation, for example, incongruity of thought and affect, errors in the timing of communication which make it seem odd or incoherent, and the attribution of meaning to an irrelevant event which reflects a mismatch of a percept and the sense of significance. Such phenomena suggest a disjunction of functional units of the brain. Likewise, several types of dysfunctional attention can be observed that indicate selection of an incorrect channel, simultaneous activation of several channels, or inadequate tuning of concentration to a level capable of registering the quantity of information required. Perseverative intrusions of previous thoughts and motor behaviours also reflect erroneous connections.

Brain imaging studies of psychotic patients provide preliminary data consistent with our proposal. They show activation of cerebral blood flow or glucose metabolism in a part of the brain inappropriate to a task, and failure to activate an appropriate region. The activity of different frontal lobe regions is less highly intercorrelated in schizophrenic patients than in normal people.

Because neurological structures and functions are grossly intact in schizophrenia, we suggest that there is a desynchronization of functional units in the brain. Those units are computational or cognitive modules that generate intact bits of complex behavior. In schizophrenia, there is a disjunction of certain cognitive modules.

Several sources of data are suggested that may help illuminate mechanisms of this neuropsychological process. (1) Widely distributed anatomical systems have been found that connect those various structures implicated in neuropathological studies of schizophrenia. These neuroanatomical systems link temporolimbic, striatal, prefrontal, and parietal cortex and are required for processing cognitive information and its emotional meaning. Abnormalities in brain tissue in all these regions have been described. (2) Pharmacologic studies demonstrate that switching mechanisms in animals' brains are subserved by dopamine, whereas tuning mechanisms are regulated by norepinephrine. Both norepinephrine and dopamine have been implicated in schizophrenia. Sustained administration of drugs that mimic norepinephrine or dopamine produce changes in motor behavior and attention similar to those seen in the emergence of psychosis. (3) A neurophysiological model is also described. It defines a scheme for the selection, activation, sequencing, and switching of compartmentalized motor programs. A similar scheme may apply to cognitive programs. Psychotic symptoms may result from disturbances in these processes that produce errors in communication between cognitive modules.

If the proposed conceptual framework for a pathological psychophysiology is valid, what are the specific mechanisms and causes of such a profound yet relatively subtle neurocognitive disorder? Some neurodevelopmental possibilities are briefly mentioned.

Acknowledgement. Supported in part by grants from Medical Research Council of Canada (MA 10214) and National Institutes of Mental Health (MH 44073).

References

1. Cleghorn JM: A neurodiagnostic approach to schizophrenia. *Can J Psychiatry* 1988;33:555–561.
2. Anscombe R: The disorder of consciousness. *Schizophr Bull* 1987;13:241–260.
3. Hoffman RE: Verbal hallucinations and language production processes in schizophrenia. *Behav Brain Sci* 1986;9:503–548.
4. Frith CD, Done DJ: Towards a neuropsychology of schizophrenia. *Br J Psychiatry* 1988;153:437–443.
5. Ciompi L: Is there really a schizophrenia? The long-term course of psychotic phenomena. *Br J Psychiatry* 1984;145:636–640.

6. Vaillant GE: The natural history of the remitting schizophrenics. *Am J Psychiatry* 1963;120:367–376.
7. Shakow D: Segmental set: a theory of the formal psychological deficit in schizophrenia. *Arch Gen Psychiatry* 1962;6:1–17.
8. Shakow D: Some Psychophysiological Aspects of Schizophrenia. First Rochester International Conference on Schizophrenia, 1972.
9. Shakow D: Some observations on the psychology (and some fewer, on the biology) of schizophrenia. *J Nerv Mental Dis* 1971;153:300–316.
10. Cleghorn JM, Brown GM, Brown PJ, et al: Growth hormone responses to apomorphine HCl in schizophrenic patients on drug holidays and at relapse. *Br J Psychiatry* 1983;142:482–488.
11. Brown GM, Cleghorn JM, Kaplan RD, et al: Longitudinal growth hormone studies in schizophrenia. *Psychiatry Res* 1988;24:123–136.
12. Vandervelde CD: Variability of schizophrenia: reflection of a regulatory disease. *Arch Gen Psychiatry* 1976;33:489–496.
13. Van Kammen D, Doherty JP, Marder SR, et al: Long-term pimozide pretreatment differentially affects behavioral responses to dextroamphetamine in schizophrenia. *Arch Gen Psychiatry* 1982;39:275–281.
14. Fodor JA: Precis of the modularity of mind. *Behav Brain Sci* 1985;8:1–42.
15. Gardner H: *Frames of Mind: The Theory of Multiple Intelligences.* New York, Basic Books, 1985.
16. Gardner H: *The Mind's New Science.* New York, Basic Books, 1985.
17. Newcombe F: Neuropsychology qua interface. *J Clin Experimental Neuropsychology* 1986;7:663–681.
18. Posner MI, Petersen, SE, Fox PT, et al: Localization of cognitive operations in the human brain. *Science* 1988;240:1627–1631.
19. Gazzaniga M: *The Social Brain.* New York, Basic Books, 1985.
20. Kovelman JA, Scheibel AB: Biological substrates of schizophrenia. *Acta Neurolog Scand* 1986;73:1–32.
21. Andrews HB, House AO, Cooper JE, et al: The prediction of abnormal evoked potentials in schizophrenic patients by means of symptom pattern. *Br J Psychiatry* 1986;147:46–50.
22. Rutter DR: Language in schizophrenia: the structure of monologues and conversations. *Br J Psychiatry* 1985;146:399–400.
23. Andreasen NC, Hoffman R, Grove W: Language abnormalities in schizophrenia, in Seeman M. Menuck M (eds): *New Perspectives in Schizophrenia.* London, Heath, 1984.
24. Bartolucci G: Nonverbal disturbances attributed to the schizophrenic psychoses. *Comp Psychiatry* 1984;25:491–502.
25. Feinberg TE, Rifkin A, Schaffer C, et al: Facial discrimination and emotional recognition in schizophrenia and affective disorders. *Arch Gen Psychiatry* 1986;43:276–279.
26. Schefen AE: *Levels of Schizophrenia.* New York, Bruner/Mazel, 1981.
27. Wynne LC, Singer MT: Thought disorder and family relations of schizophrenics: II. A classification of forms of thinking. *Arch Gen Psychiatry* 1963;9:199–206.
28. Wagener DK, Hogarty GE, Goldstein M, et al: Information processing and communication deviance in schizophrenic patients and their mothers. *Psychiatry Res* 1986;18:365–377.

29. Lecours AR: The language of psychotics and neurotics, in Lecours AR, Lhermitte F, Bryans B (eds): *Aphasiology*. New York, Saunders, 1983.
30. Bartolucci GL, Fine J: The frequency of cohesion weakness in psychiatric syndromes. *Applied Psycholinguistics* 1987;8:67–74.
31. Gould LH: Auditory hallucinations in subvocal speech. *J Nerv Mental Dis* 1949;109:418–427.
32. Bick PA, Kinsbourne M: Auditory hallucinations and subvocal speech in schizophrenic patients. *Am J Psychiatry* 1987;144:222–225.
33. Frith CD: The positive and negative symptoms of schizophrenia reflect impairments in the perception and initiation of action. *Psych Med* 1987;17:631–648.
34. Sandson J, Albert ML: Varieties of perseveration. *Neuropsychologia* 1984;22:715–732.
35. Baribeau J, Perton T, Gosselin JY: A neurophysiological evaluation of abnormal information processing. *Science* 1983;219:874–876.
36. Saccuzzo DP, Braff DL: Information-processing abnormalities: trait- and state-dependent components. *Schizophr Bull* 1986;12:447–459.
37. Knight RT: Converging models of cognitive deficit in schizophrenia, in Spaulding WD, Cole JK (eds): *Theories of Schizophrenia and Psychosis*. Lincoln, University of Nebraska Press, 1984.
38. Pritchard WS: Cognitive event-related potential correlates of schizophrenia. *Psych Bull* 1986;86:43–66.
39. Zubin J: Negative symptoms: are they indigenous to schizophrenia? *Schizophr Bull* 1985;11:461–470.
40. Morstyn R, Duffy FH, McCarley RW: Altered P300 topography in schizophrenia. *Arch Gen Psychiatry* 1983;40:729–734.
41. Holzman PS. Eye movement dysfunctions and psychoses. *Int Rev Neurobiology* 1985;27:179–225.
42. Kaplan RD, Cleghorn J, Brown G, et al: Clinical and regional cerebral glucose metabolism correlates of neuropsychological deficits in acutely ill and ambulatory schizophrenic men. *J Clin Exp Neuropsychol* 1988;1:20.
43. Asarnow RF, Steffy RA, MacCrimmon DJ, et al: An attentional assessment of foster children at risk for schizophrenia. *J Abnorm Psychol* 1977;86:267.
44. Asarnow RF, MacCrimmon DJ: Residual performance deficit in clinically remitted schizophrenics: A marker for schizophrenia? *J Abnorm Psychol* 1978:87:597–608.
45. Asarnow RF, MacCrimmon DJ: Attention/information-processing, neuropsychological functioning, and thought disorder during the acute and partial recovery phases of schizophrenia: A longitudinal study. *Psychiatry Res* 1982;7:309.
46. Nuechterlein KH, Dawson ME: Information processing and attentional functioning in the developmental course of schizophrenic disorders. *Schizophr Bull* 1984;10:160–203.
47. Kristofferson MW: Shifting attention between modalities: a comparison of schizophrenics and normals. *J Abnormal Psych* 1967;72:388–394.
48. Allen LG: The attention switching model: implications for research in schizophrenia, in Wynne LC, Cromwell RL, Matthysse S (eds): *The Nature of Schizophrenia*. New York, John Wiley & Sons, 1978.
49. Alpert M: The signs and symptoms of schizophrenia. *Comp Psychiatry* 1985;26:103–112.

50. Seidman LJ: Schizophrenia and brain dysfunction: an integration of recent neurodiagnostic findings. *Psych Bull* 1983;94:195–238.
51. Shagass C: Contingent negative variation and other slow potentials in adult psychiatry, in Hughes JR, Wilson WP (eds): *EEG and Evoked Potentials in Psychiatry and Behavioral Neurology*. New York, Butterworths, 1983.
52. Calloway E, Naghdi S: An information processing model of schizophrenia. *Arch Gen Psychiatry* 1982;39:339–347.
53. Posner MI: Hierarchical distributed networks in the neuropsychology of selective attention, in Caramazza A (ed): *Advances in Cognitive Neuropsychology*. New York, Erlbaum Associates, 1986.
54. Mesulam M-M: *Principles of Behavioral Neurology*. Philadelphia, F.A. Davis, 1985.
55. Goldman-Rakic PS: Topography of cognition: parallel distributed cortical networks in primate association cortex. *Ann Rev Neurosci* 1988;11:137–156.
56. Cleghorn JM, Garnett ES, Nahmias C, et al: Increased frontal and reduced parietal glucose metabolism in acute untreated schizophrenia. *Psychiatry Res,* 1989;28:119–133.
57. Szechtman H, Nahmias C, Garnett ES, et al: Effect of neuroleptics on altered cerebral glucose metabolism in schizophrenia. *Arch Gen Psychiatry* 1988;45:523–532.
58. Wiesel FA, Wik G, Sjorgen I, et al: Regional brain glucose metabolism in drug free schizophrenic patients and clinical correlates. *Acta Psychiatr Scand* 1987;76:628–641.
59. Kishimoto H, Kuwahara H, Ohno S, et al: Three subtypes of chronic schizophrenia identified using ^{11}C-glucose positron emission tomography. *Psychiatry Res* 1987;21:285–292.
60. Weinberger DR, Berman KF, Zec RF: Physiologic dysfunction of dorsolateral prefrontal cortex in schizophrenia. Arch Gen Psychiatry 1986;43:114–135.
61. Berman KF, Weinberger DR, Shelton RC, et al: A relationship between anatomical and physiological brain pathology in schizophrenia: lateral cerebral ventricular size predicts cortical blood flow. *Am J Psychiatry* 1987;144:1277–1282.
62. Gur RE, Skolnick BE, Gur RC, et al: Brain function in psychiatric disorders. *Arch Gen Psychiatry* 1983;40:1250–1254.
63. Holcomb HH, Semples WE, Birchsbaum MS, et al: Evolved potential and brain metabolism correlations, abstract. Washington, DC, American Psychiatric Association Press, 1986.
64. Clark CM, Kessler R, Buchsbaum MS, et al: Correlational methods for determining regional coupling of cerebral glucose metabolism: a pilot study. *Biol Psychiatry* 1984;19:663–678.
65. Volkow ND, Wolf AP, Brodie JD, et al: Brain interactions in chronic schizophrenics under resting and activation conditions. *Schizophr Res* 1988;1:47–54.
66. Kennedy D: The control of output by central neurons, in Brazier MAB (ed): *The Interneuron*. Los Angeles, University of California Press, 1969.
67. Mountcastle VB, Lynch JC, Georgopoulos A, et al: Posterior parietal association cortex of the monkey: command functions for operations within extrapersonal space. *J Neurophysiol* 1975;38:871–908.

68. Nauta WJH: Circuitous connections linking cerebral cortex, limbic system, and corpus striatum, in Doane BK, Livingstone KE (eds): *The Limbic System*. New York, Raven Press, 1986.
69. McKenzie JS, Kemin RI, Wilcock L: *The Basal Ganglia, Structure and Function*. New York, Plenum Press, 1984.
70. Manshreck TC, Maher BA, Waller NG, et al: Deficient motor synchrony in schizophrenic disorders: clinical correlates. *Biol Psychiatry* 1985;20:990–1002.
71. Swerdlow NR, Koob GF: Dopamine, schizophrenia, mania and depression: toward a unified hypothesis of cortical, striatal-pallido-thalamic function. *Behav Brain Sci* 1987;10:197–208.
72. Oke AF, Adams RN: Elevated thalamic dopamine: possible link to sensory dysfunctions in schizophrenia. *Schizophr Bull* 1987;13:589–604.
73. Hornykiewicz O: Brain catecholamines in schizophrenia—A good case for noradrenaline. *Nature* 1982;299:454–456.
74. Iversen S, Iversen L: *Behavioural Pharmacology*. London, Oxford University Press, 1984.
75. Antelman SM, Caggiula AR: Norepinephrine–dopamine interactions and behavior. *Science*. 1977;195:646–653.
76. Oades RD: The role of noradrenaline in tuning and dopamine in switching between signals in the CNS. *Neurosci Biobehav Rev* 1985;9:261–282.
77. Bruto V, Kokkinidis L, Anisman H: Attenuation of perseverative behavior after repeated amphetamine treatment: tolerance or attentional deficits? *Pharmacol Biochem Behav* 1983;19:497–504.
78. Kokkinidis L, Anisman H: Amphetamine models of paranoid schizophrenia: an overview and elaboration of animal experimentation. *Psych Bull* 1980;88:551–579.
79. Ellinwood EH, Sudilovsky A: Chronic amphetamine intoxication: behavioral model of psychoses, in Cole JO, Freedman AM, Friedhoff AJ (eds): *Psychopathology and Psychopharmacology*. Baltimore, Johns Hopkins University Press, 1973.
80. Robertson A, MacDonald C: Opposite effects of sulpiride and metoclopramide on amphetamine-induced stereotypy. *Eur J Pharmacol* 1985;109:81–89.
81. Rebec GV, Bashore TR: Critical issues in assessing the behavioral effects of amphetamine. *Neurosci Biobehav Rev* 1984;8:153–159.
82. Matthysse S: Animal models in psychiatric research, in van Ree JM, Matthysse S (eds): *Progress in Brain Research*. Amsterdam, Elsevier Science Publishers, 1986.
83. Szechtman H, Ornstein K, Teitlebaum P, et al: The morphogenesis of stereotyped behaviour induced by the dopamine receptor agonist apomorphine in the laboratory rat. *Neuroscience* 1985;14:783–798.
84. Ciompi L: Is there really a schizophrenia?—The long-term course of psychotic phenomena. *Br J Psychiatry* 1984;145:636–640.
85. Ellinwood EH: Amphetamine psychosis. I. Description of the individuals and process. *J Nerv Mental Dis* 1967;44:273–283.
86. Friedhoff AJ: Restitutive processes in the regulation of behavior, in Alpert M (ed): *Controversies in Schizophrenia*. New York, Guilford Press, 1985.
87. Cleghorn JM, Brown GM, Brown PJ, et al: Longitudinal instability of hormone responses in schizophrenia. *Prog Neuro-Psychopharm Biol Psychiatry* 1983;7:545–549.

88. Raese JD, King RJ, Barnes D, et al: Retinal oscillatory potentials in schizophrenia. *Psychopharmacol Bull* 1982;18:72–78.
89. Pycock CJ, Kerwin RW, Carter CJ: Effect of lesion of cortical dopamine terminals on subcortical dopamine in rats. *Nature* 1980;286:74–77.
90. Morency MA, Stewart RJ, Beninger RJ: Effects of unilateral microinjections of sulpiride into the medial prefrontal cortex on circling behavior of rats. *Prog Neuro-Psychopharmacol Biol Psychiatry* 1985;9:735–738.
91. Stewart RJ, Morency MA, Beninger RJ: Differential effects of intrafrontocortical microinjections of dopamine agonists and antagonists on circling behavior of rats. *Behav Brain Res* 1985;17:67–72.
92. Brozoski TJ, Brown RM, Rosvold HE, et al: Cognitive deficit caused by regional depletion of dopamine in prefrontal cortex of rhesus monkey. *Science* 1979;205:929–932.
93. Cleghorn JM, Garnett ES, Nahmias C, et al: Temporal lobe metabolism in schizophrenia. *Am J Psychiatry* 1988, submitted.
94. Benes FM, Davidson J, Bird E: Quantitative cytoarchitectural studies of the cerebral cortex of schizophrenics. *Arch Gen Psychiatry* 1986;43:31–35.
95. Morihisa J, Weinberger DR: Is schizophrenia a frontal lobe disease?—An organizing theory of relevant anatomy and physiology, in Andreasen N (ed): *Can Schizophrenia Be Localized in the Brain?* Washington, DC, American Psychiatric Association Press, 1986.
96. Benes FM, Bird E: An analysis of the arrangement of neurons in cingulate cortex of schizophrenics. *Arch Gen Psychiatry* 1987;44:608–616.
97. Davison K, Bagley CR: Schizophrenia like psychoses associated with organic disorders of the central nervous system: a review of the literature, in Herrington RN (ed): *Current Problems in Neuropsychiatry*. London, Headley Brothers, 1969.
98. Stevens JR, Bigelow L, Denney D, et al: Telemetered EEG-EOG during psychotic behaviors of schizophrenia. *Arch Gen Psychiatry* 1979;36:251–262.
99. Nishikawa T, Takashima M, Toru M: Increased [³H] kainic acid binding in the prefrontal cortex in schizophrenia. *Neuroscience Lett* 1983;40:245–250.
100. Levin S: Frontal lobe dysfunctions in schizophrenia. II: Impairments of psychological and brain function. *J Psychiatr Res* 1984;18:57–72.
101. Müller HF: Prefrontal cortex dysfunction as a common factor in psychosis. *Acta Psychiatr Scand* 1985;71:431–440.
102. Nauta WJH: The problem of the frontal lobe: a reinterpretation. *J Psychiatr Res* 1971;8:167–187.
103. Brown R, Colter N, Corsella N, et al: Postmortem evidence of structural brain changes in schizophrenia. *Arch Gen Psychiatry* 1986;43:36–42.
104. Early TS, Reiman ER, Raichle ME, et al: Left globus pallidus abnormality in never-medicated patients with schizophrenia. *Proc Natl Acad Sci* 1987;84:561–563.
105. Markowitsch HJ: Thalamic mediodorsal nucleus and memory: a critical evaluation of studies in animals and man. *Neurosci Biobehav Rev* 1982;6:351.
106. Nasrallah HA: Is schizophrenia a left hemisphere disease?, in Andreasen N (ed): *Can Schizophrenia be Localized in the Brain?* Washington, DC, American Psychiatric Association Press, 1986.
107. Snider SR: Cerebellar pathology in schizophrenia: cause or consequence? *Neurosci Biobehav Rev* 1982;6:47–53.

108. Buchsbaum MS, DeLisi LE, Holcomb HH, et al: Anteroposterior gradients in cerebral glucose use in schizophrenic and affective disorders. *Arch Gen Psychiatry* 1984;41:1159–1168.
109. Cleghorn JM, Garnett ES, Nahmias C, et al: Temporal lobe metabolism in schizophrenia, abstract. *Schizophr Res* 1988.
110. Kraepelin E: Dementia praecox and paraphrenia. New York, RE Krieger, 1971.
111. Stuss DT, Benson DF: *The Frontal Lobes*. New York, Raven Press, 1986.
112. Goldman-Rakic PS: Topography of cognition: parallel distributed cortical networks in primate association cortex. *Ann Rev Neurosci* 1988.
113. Goldman-Rakic PS: Circuitry of the prefrontal cortex and the regulation of behaviour by representational knowledge, in Plum F, Mountcastle V (eds): *Handbook of Physiology*. American Physiological Society, 1987.
114. Steffy RA, Asarnow RF, Asarnow JR, et al: The McMaster-Waterloo high-risk project: multifaceted strategy for high-risk research, in Watt NF, Anthony J, Wynne LC, Rolf JE (eds): *Children at Risk for Schizophrenia: A Longitudinal Perspective*. New York, Cambridge University Press, 1984.
115. Watt NF: In a nutshell: the first two decades of high-risk research in schizophrenia, in Watt NF, Anthony J, Wynne LC, Rolf JE (eds); *Children at Risk for Schizophrenia: A Longitudinal Perspective*. New York, Cambridge University Press, 1984.
116. Itil TM, Hegue MF, Shapiro DM, et al: Computer-analyzed EEG findings in children of schizophrenic parents. *Integrative Psychiatry*, 1983;1:71–80.
117. McNeil TF, Kaij L: Offspring of women with nonorganic psychoses, in Watt NF, Anthony J, Wynne LC, Rolf JE (eds): *Children at Risk for Schizophrenia: A Longitudinal Perspective*. New York, Cambridge University Press, 1984.
118. Hamilton M: *Fish's Schizophrenia*. New York, John Wright & Sons, 1984.
119. MacCrimmon DJ, Cleghorn JM, Asarnow RF, et al: Children at risk for schizophrenia. *Arch Gen Psychiatry* 1980;37:671–674.
120. Rakic P: Specifics of cerebral cortical areas. *Science* 1988;241:170–176.
121. Mednick SA, Machon RA, Huttunen MO, et al: Adult schizophrenia following prenatal exposure to an influenza epidemic. *Arch Gen Psychiatry* 1988;45:189–192.
122. Weinberger DR: Implications of normal brain development for the pathogenesis of schizophrenia. *Arch Gen Psychiatry* 1987;44:660–670.
123. Etienne P, Baudry M: Calcium dependent aspects of synaptic plasticity, excitatory amino acid neurotransmission, brain aging and schizophrenia: a unifying hypothesis. *Neurobiology of Aging* 1988;8:362–366.

4
Meaning of Structural Changes in the Brain in Schizophrenia

Timothy J. Crow

Schizophrenia is often described as a "functional" psychosis with the implication that, along with manic-depressive disease, the illness is distinguishable on pathological grounds from the "organic" psychoses, for example, the dementias, in which brain changes can be identified. A psychological distinction also drawn is that impairments of learning, manifest as disorders of orientation, characteristic of the organic psychoses, are absent in the "functional" psychoses.

Work during the past 15 years casts doubt on both these assumptions. Structural brain changes are present in schizophrenia, as a number of radiological studies have shown. "Organic" type cognitive deficits are also sometimes seen in the chronic forms of the disease, and may be severe. This chapter considers the implications of these findings. What sort of a disease is schizophrenia? What is the meaning of the changes in the brain? What is their relationship to the psychological changes? The answers to these questions bring us to a specific and novel concept of aetiology.

Age Disorientation

Both Kraepelin and Bleuler appear to have believed that true impairments of memory and learning do not occur in the conditions they referred to as dementia praecox or the group of schizophrenias, respectively. Thus, Bleuler[1] wrote that "In contrast to the organic psychoses, we find in schizophrenia . . . that sensation, memory and consciousness . . . are not directly disturbed" (p 55) and "memory as such does not suffer in this disease" (p 59), and Kraepelin[2] asserted that "memory is comparatively little disordered. The patients are able, when they like, to give a correct detailed account of their past life, and often know accurately to a day how long they have been in the institution" (p 18).

These views are challenged by the phenomenon of "age disorientation." Aspects of this phenomenon have been noted in patients with chronic schizophrenia by a number of workers. Lanzkron and Wolfson[3] in 1958 described a "perceptual distortion of temporal orientation" in a group of 50 chronic patients, and Dahl[4] replicated the finding in a population of 500 institutionalized patients and claimed that this "singular distortion of temporal orientation" occurred only in schizophrenia. Ehrenteil and Jenney[5] found a number of hospitalized schizophrenic patients gave ages younger than their true age and asked "Does time stand still for some psychotics?" Michelson[6] also apparently unaware of previous findings, described systematic errors made by 62 patients in estimating their ages over a 6-year period.

In the course of a survey of inpatients with schizophrenic illnesses of long standing, Crow and Mitchell[7] were impressed by the frequency with which such subjects believed themselves to be an age widely different from their true age. In a sample of 237 patients in the wards of four mental hospitals in Scotland, they found that approximately 25% believed themselves to be 5 or more years younger than they really were. Twelve percent believed themselves to be within 5 years of their age on admission, although on average they were 28 years older than this. Similar findings were obtained in other surveys. Thus, Stevens et al[8] surveyed the population of patients with a diagnosis of schizophrenia in Shenley Hospital in Northwest London and found that age disorientation (defined as a 5-year discrepancy between subjective and true age) was present in 25% of this sample, and a similar figure was arrived at for patients in the Harlem Valley Psychiatric Center in New York by Smith and Oswald.[9] Stevens et al[8] found that patients with age disorientation were younger at first admission than age-matched patients without age disorientation; it seemed that age disorientation might be a feature of a type of schizophrenic illness with early onset and poor outcome.

Age disorientation cannot be attributed to past physical treatments. Patients with age disorientation are no more likely than patients in the same institution with a diagnosis of schizophrenia but without such cognitive deficits to have received electroconvulsive or insulin coma therapy, a combination of these treatments, or leukotomy.[10] Nor are they more likely to have received neuroleptic or anticholinergic medication.[11]

Temporal Disorientation or Global Intellectual Impairment?

The question arises whether age disorientation is an isolated psychopathological deficit, part of a wider pattern of impairments of temporal orientation, or an aspect of a more general loss of intellectual capacity. Crow and Stevens[12] found that patients with age disorientation were much less likely than those without age disorientation to be able to give correct answers to simple questions about dates and the passage of time (eg, the present year and the duration of their hospital stay). The errors that individual patients made in their answers to these questions were consistent with their concept of their own age. Thus, age disorientation is part of a constellation of deficits of temporal orientation—for these patients "time stands still."

Liddle and Crow[13] addressed the question of whether temporal orientation is associated with general deficits of intellectual function. A series of 21 patients with age disorientation (each of whom believed himself to be within 5 years of his age on admission) were compared on a battery of tests of cognitive function with a group of patients without age disorientation matched for age and duration of hospital stay. On all tests age-disoriented patients were more impaired. This was true of tests of orientation and general knowledge as well as tests of new learning (face-name learning and the digit-symbol test of the WAIS), problem solving (Raven's matrices), tests of previous learning (Peabody picture vocabulary test and the famous personalities test), and dysphasia (Boston naming test). Thus, age disorientation is but part of a global impairment of intellectual function.

The pattern of intellectual deficits in these patients with schizophrenia is difficult to distinguish from that seen in Alzheimer's disease. Indeed their performance on the Peabody picture vocabulary test (intended to tap premorbid intellectual function) did not establish that these patients had ever functioned at an adequate level. However, further inquiry[11] indicated that in terms of their academic and occupational records, these patients did not have significantly greater deficits than other institutionalized patients with schizophrenia; some at least had functioned at an entirely adequate level.

When Do the Cognitive Deficits Occur?

There have been a number of reports of intellectual deficits preceding the onset of psychosis. For example school performance[14] and intelligence[15] have been found lower in subjects who later developed schizophrenic illnesses than in their siblings. That cognitive impairments also sometimes progress with progression of the disease is suggested by the following: (1) some patients who later developed profound intellectual losses apparently functioned at an adequate academic level before the onset of their illness, as noted; and (2) in a comparison of groups of patients with schizophrenia, nonschizophrenic psychiatric illnesses, and normal controls, Garside[16] found that schizophrenic patients showed significant intellectual deterioration on the Wechsler-Bellevue scales relative to the school grading these subjects had received years earlier, this deterioration being greatest in those with hebephrenic forms of the disease. Somewhat similar findings were reported by Rappaport and Webb.[17]

It can be concluded that, contrary to the views of Kraepelin and Bleuler, intellectual impairments are sometimes seen in patients with schizophrenia and may be profound. In some patients they precede the onset of the psychosis, apparently by many years. In other (perhaps sometimes the same) patients these impairments progress, although whether such progression occurs in episodes of illness is unclear.

Structural Brain Changes

Temporal disorientation in chronic schizophrenia formed part of the background to the first computed tomographic (CT) scan study.[18] There had been earlier pneumoencephalographic investigations. In particular, Haug,[19] Asano,[20] and Huber[21] reported that patients with the more chronic and deteriorating forms of illness were more likely to have abnormalities, including ventricular enlargement, than other patients. In our CT scan investigation[18] we found that a group of 17 patients with chronic schizophrenia had significant enlargement of the lateral ventricles by comparison with a group of normal individuals matched for age and premorbid occupational status. Within the patient group lateral ventricular size was significantly related to intellectual status assessed on the Withers and Hinton tests of the sensorium.

Although these findings generated controversy, subsequent work has confirmed that when groups of patients studied are sufficiently large and include those with the more chronic and deteriorating forms of illness, mean ventricular size is modestly but significantly increased by comparison with normal controls and with some other (eg, neurotic) patient samples. For example, Weinberger and colleagues[22] studied chronic patients in St. Elizabeth's Hospital in Washington, D.C., and included a range of ages that was wider and younger than ours with substantially similar findings. Of particular note is that one group of workers who, in an earlier carefully controlled study of ventricular volume had failed to detect differences between patients with schizophrenia and normal controls,[23] were later able to detect such differences when they included in their patient sample groups of severely ill chronic hospitalized patients.[24]

An important question is whether these changes can be attributed to past physical treatment. Both our own[18] and the National Institute of Mental Health (NIMH) study[22] addressed this question and found no evidence that the changes were more marked in patients who had received significant amounts of physical treatments, including electroconvulsive therapy (ECT), insulin coma treatment, or neuroleptic medication. Ventricular size was as large in patients who had received little or none of these treatments. This conclusion is reinforced by a subsequent study[25] that included more than 100 hospitalized patients with chronic schizophrenia, and compared groups matched by age, sex, and duration of illness, that had received none or much of each of the three treatments of neuroleptic medication, ECT, and insulin coma therapy. Lateral ventricular size was no greater in patients who had received much of each of these treatments. The conclusion is that the structural differences between the brains of patients with schizophrenia and various comparison groups are not to be attributed to physical treatments. These changes tell us something about the disease process.

Clinical Correlates of Structural Change: The Two Syndrome Concept

The clinical correlates of ventricular enlargement are of particular interest. One attempt to understand the variety of manifestations of the disease and their pathological correlates is the two syndrome concept (Table 4.1).

The two syndrome concept[26,27] was an attempt to assimilate the findings of three studies which my colleagues and I had completed by 1980: (1) The CT scan investigation in chronic patients described above.[18] (2) A study in patients with acute schizophrenia of the mechanism of the antipsychotic effect of neuroleptic drugs making use of the two stereoisomers of flupenthixol.[28] The findings were compatible with the hypothesis that dopamine antagonism is the critical ingredient in the antipsychotic effect; they suggested also that the beneficial effects of such medication were relatively selective to positive symptoms; negative symptoms (narrowly defined) were less affected.
(3) A postmortem investigation[29] of schizophrenics in which presynaptic dopaminergic function in the basal ganglia was unchanged but numbers of D2 dopamine receptors were increased. Whether this change is disease- or medication-related remains uncertain.

The essence of the concept is that there are at least two components of the disease process—a drug responsive element that includes the positive

TABLE 4.1. The two syndrome concept.

	Type I	Type II
Characteristic symptoms	Delusions, hallucinations, thought disorder (positive symptoms)	Affective flattening, poverty of speech, loss of drive (negative symptoms)
Type of illness in which most commonly seen	Acute schizophrenia	Chronic schizophrenia, the "defect" state
Response to neuroleptic medication	Good	Poor
Outcome	Reversible	? irreversible
Intellectual impairment	Absent	Sometimes present
Postulated pathological process	Increased dopamine receptors	Cell loss and structural changes in the brain

Reprinted with permission from Crow.[25]

symptoms and is perhaps related to dopaminergic transmission, and a less readily reversible component that includes the features of the defect state. According to this concept, an association between the latter component and the structural anomalies in the brain is predicted.

The findings with respect to this prediction have been mixed. Although there is a general trend in radiological studies for ventricular size to relate to behavioral deterioration and more chronic forms of disease, significant associations with individual features of the defect state are not always found.[30] Thus, correlations with affective flattening and other negative symptoms, and with intellectual impairment are found in some studies but not in others. In our own recent investigation[25] lateral ventricular size was significantly related to behavioral deterioration and the presence of dyskinesias, but not to negative symptoms or intellectual impairment. Although such correlations have been reported in some other CT scan studies,[31-34] and in one postmortem investigation,[35] the absence of a consistent relationship is puzzling. In particular in our own study,[25] in which groups of patients with and without features of the defect state were matched for other relevant variables, no difference in lateral ventricular size was detected.

Age of Onset as a Predictor

Some light is thrown on this issue by examination of age of onset as a predictor of outcome and of the relationship between brain structure and cognitive function.[36] In our chronic patients we found that when other relevant variables (eg, age and duration of illness) were controlled, age of onset predicted a number of aspects of outcome. Thus, patients who were first admitted to a hospital at an age below the mode for the group as a whole (25 years for males and 28 years for females) were more likely than those who were first admitted at a later age to show negative symptoms, intellectual impairment (eg, age disorientation), and behavioral deterioration.

In this study we found three major structural variables: lateral ventricle-to-brain ratio (VBR), third ventricular area, and brain area, that distinguished patients with schizophrenia from the psychiatric comparison groups (Table 4.2). Lateral and third ventricular enlargement have been noted in a number of studies. In this investigation we found that various indices of ventricular enlargement were intercorrelated; there was no in-

TABLE 4.2. Schizophrenic ($N = 127$) vs nonschizophrenic psychiatric patients ($N = 45$).

VBR	Increased by 10%	$P < 0.05$
Third ventricle area	Increased by 16%	$P < 0.05$
Brain area	Decreased by 3%	$P < 0.01$

dication that the components were varying independently. A reduction in brain area has not previously been emphasized. Although the magnitude of the change was relatively small, it was significant at the 1% level. Whereas ventricular enlargement might well be regarded as a consequence of a degenerative process, a reduction in brain area is less easily explained in this way. Such reduction might be a result of a failure of development. In support of this view we found that although in the schizophrenic patient group as a whole there were few significant relationships between structural changes and psychological impairments, such correlations were present in the subgroup with ages of onset before the mean (25 years for males and 28 years for females). When present, these correlations were with brain area rather than ventricular size.

The findings suggest that the relationship between brain structure and the cognitive impairments that are one consequence of the schizophrenic disease process are established early in the course of the illness. They are compatible with the notion that the disease is an anomaly of development rather than a degenerative process caused by an exogenous pathogen.

On this basis it might be expected that age of onset would be a determinant of the structural changes in schizophrenia. Surprisingly, we found that the three measures (lateral and third ventricular areas and brain area) that distinguished patients with schizophrenia from other subjects did not separate patients with early from those with late age of onset. However, a further structural index, the difference between the widths of the two sides of the brain in the posterior segments, did distinguish these groups. Patients with early onset had significant ($P < .01$) reductions in the relative width of the left hemisphere in measures taken in the occipital and temporal regions.[37] It seemed that early onset arrests the development of the normal asymmetries in the posterior part of the brain.

Postmortem Brain Studies

The nature of the brain changes and their location is further elucidated by two recent postmortem studies. The first study[38] compared patients with schizophrenia with those with affective disorder who had died in the same institution. Brains were excluded from both groups if there was identifiable microscopic pathology (eg, Alzheimer-type changes or vascular disease). Brain structures were assessed on a photograph of a coronal brain section at the level of the interventricular foramina. The main findings were that when age, sex, and year of birth were controlled: (1) brain weight was reduced (by 5 to 6%) in the patients with schizophrenia; (2) lateral ventricular area was modestly (by 15%), but not significantly, increased; (3) temporal horn area was significantly ($P < .01$) increased, the relative increase being more than 80%; and (4) the width of the parahippocampal gyrus was reduced ($P < .01$). Reduction of parahippocampal gyrus width was reported in another recent postmortem study.[39] Of particular interest was a diagnosis by side interaction, the differences between the groups being significantly ($P < 0.02$) greater on the left side.[38]

The second postmortem study[40] further emphasizes the relevance of asymmetry. Brains of patients with schizophrenia were compared with age-matched controls. The components of the lateral ventricle were assessed radiologically after infusion of radio-opaque medium into the ventricular spaces following formalin fixation. The posterior and particularly the temporal horns of the lateral ventricles were increased in patients with schizophrenia, in the latter case by a factor of 80% relative to the control group. In cases of Alzheimer-type dementia studied at the same time, ventricular enlargement was more generalized, affecting the anterior horns and body as well as the temporal and posterior horns of the ventricle. The findings in schizophrenia therefore are most marked in the temporal lobe. Of particular interest was the finding that the change in schizophrenia was selective to the left side of the brain (ANOVA $P < .001$), while in the Alzheimer cases there was no such lateralization.

There have been previous reports of lateralized changes. In a pneumoencephalographic comparison of acute and chronic patients, Haug[41] found the changes in his chronic cases to be more marked in the left temporal horn, and in a CT scan investigation of monozygotic twins discordant for schizophrenia Reveley et al[42] demonstrated a reduction in scan density in the ill twin on the left side. Such density reduction probably reflects enlargement of cerebrospinal fluid (CSF) spaces. Therefore, the structural changes in the brain in schizophrenia are more pronounced on the left side. Lateralized chemical changes also have been reported. Thus, Reynolds[43] found the content of dopamine was increased in the amygdala of patients with schizophrenia on the left but not on the right side, and in a PET scan study of patients in the acute phase of illness, Early and colleagues[44] reported a relative increase in glucose metabolism in the left globus pallidus.

The question raised by these findings is whether the laterality of the change relates to the disease process or to the normal asymmetries in the human brain (ie, do they indicate that the disease process itself is lateralized or do they reflect an interaction between a bilateral process and normal anatomical and chemical asymmetries)? The findings of the second postmortem study[40] answer this question. Temporal horn enlargement is present in Alzheimer-type dementia but it is not lateralized; when present in schizophrenia it is selective to the left hemisphere.

What could such lateralization mean? If the disease is genetic in origin it seems that the genes that determine the normal asymmetries in the brain are relevant. Such asymmetries were first postulated by Dax[45] and Broca[46] to account for clinical observations on aphasia; their anatomical reality has been established by the work of Geschwind.[47]

Interest in the left brain in schizophrenia in recent years dates from Flor-Henry's report[48] that when psychotic changes are seen in association with temporal lobe epilepsy the form of the psychosis is schizophrenia-like when the focus is on the left side. However, the concept has a history that extends back to not long after Broca's confirmation of Dax's localization of speech to the left hemisphere. Thus, in 1879 Crichton-Browne[49] wrote that "the cortical centers which are last organized, which are the most highly evolved and voluntary, and which are supposed to be located on the left side of the brain, might suffer first in insanity. . . ." Both Crichton-Browne and Luys[50] conducted postmortem studies to determine the relative weights of the two hemispheres in patients with mental illness. The findings are not easy to interpret (in part because of the diagnoses employed), but Luys thought that whereas in his normal sample the left hemisphere was generally heavier than the right, in his ill population the reverse was the case. In 1915 Southard[51] summarized his own studies of the pathology of schizophrenia as showing that "the atrophies and aplasias when focal show a tendency to occur in the left cerebral hemisphere." He added that "aside from the left-sidedness of the lesions, very striking is the preference of these changes to occupy the association centers of Flechsig" and "for this there is probably good a priori reason in the structure, late evolutionary development, and consequent relatively high lability of these regions."

The Genetics of Laterality and Psychosis

Thus, the notion that the left side of the brain is particularly affected in the psychoses has a long pedigree. The findings summarized in this chapter suggest that the structural anomalies in schizophrenia occur particularly in the left hemisphere. Perhaps it is not merely that the left temporal lobe is selectively vulnerable to the disease process, but that the pathogen is intrinsic to the genetic mechanism that controls the differential development of the two hemispheres.[52] Asymmetries of the temporal lobe presumably relate to the human capacity for speech and to hand preference. The mode of genetic transmission may be relatively simple. It is suggested[53,54] that handedness is decided by the presence or absence of a single autosomal dominant factor, the right shift factor or cerebral dominance gene. Brain asymmetries probably developed late in primate evolution; certainly they are more prominent in humans than in lower primates, and may be absent in some primate species.[55] Perhaps the cerebral dominance gene is subject to a high degree of variation and some of these variations are associated with pathology.

There is a case[56] that the genes for psychosis are located in the pseudo-autosomal region of the sex chromosomes, that is, that segment of the short arms of the X and Y chromosomes within which crossing over occurs in male meiosis. There are reasons for considering that genetic determinants of cerebral asymmetry are also located in this region. For example, in sex chromosome aneuploidies psychological deficits are described that may be lateralized. Thus, in XO (Turner's) syndrome, a deficit of perceptual organization relative to verbal comprehension has been described as a degree of "space–form blindness"[57] and diminished hemispheric specialization is reported.[58] In Klinefelter's (XXY) syndrome verbal deficits are present.[59] Because in normal females one X chromosome is inactivated, and this is probably also true of Klinefelter's syndrome, the deficits in Turner's and Klinefelter's subjects may relate to that segment of the X chromosome that is not inactivated (ie, the pseudoautosomal region).

Further evidence that determinants of asymmetry are located on the short arm of the X chromosome comes from Rett's syndrome. In this condition progressive loss of intellectual function is associated with a shift from left to right handedness at the age of 7 years.[60] The disorder is seen only in females and has been observed in association with a deletion of the short arm of the X chromosome;[61] the gene may therefore be X-linked and lethal to males. It may provide a clue to the location of the cerebral dominance gene.

Conclusions and Summary

1. The fact that some patients with schizophrenia develop "organic" type psychological impairments (eg, temporal disorientation) challenges the definition of the disease as a "functional" psychosis. In some patients intellectual deficits precede onset and in others they progress with disease progression. Intellectual functions are closer to the core of the disease process than is often thought.

2. Age at onset is a determinant of outcome—patients with early onset are more likely to develop intellectual impairments, negative symptoms, and behavioral deterioration than those with later onset. Moreover, age at onset is relevant to the relationship between intellectual impairments and brain structure; significant correlations between cognitive function and brain area are seen in early but not late onset patients. These findings are consistent with the view that anomalies in the brain in schizophrenia are at least in part developmental, that is, they occur at a time when the structure of the brain is still being formed.

3. Some structural changes in the brain in schizophrenia are lateralized. Asymmetries in the posterior part of the brain are significantly reduced in patients with an early onset of illness; thinning of the parahippocampal gyrus is greater on the left side; and temporal horn enlargement in schizophrenia (by contrast with that seen in Alzheimer-type dementia) is selective to the left hemisphere. The disease may be a disorder of the determinants of cerebral asymmetry (ie, of those genetic mechanisms that are responsible for the human capacity for speech and communication).

4. There is a case that the genes for psychosis (and perhaps also for cerebral asymmetry) are located in the pseudoautosomal region of the sex chromosomes, that region within which there is genetic exchange between X and Y chromosomes in male meiosis.

5. To account not only for developmental aspects and persisting impairments, but also for episodes of illness, it is necessary to postulate that the relevant genes possess a degree of autonomy, that is, a capacity to break free of cellular controls. For this reason it is suggested that the psychosis gene may have some characteristics of an unstable element or "virogene."[62]

References

1. Bleuler E: *Dementia Praecox or the Group of Schizophrenias*, J Zinkin (trans). New York, International Universities Press, 1950.
2. Kraepelin E: *Dementia Praecox and Paraphrenia*, RM Barclay, GM Robertson (trans). New York, RE Krieger, 1919.
3. Lanzkron J, Wolfson W: Prognostic value of perceptual distortion of temporal orientation in chronic schizophrenics. *Am J Psychiatry* 1958;114:744–746.
4. Dahl M: A singular distortion of temporal orientation. *Am J Psychiatry* 1958;115:146–149.
5. Ehrenteil OF, Jenney PB: Does time stand still for some psychotics? *Arch Gen Psychiatry* 1960;3:1–3.
6. Michelson M: A note on age confusion in psychosis. *J Consult Psych* 1968;42:331–338.
7. Crow TJ, Mitchell WS: Subjective age in chronic schizophrenia: evidence for a subgroup of patients with defective learning capacity? *Br J Psychiatry* 1975;126:360–363.
8. Stevens M, Crow TJ, Bowman MJ, et al: Age disorientation in chronic schizophrenia: a constant prevalence of 25% in a chronic mental hospital population. *Br J Psychiatry* 1978;133:130–136.
9. Smith JW, Oswald WT: Subjective age in chronic schizophrenia. *Br J Psychiatry* 1976;128:100.
10. Crow TJ: Temporal disorientation in chronic schizophrenia: the implications of an "organic" psychological impairment for the concept of "functional" psychosis, in Kerr A, Snaith P (eds): *Contemporary Issues in Schizophrenia*. London, Gaskell, 1986, pp. 168–174.
11. Buhrich N, Crow TJ, Johnstone EC, et al: Age disorientation in chronic schizophrenia is not associated with premorbid intellectual impairment or past physical treatment. *Br J Psychiatry* 1988;152:466–469.
12. Crow TJ, Stevens M: Age disorientation in chronic schizophrenia: the nature of the cognitive deficit. *Br J Psychiatry* 1978;133:137–142.
13. Liddle P, Crow TJ: Age disorientation in chronic schizophrenia is associated with global intellectual impairment. *Br J Psychiatry* 1984;144:193–199.
14. Pollack M, Woerner MG, Goodman W, et al: Childhood developmental patterns of hospitalized adult schizophrenic and nonschizophrenic patients and their siblings. *Am J Orthopsychiatry and Psychiatry* 1966;36:510–517.
15. Lane E, Albee G; Early childhood intellectual differences between schizophrenic adults and their siblings. *J Abn Soc Psych* 1964;68:193–195.

16. Garside RF: The relationship between schizophrenia and intelligence, PhD thesis. University of Newcastle-upon-Tyne, UK 1969.
17. Rappaport SR, Webb WB: An attempt to study intellectual deterioration by premorbid testing. *J Consult Psych* 1950;14:95–98.
18. Johnstone EC, Crow TJ, Frith CD, et al: Cerebral ventricular size and cognitive impairment in chronic schizophrenia. *Lancet* 1976;ii:924–926.
19. Haug JO: Pneumoencephalographic evidence of brain atrophy in acute and chronic schizophrenic patients. *Acta Psychiatrica Scandinavica,* 1982; 66:374–383.
20. Asano N: Pneumoencephalographic study of schizophrenia, in Mitsuda H (ed): *Clinical Genetics in Psychiatry.* Tokyo, Igaku-Shoin, 1967, pp. 209–219.
21. Huber G: Neuroradiologie und Psychiatrie, in Gruhle HW, Jung R, Mayer-Gross W, Muller M (eds): *Psychiatrie der Gegenwart, Forschung und Praxis, vol 1/1B Grundlagenforschung zur Psychiatrie Part B.* Berlin, Springer-Verlag, 1964.
22. Weinberger DR, Torrey EF, Neophytides AN, et al: Lateral cerebral ventricular enlargement in chronic schizophrenia. *Arch Gen Psychiatry* 1979;36:735–739.
23. Jernigan TL, Zatz LM, Moses JA, et al: Computer tomography in schizophrenics and normal volunteers: I. fluid volume. *Arch Gen Psychiatry* 1982;39:765–770.
24. Stahl SM, Jernigan T, Pfefferbaum A, et al: Brain computerized tomography in subtypes of severe chronic schizophrenia. *Psychol Med* 1988;18:73–77.
25. Owens DGC, Johnstone EC, Crow TJ, et al: Cerebral ventricular enlargement in schizophrenia: relationship to the disease process and its clinical correlates. *Psychol Med* 1985;15:27–41.
26. Crow TJ: Molecular pathology of schizophrenia: more than one dimension of pathology? *Br Med J* 1980;280:66–68.
27. Crow TJ: The two-syndrome concept—origins and current status. *Schizophrenia Bulletin* 1985;11:471–486.
28. Johnstone EC, Crow TJ, Frith CD, et al: Mechanism of the antipsychotic effect in the treatment of acute schizophrenia. *Lancet* 1978;i:848–851.
29. Owen F, Cross AJ, Crow TJ, et al: Increased dopamine receptor sensitivity in schizophrenia. *Lancet* 1978;ii:223–226.
30. Crow TJ, Johnstone EC: Schizophrenia: nature of the disease process and its biological correlates, in VB Mountcastle, F Plum (eds): *Handbook of Physiology—The Nervous System V.* Washington, American Physiological Society, 1986, pp. 843–869.
31. Kemali D, Maj M, Galderisi S, et al: Clinical, biological, and neuropsychological features associated with lateral ventricular enlargement in DSM-III schizophrenic disorder. *Psychiatry Res* 1987;21:137–149.
32. Kling AS, Kurtz N, Tachiki K, et al: CT scans in subgroups of chronic schizophrenics. *J Psychiatric Res* 1983;17:375–384.
33. Takahashi R, Inanaga V, Kato N, et al: CT scanning and the investigation of schizophrenia, in C Perris, G Struwe, B Jansson (eds): *Biological Psychiatry, 1981.* Amsterdam, Elsevier-North Holland, 1982, pp 259–268.
34. Williams AO, Reveley MA, Kolakowska T, et al: Schizophrenia with good and poor outcome: II Cerebral ventricular size and its clinical significance. *Br J Psychiatry* 1985;146:239–246.

35. Pakkenberg B: Postmortem study of chronic schizophrenic brains. *Br J Psychiatry* 1987;151:744–752.
36. Johnstone EC, Owens DGC, Colter N, et al: The spectrum of structural changes in the brain in schizrenia: age of onset as a predictor of clinical and cognitive impairments and their cerebral correlates. *Psychological Medicine,* 1989;19:91–103.
37. Crow TJ, Colter N, Frith CD, et al: Early onset schizophrenia arrests the development of cerebral asymmetries. *Psychiatry Res* in press.
38. Brown R, Colter N, Corsellis JAN, et al: Postmortem evidence of structural brain changes in schizophrenia. *Arch Gen Psychiatry* 1986;43:36–42.
39. Bogerts B, Meertz E, Schonfeldt-Bausch R: Basal ganglia and limbic system pathology in schizophrenia. *Arch Gen Psychiatry* 1985;42:784–791,
40. Crow TJ, Colter N, Brown R, et al: Lateralized asymmetry of temporal horn enlargement in schizophrenia. *Schizophrenia Research* 1988;1:155–156.
41. Haug JO: Pneumoencephalographic studies in mental disease. *Acta Psychiatrica Scandinavica* 1962;38 suppl:165.
42. Reveley MA, Reveley AM, Baldy R: Left hemisphere hypodensity in discordant schizophrenic twins: a controlled study. *Arch Gen Psychiatry* 1987;44:625–632.
43. Reynolds GP: Increased concentrations and lateral asymmetry of amygdala dopamine in schizophrenia. *Nature* 1983;305:527–529.
44. Early TS, Reiman ER, Raichle ME, et al: Left globus pallidus abnormality in never-medicated patients with schizophrenia. *Proc Nat Acad Sci* 1987;84:561–563.
45. Dax M: Lesions de la moitié gauche d l'encéphale coincident avec l'oubli des signes de la pensée, lu au congres meridional tenu a Montpellier en 1836. *Gaz Hebdom de Med et Chir* 1865;11:259–260.
46. Broca P: Nouvelle observations d'aphemie produit par un lesion de la moitié posterieure des deuxieme et troisieme circonvolutions frontales. *Bull Soc Anat* 1861;6:398–407.
47. Geschwind N, Levitsky W: Left-right asymmetry in temporal speech region. *Science* 1968;161:186–187.
48. Flor-Henry P: Psychosis and temporal lobe epilepsy: a controlled investigation. *Epilepsia* 1969;10:363–395.
49. Crichton-Browne J: On the weight of the brain and its component parts in the insane. *Brain* 1897;2:42–67.
50. Luys MJ: Contributions a l'étude d'une statistique sur le poids des hemispheres cerebraux à l'état normal et à l'état pathologique. *L'Encephale* 1881;1:644–646.
51. Southard EE: On the topographic distribution of cortex lesions and anomalies in dementia praecox with some account of their functional significance. *Am J Insanity* 1915;71:603–671.
52. Crow TJ: A reevaluation of the viral hypothesis: is psychosis the result of retroviral integration at a site close to the cerebral dominance gene? *Br J Psychiatr* 1984;145:243–253.
53. Annett M: Left, right, hand and brain: the right shift theory. *London,* L Erlbaum, 1985.
54. McManus IC: Handedness, language dominance, and aphasia: a genetic model. *Psychol Med* 1985;8 suppl:1–40.

55. Holloway R, de Lacoste MC: Brain endocast asymmetry in pongids and hominids: some preliminary findings on the palaeontology of cerebral dominance. *Am J Phys Anthropol* 1982;58:101–110.

56. Crow TJ: Sex chromosomes and psychosis; the case for a pseudoautosomal locus. *Br J Psychiatry* 1988;153;675–683.

57. Money J: Cytogenetic and psychosexual incongruities with a note on space-form blindness. *Am J Psychiatry* 1963;119:820–827.

58. Netley C, Rovet J: Atypical hemispheric lateralization in Turner syndrome subjects. *Cortex* 1982;18:377–384.

59. Ratcliffe, SG, Murray L, Teague P: Edinburgh study of growth and development of children with sex chromosome abnormalities III. *Birth Defects,* 1986;3(22),:73–118.

60. Olsson B, Rett, A: Shift to right handedness in Rett syndrome around age 7. *Am J Med Genetics* 1986;24:133–141.

61. Wahlstrom J, Anvret M: Chromosome findings in the Rett syndrome and a test.of a two-step mutation theory. *Am J Med Genetics* 1986;24:361–368.

62. Crow TJ; The viral theory of schizophrenia. *Br J Psychiatry* 1988;153:564–566.

5
Conceptual Approaches to the Study of Schizophrenia

WILLIAM T. CARPENTER, JR., BRIAN KIRKPATRICK, AND ROBERT W. BUCHANAN

In this chapter, we offer a general overview of relevant conceptual approaches to schizophrenia and illustrate their importance by discussing their application to the treatment of schizophrenia. The concepts to be presented are:

1. The medical model most capable of defining the range of relevant data for the care of the schizophrenic patient and the understanding of the disorder.
2. The syndromal nature of schizophrenia nosology.
3. Models of psychopathology identifying specifiable dimensions or domains of relevance to schizophrenia.
4. Constructs for integrating data defining natural history and course of schizophrenia.
5. Concepts of clinical intervention aimed at prevention of relapse.
6. The relevance of the above constructs for the integration of therapeutic strategies.

The Medical Model

Understanding of the complexity of human behavior has expanded enormously during the past 20 years. The biopsychosocial medical model, as espoused by Engel,[1,2] was developed in response to the limitations of the traditional biomedical model in integrating all of the relevant data for a particular disease. The biopsychosocial model is derived from general systems theory, and has as an essential tenet a hierarchical organization of a reverberating system.

The left side of Figure 5.1 illustrates the multiple levels of the hierarchical organization of a person, with the interactive arrows implying that perturbations at any one level have influence at levels located at both lower and higher positions in the hierarchy. Unlike the biomedical model or other reductionistic models, the biopsychosocial model does not, *a priori,* discount information from any level of the hierarchy. Engel has

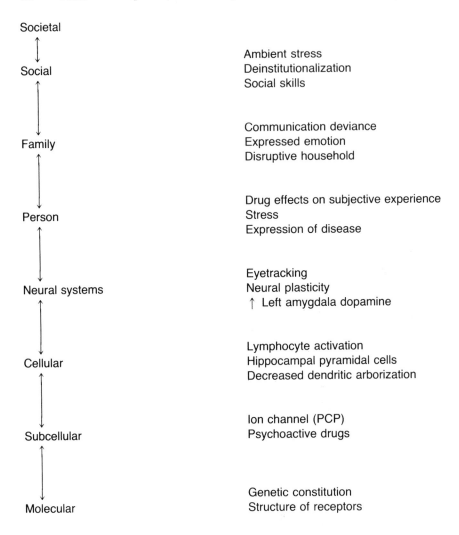

FIGURE 5.1. The biopsychosocial hierarchical model (left) and relevant areas of clinical investigation (right). Based on Engel's biopsychosocial medical model.[1]

argued such an approach is the most scientifically valid model for defining the range of information relevant to understanding disease and providing care to patients. The right side of Figure 5.1 illustrates present areas of clinical investigation relevant to each of these levels in the hierarchy. Although not exhaustive, this material readily demonstrates the neglect of important areas that occurs with acceptance of a model defining a more narrow range of relevant data. Figure 5.2 illustrates how currently used therapeutic approaches can be characterized at the hierarchical level of initiation. The broad biopsychosocial model is necessary for studying the effects of any intervention at the multiple levels of human functioning. This figure illustrates, within the person, the intimate relationship between different therapeutic techniques.

The use of this model in the integration of therapeutic approaches is further illustrated by the following example. A patient under considerable pressure for social and occupational performance begins manifesting insomnia, anxiety, and heightened suspiciousness. At this point, the family therapist will wish to enhance support and diminish intensity of expectation. The psychosocial therapist will wish to diminish the stimulating qualities in the environment. The individual therapist will choose to be supportive in a realistic context aimed at enhancing coping skills and diminishing idiosyncratic responses to environmental events. The pharmacotherapist will wish to initiate or increase medication. Each of these functions can be articulated in the context of the biopsychosocial medical model, and implications for the integration of these therapeutic approaches and for understanding their impact on the person are defined by that model. For example, because the family may be a key source of information regarding increased suspiciousness and anxiety, the family therapist must understand the relevance of this information for pharmacotherapy.

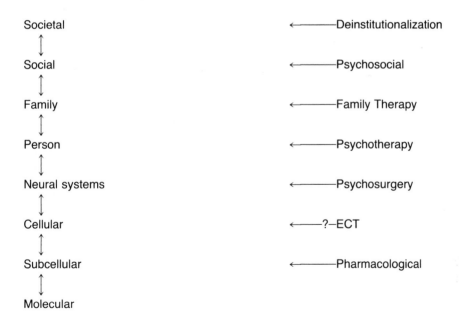

FIGURE 5.2. Therapeutic intervention, organized according to biopsychosocial hierarchical model.

The Syndromal Status of Schizophrenia

The conceptualization of schizophrenia as a heterogeneous disorder or syndrome is derived from the marked diversity in clinical presentation. Age and rate at onset, premorbid features, symptoms and signs, severity of interepisode impairments, treatment response, laboratory assessments, and brain imaging characteristics all vary so much as to bring into question the hypothesis that schizophrenia is a single disease entity. If schizophrenia is a syndrome rather than a single disease, the problem remains, however, as to how many forms of schizophrenia are present within the syndrome, and to what extent these forms have distinct etiologies and pathophysiologies. Many workers propose a multifactorial approach to etiology and pathophysiology of schizophrenia, and this seems useful heuristically until proven otherwise. However, the fact that distinguishable risk factors are associated with the syndrome (eg, genetic risk, pregnancy and birth complications, and excess in winter births) does not answer the question as to whether each specific disease entity will have multiple factors contributing to etiology. In addition, the concept of schizophrenia as a clinical syndrome has important implications for research methodology. If multiple pathophysiological processes underlie schizophrenia, studying heterogeneous groups will obscure these processes; whereas if there is a unitary pathophysiology, studying clinically homogeneous groups will not undermine the elucidation of that single process. A key research strategy issue is definition of study and comparison groups. The heterogeneity assumption will lead to comparisons of schizophrenia subdivisions (eg, family history positive *vs* negative), whereas the unitary pathophysiology hypothesis leads to schizophrenia *vs* nonschizophrenia comparisons.

The heuristic assumption of clinical variability and pathophysiological heterogeneity has important treatment implications. The development of treatment-relevant subtypes based on differences in symptom, personality, and family characteristics has been proposed,[3] and associated features are often explored for treatment relevance (eg, CT findings and family history). Patients who do not respond to the classical neuroleptics may have important differences in the pathophysiology of their illness. Moreover, the controversy over the responsiveness of negative symptoms to neuroleptics[4,5] can be related to a failure to take into account the multiple etiologies of negative symptoms.[6]

Domains of Psychopathology

Kraepelin, in his original description of dementia praecox, proposed the existence of two distinct psychopathologic processes.[7] The first process is characterized by "weakening of those emotional activities which permanently form the mainsprings of volition"[7] and would result in symptoms analogous to negative symptoms. The second process is characterized by the "loss of inner unity"[7] and would be manifested as the positive symptoms of schizophrenia. In 1974, Strauss and co-workers[8] subdivided the manifestations of schizophrenia into positive and negative symptom types, roughly corresponding to Kraepelin's two groups of disorders. In addition, they added a third category of interpersonal psychopathology to account for illness manifestations in the social sphere, symptoms not readily classified as either positive or negative. More recently, we have introduced the concept of domains of psychopathology as a framework for studying the heterogeneity of schizophrenia.[9] A psychopathological domain is a cluster of signs and symptoms that vary together and can be delineated clinically from other such groupings. We have proposed five domains of psychopathology which we believe merit separate scrutiny in the study of schizophrenia: (1) hallucinations and delusions, (2) cognitive impairments, (3) dissociative affective processes, (4) deficit symptoms, and (5) neurological impairment.

Hallucinations and delusions have traditionally been conceptualized as being closely associated. Family studies have suggested that they are transmitted somewhat independently from other features of schizophrenia.[10-12] Furthermore, they have been shown to have only a modest or insignificant correlation with important prognostic, course, and other symptom domains.[13-15] The second domain, cognitive impairment, may most usefully be subdivided into deficits in information processing and formal thought disorder.[16] Deficits in information processing may serve as potential vulnerability markers to the development of schizophrenia,[17-20] whereas formal thought disorder has been demonstrated to run in families, including relatives who do not manifest clinical schizophrenia.[21,22] The third domain, dissociative affective processes, that is, the dissociation of affect and behavior or thought, has tended to be correlated with certain positive symptoms, but not with deficit features.[6] The fourth domain, that of the deficit syndrome, refers to primary, enduring negative symptoms, ie, blunted affect, diminished emotional range, poverty of speech, diminished curiosity, diminished sense of purpose, and diminished social drive. A subgroup of schizophrenics is defined by deficit features characterized by: premorbid asociality; anhedonia; and specific neurological, neuropsychological, and eye-tracking deficits.[23,24] The final domain, neurological impairment, refers to the frequently observed clinical neurological manifestations observed in schizophrenia. The relationship between these impairments and other neurologically based abnormalities (eg, eye-tracking and neuroanatomical findings, including enlarged ventricles), as well as other domains, remains to be elucidated.

The importance of the domains model is threefold. First, in the care and study of schizophrenic patients, we must identify and observe those phenomena that seem most important in characterizing the manifestations of illness. It has been demonstrated that certain domains have a relatively low relationship to other domains within the patient, and that persons with schizophrenia may not have psychopathology drawn from all the domains.[25] Hence, to generate data of specific relevance to the domain, each domain must be specifically assessed. Failure to do so has already brought about a remarkable shortfall in our knowledge. For example, after 36 years of studying the therapeutic effects of neuroleptic medication, we still do not know if, in the long-term, these drugs are either therapeutic, have no effect, or have an adverse effect on neurological manifestations and deficit symptoms. Second, clinical manifestations of schizophrenia are not pathognomonic. It will be important to have a clear view as to which pathological attributes are found across disease categories and merely vary in proportion, and which may be relatively specific to schizophrenia. For example, do the 10 to 20% of major affective disorder patients who run a chronic and unremitting course have personality deterioration similar to the deficit syndrome of schizophrenia, or is the nature of chronicity in this class qualitatively different? Third, it is possible that the domains are distinguishable in their etiology, pathophysiology, and neural substrates. If this is the case, then studies should focus on specific domains rather than on diagnostic class. For instance, if schizophrenia with the deficit syndrome is distinguished from other forms of schizophrenia, the etiology and pathophysiology of deficit symptoms can be studied with more robust designs than when this type of categorical distinction is not made.

Course of Illness

Long-Term Course

An Overview of Long-term Course

Patients with schizophrenia are strikingly heterogeneous in virtually every clinical feature. The variability in long-term course is also striking. A considerable variability in long-term course has been well documented, even in the relatively chronic category of DSM-III schizophrenia.[26-29] Moreover, family aggregation studies also suggest that chronicity is an arbitrary guide to the separation of schizophrenia and other mental illnesses.[11]

There have been several attempts to define subtypes of schizophrenia based on long-term course. Huber described 12 patterns of course of illness, Bleuler 7, and Ciompi 8.[30-35] A summary and integration of the results from these studies is presented in Table 5.1.

We have argued for a new classification system for putative schizophrenic subtypes defined by course.[36] This classification is based on the following considerations:

TABLE 5.1. A summary of patterns of course in schizophrenia.

Pattern	Onset	Nature of psychotic episodes	Improvement late in life
1	Insidious	Chronic	Present
2	Insidious	Chronic	Absent
3	Insidious	Episodic	Present
4	Insidious	Episodic	Absent
5	Acute	Chronic	Present
6	Acute	Chronic	Absent
7	Acute	Episodic	Present
8	Acute	Episodic	Absent

These are a summary and integration of the eight long-term course subtypes of Ciompi.[34] Summarizing the course subtypes in this way demonstrates that his eight subtypes are generated from a dichotomization within each of three course epochs.

1. Although long-term course has been shown to be a powerful predictor of other clinical features,[37–40] the most powerful discriminations usually have been based on the combination of several features of course. Consequently, which features account for the variance remains unclear.
2. In the definition of course subtypes, researchers should distinguish between psychosis per se and nonpsychotic impairments such as deficit symptoms.
3. It may be useful to distinguish along three epochs of the lifetime course of schizophrenia: onset, middle course, and late course.

A Strategy for Research on Long-term Course

We propose that distinguishing among the epochs of long-term course will be useful in understanding the heterogeneity of schizophrenia. The onset epoch is concerned with psychotic and psychotic-like symptoms, such as perceptual aberrations, as well as nonpsychotic personality abnormalities, such as childhood asociality, that often precede the appearance of psychotic symptoms.[41–45] The middle course epoch includes episodic or unremitting psychosis and, in many patients, persistent nonpsychotic (personality) impairments. The third epoch refers to late outcome: a pattern of improvement or recovery in psychosis is observed in some patients late in adulthood, whereas persistence is seen in others. There also may be improvement in nonpsychotic impairments such as the deficit syndrome.[26,27,32,33,46]

It is important to make these distinctions for the purposes of research. To illustrate, suppose a biological marker distinguished classic "process" schizophrenia (with an insidious onset and unremitting psychotic symptoms) from classic "good prognosis" patients (with an acute onset and an episodic course of psychotic symptoms). It would be difficult to interpret such a finding, as the marker could be associated with the prepsychotic abnormality or with the course of the psychotic symptoms. However, if the two study groups differed in the nature of their onset but not relative to the course of their psychotic symptoms, a correlation with a marker would have a more specific interpretation.

The Epoch of Onset

Researchers have long divided schizophrenic groups according to premorbid, early morbid, and onset characteristics. The dichotomies of good *vs* poor premorbid, reactive *vs* process schizophrenia, and acute *vs* insidious onset are examples of groups defined by the features of the epoch of onset. These dichotomies have been validated by assessing short- and long-term outcome, association with precipitating stressors, prediction of treatment response, familial aggregation of distribution of schizophrenia spectrum features, and, with less consistency, age at onset, psychophysiologic and biochemical markers, and structural alterations in the brain.[37–40,47]

However, there has been some confounding of the clinical features used to define such cohorts. Some workers have focused on the rate of evolving psychosis (ie, acute *vs* insidious), whereas others distinguish the groups on the basis of developmental personality impairments (eg, asocial *vs* social). Predictive power is enhanced by combining features of both psychotic and nonpsychotic features, and clinicians appropriately base prognosis on data from both developmental history and the onset of psychosis. However, to study specific psychopathologic processes, it is useful and probably valid to consider personality pathology separately from psychosis and its rate of onset.[11,48,49]

Middle Course

A number of terms in the literature such as chronic, treatment-refractory, and residual symptoms have been used to delineate putative groups on the basis of the features of the middle course epoch. However, such approaches do not make clear whether the putative subgroups are based on interepisode personality pathology, sometimes referred to as residual symptoms, or on the persistence of psychosis per se. It may be important to distinguish the course of psychosis from enduring nonpsychotic personality pathology in the study of pathophysiology and treatment effects.

Some data already support the validity of distinguishing course of psychosis from personality impairments. Deficit syndrome patients appear to differ from other chronic schizophrenics on the basis of eyetracking features, neuropsychological test results, premorbid adjustment, neurologic signs, and self-report of anhedonia[24,50] (Buchanan et al, unpublished data; Kirkpatrick et al, unpublished data). Family aggregation studies[11,51] also support the view that the factors involved in the pathogenesis of psychotic symptoms (hallucinations, delusions, and formal thought disorder) may be different from factors involved in the pathogenesis of long-standing, interepisode impairments of personality.

Late Course

One influential school of thought has viewed schizophrenia as a chronic, deteriorating illness. Consequently, long-term outcome has been proposed as a definitive diagnostic tool. Recovery or very substantial improvement is not considered consistent with the diagnosis of schizophrenia, and diagnoses such as schizophreniform psychosis were introduced for the nonprogressive cases.[52-54] However, studies from several countries have documented variability in course regardless of diagnostic criteria;[26-29,32-35,55-58] a substantial number of patients manifest a sustained and significant improvement in psychopathology late in the course of illness, the proportion of such cases depending on factors such as population sample, treatment, and environmental circumstances.[59] This improvement reflects a decreased intensity of psychosis and may involve improvement in nonpsychotic impairments as well. These findings hold even with the application of DSM-III criteria.[26,27,60] Predictors of improvement in this epoch have not yet been well validated, but preliminary findings suggest premorbid family "closeness" and schizotypal personality merit further study.[46]

Research on late course improvement should distinguish between improvement in psychotic and nonpsychotic impairments. When investigating improvement in the deficit syndrome, it may also prove very interesting to differentiate between cases with early onset (ie, deficit impairments were apparent before the onset of psychosis) and those in which the deficit syndrome developed only after the appearance of psychosis.

Short-Term Course

In most patients with schizophrenia it is possible to discern episodes of illness, even in the presence of persistent hallucinations and delusions. Research has demonstrated that neuroleptics and certain psychosocial treatments are clearly more effective than placebo in treating acute episodes and preventing relapse. Recent research has focused on strategies for the reduction of neuroleptic exposure, with the goal of minimizing neuroleptic side effects.[61-63] Both a decrease in maintenance neuroleptic doses and the use of drug-free periods in stable patients have been part of this effort. Drug reduction strategies would be enhanced if clinicians could identify cases at high risk for relapse.

Clinical Features

Several clinical features appear to predict early relapse. One predictor of relapse after drug discontinuation is the severity of psychotic symptoms during neuroleptic treatment.[64,65] It is not always clear if patients with more severe symptoms are in relative remission, and decreasing treatment may simply allow more symptom expression. A related predictor is neuroleptic dose; patients with early relapse were found to have higher neuroleptic doses before drug discontinuation.[66-68] However, as neuroleptic dose was not assigned randomly, this relationship also may reflect severity of psychotic symptoms. There are also some data suggesting tardive dyskinesia manifested during neuroleptic treatment is a risk factor for early relapse after drug discontinuation. The dyskinesia and neuroleptic dose findings have contributed to the controversial "supersensitivity psychosis" hypothesis.[69]

"Expressed emotion" (EE), a measure from which family interactions are inferred, also may be a factor for relapse, although these findings have not always been replicated.[70,71] High EE is characterized by intrusiveness, hostility, and criticism directed toward the patient. It has long been noted that psychosocial stress appears to increase the risk of relapse in schizophrenic patients, and EE data may support the view. However, these results are open to alternative explanations. Most important is that very severely ill patients, who are prone to frequent relapses, may elicit high EE characteristics in their caretakers.[72] However, a recent small study found family treatment decreased the frequency of relapse in patients with high EE families, and this improvement was related to a decrease in EE.[73] The mode of therapeutic action may have been the reduction of EE. This study also supports others in demonstrating that certain psychosocial treatments are effective in reducing relapse rates.

Pharmacological Measures

There has been a great deal of interest in measures related to dopaminergic function as possible predictors of early relapse. These have included responses to pharmacological agents (eg, methylphenidate and amphetamine) and neuroendocrine measures (eg, prolactin and growth hormone). An increase in psychotic symptoms after infusion of methylphenidate and amphetamine has been shown to predict early relapse.[74-77] As these agents are dopaminergic agonists, it has been presumed that these behavioral measures revealed the functional "set point" of brain dopaminergic systems.

Low prolactin concentration during neuroleptic treatment also has been found to predict relapse in a subsequent drug-free period by two of three groups.[78-80] Dopamine has a tonic inhibitory effect on hypothalamic release of prolactin, and neuroleptic treatment results in an increase in plasma prolactin concentration. Prolactin concentration also predicted relapse in a dose-reduction paradigm,[81] as well as in two studies in which the patients' doses were left unchanged (Wilkins et al, unpublished data).[82,83]

One group did not find a relationship between prolactin concentration and time to relapse in a drug discontinuation study.[80] That study differed from the drug discontinuation studies[78,79] that did find such a relationship in that relapse was examined over a year-long period rather than a period of several weeks. In addition, patients in the negative study had less past neuroleptic drug exposure than did the patients in the other studies. These population differences, if confirmed, raise questions about differing mechanisms in the patient groups.

The relationship between prolactin and early relapse is interesting because of the mechanistic questions it raises. One interpretation of this evidence is that it lends some support to the "supersensitivity psychosis" hypothesis. Because neuroleptic drugs raise prolactin concentrations, low concentrations may identify a subgroup with an "excessive" adaptation to the neuroleptic-induced dopamine receptor blockade.

Another neuroendocrinological measure that has been investigated as a predictor of relapse is growth hormone. One group found that a robust growth hormone response to apomorphine infusion predicted relapse in drug-free patients.[84] This relationship has not yet been replicated by others.

These endocrinological measures are still in the research stage. However, the clinical features and pharmacologic data already offer guidance to clinicians. Based on the above material and clinical reasoning discussed elsewhere,[85] we regard it as prudent to consider the following as increased risk of relapse indicators:

1. Unstable course, recent psychotic exacerbation, severe psychotic symptoms, and presence of prodromal symptoms (see below).
2. High neuroleptic dose and recent history of early relapse on drug reduction.
3. Overly stimulating or stressful living circumstances.

Prevention of Relapse

Occasionally, a schizophrenic patient with a psychotic episode will recover and not have subsequent psychotic episodes. More often, a patient develops psychosis and never fully recovers from the initial psychotic episode. The most frequently occurring pattern, however, is the course of illness that includes multiple episodes of psychotic exacerbation, sometimes springing from a psychosis-free baseline and sometimes springing from the clinically stable baseline that includes a degree of psychotic symptomatology. The prevention of relapse is a key component in the therapeutics of this most common form of schizophrenia. It has been empirically demonstrated that the number of exacerbations is diminished when patients are on neuroleptic medication.[86–89] This beneficial effect may be even greater in patients living in stressful environments.[90,91]

The pharmacological strategy for relapse prevention has, for many years, relied exclusively on the use of continuous maintenance medication at a substantial dose level. More recent work, springing from the concern of adverse effects of the drugs and from the desire to find alternative strategies for treatment of noncompliant patients, has placed emphasis on dose reduction strategies. One such strategy relies on continuous medication, but at doses that are in the range of 10 to 20% of standard doses. These strategies are effective at relapse prevention, but somewhat less so than standard doses.[61–63,73,92–94] The decreased effectiveness of low-dose strategies is offset by the reduced dyskinesia, increased compliance, decreased drug interference with social and cognitive functioning, and greater sense of well-being associated with these strategies.[62,63,73] Furthermore, much of the disadvantage of the increase in symptom exacerbations with low-dose strategies may be successfully treated by procedures that rapidly increase medication at the time of exacerbation, while decreasing medication to the low-dose continuous strategy levels after stabilization.

An alternative treatment strategy for relapse prevention presumes that early warning signs of relapse can be noted by patient and clinician and that neuroleptic drug intervention targeted to those warning signs will be effective in preventing the full manifestations of relapse.[95,96] This targeted or intermittent strategy has been demonstrated to be a successful therapeutic strategy associated with less dyskinesia, more symptom exacerbation, and similar course of occupational and social functioning as well as global assessments of illness.[97–100] The clinician may find this approach particularly useful in patients who are actively noncompliant with drugs because of the subjective discomfort of adverse side effects. These effects will be minimized if drugs are used only at times of symptom exacerbation.

These several strategies allow clinicians to individualize treatment according to the particular risks and benefits judged to be most preferable for any given patient. For example, patients with relatively infrequent relapse or with early warning signs that enable successful intervention will be good candidates for a drug-reduction strategy. The targeted patients with frequent or severe relapses, or who are noncooperative at times of exacerbation, may be good candidates for continuous standard-dose medication approaches.

Another approach to relapse prevention may be the use of antianxiety drugs, in an attempt to treat prodromal symptoms when they occur. Prodromal symptoms typically include agitation, insomnia, anxiety, and depression—symptoms often responsive in other circumstances to antianxiety medication. Furthermore, these drugs may diminish the impact of stress in promulgating relapse phenomena. Finally, such drugs may be effective through GABAergic interconnections that modulate dopaminergic functioning in mesolimbic and mesocortical neurons.

A final approach to relapse prevention depends on interpersonal therapeutic strategies; psychosocial interventions have been shown to be efficacious. Furthermore, the ability to identify early warning signs and to facilitate patient collaboration, central to the application of the targeted strategy, will be dependent on the centrality and continuity of the personal clinical relationship.

Conclusions and Summary

An appreciation of the natural history of schizophrenia and the relevant medical and scientific concepts has direct implications for the care and study of patients with the disorder.

1. Consonant with the biopsychosocial medical model is the principle that therapeutic strategies will be derived from multiple levels of intervention. These interventions must be integrated for optimal impact on the individual patient. It is integration of multiple therapies that is most desirable. Evaluation of therapeutic efficacy can be simultaneously addressed at the social, psychological, and biological levels of function.
2. As a heterogeneous clinical syndrome, individual patients with schizophrenia will vary considerably from each other in their specific treatment requirements.
3. Domains of psychopathology have discrete attributes that require focused therapeutics and specific ascertainment of treatment effect. This is necessary if we are to provide an empirical literature on the effectiveness of treatment for all major aspects of schizophrenia. It is necessary if the clinician is to appreciate fully treatment effects in each patient.
4. The variability in the course of illness between patients, and the fact that any given patient will be in quite different phases of illness at different times, means that the clinician must continually evaluate the phase of illness with a view toward altering the therapeutic strategy accordingly. This evaluation must extend to the psychosocial environment in which the patient is being treated.
5. Consideration of the episodic course of psychosis places special emphasis on ascertainment of vulnerability to relapse. The clinician can presently use clinical features, recent history, neuroleptic dose, and environmental factors in determining risk for relapse. Research developments promise new tools drawn from endocrine markers and pharmacologic probes.

6. Early warning signs of relapse provide a focus for relapse prevention, and strategies of prevention will necessarily include interpersonal and pharmacologic treatment.

References

1. Engel GL: The need for a new medical model: a challenge for biomedicine. *Science* 1977;196:129–136.
2. Engel GL: The clinical application of the biopsychosocial model. *Am J Psychiatry* 1980;137:535–544.
3. Carpenter WT, Heinrichs DW: Treatment relevant subtypes of schizophrenia. *J Nerv Ment Dis* 1981;169:113–119.
4. Breier A, Wolkowitz OM, Doran AR, et al: Neuroleptic responsivity of negative and positive symptoms in schizophrenia. *Am J Psychiatry* 1987;144:1549–1555.
5. Goldberg SC: Negative and deficit symptoms in schizophrenia do respond to neuroleptics. *Schizophr Bull* 1985;11:453–456.
6. Carpenter WT, Heinrichs DW, Alphs LD. Treatment of negative symptoms. *Schizophr Bull* 1985;11:440–452.
7. Kraepelin E: *Dementia Praecox and Paraphrenia,* Barclay RB (ed). Edinburgh, ES Livingston, Ltd, 1919.
8. Strauss JS, Carpenter WT, Bartko JJ: Speculations on the processes that underlie schizophrenic symptoms and signs. *Schizophr Bull* 1974;11:61–75.
9. Carpenter WT, Buchanan RW: Domains of psychopathology relevant to the study of etiology and treatment in schizophrenia, in Schulz SC, Tamminga CA (eds): *Schizophrenia: Scientific Progress*. New York, Oxford University Press, 1989, pp 13–23.
10. Kendler KS, Gruenberg AM, Tsuang MT: Psychiatric illness in first-degree relatives of schizophrenic and surgical control patients: a family study using DSM-III criteria. *Arch Gen Psychiatry* 1985;42:770–779.
11. Kendler KS, Gruenberg AM, Tsuang MT: A DSM-III family study of the nonschizophrenic psychotic disorders. *Am J Psychiatry* 1986;143:1098–1105.
12. McGuffin P, Farmer AE, Gottesman II, et al: Twin concordance for operationally defined schizophrenia. *Arch Gen Psychiatry* 1984;41:541–545.
13. Bilder RM, Sukdeb M, Rieder RO, et al: Symptomatic and neuropsychological components of defect states. *Schizophr Bull* 1985;11:409–417.
14. Andreasen NC: Positive *vs* negative schizophrenia: a critical evaluation. *Schizophr Bull* 1985;11:380–389.
15. Crow TJ: The two-syndrome concept: origins and current status. *Schizophr Bull* 1985;11:471–486.
16. Neuchterlein KH, Edell WS, Norris M, et al: Attentional vulnerability indicators, thought disorder and negative symptoms. *Schizophr Bull* 1986;12:408–426.
17. Asarnow RF, Steffy RA, MacCrimmon DJ, et al: An attentional assessment of foster children at risk for schizophrenia. *J Abnormal Psychol* 1977;86:267–275.
18. Erlenmeyer-Kimling L: Biological markers for the liability to schizophrenia. Presented at the Dahlen Workshop on Biological Perspectives in Schizophrenia. Berlin, October, 1986.

19. Erlenmeyer-Kimling L, Cornblatt B, Friedman D, et al: Neurological, electrophysiological, and attentional deviations in children at risk for schizophrenia, in Henn FA, Nasrallah HA (eds): *Schizophrenia As A Brain Disease*. New York, Oxford University Press, 1982, pp 61–98.
20. Neuchterlein KH, Dawson ME: Information processing and attentional functioning in the developmental course of schizophrenic disorders. *Schizophr Bull* 1984;10:160–203.
21. Rosvold HE, Mirsky A, Sarason I, et al: A continuous performance test of brain damage. *J Consult Psych* 1956;20:343–350.
22. Singer MT, Wynne LC, Toohey ML: Communication disorders and the families of schizophrenics, in Wynne LC, Cromwell RL, Matthysse S (eds): *The Nature of Schizophrenia*. New York, John Wiley & Sons, 1978, pp 499–511.
23. Buchanan RW, Heinrichs DW, Kirkpatrick B: Neurological signs in schizophrenia. Presented at the International Congress on Schizophrenia Research, Clearwater, Florida, March, 1987.
24. Thaker G, Buchanan RW, Kirkpatrick B, et al: Eye movements in schizophrenia: clinical and neurobiological correlates. Abstracts of the Society for Neuroscience, 1988;14:141.2
25. World Health Organization: The International Pilot Study of Schizophrenia, Vol. 1. Geneva, World Health Organization, 1973.
26. Harding CM, Brooks GW, Ashikaga T, et al: The Vermont longitudinal study of persons with severe mental illness, I: Methodology, study sample, and overall status 32 years later. *Am J Psychiatry* 1987;144:718–726.
27. Harding CM, Brooks GW, Ashikaga T, et al: The Vermont longitudinal study of persons with severe mental illness, II: Longterm outcome of subjects who retrospectively met DSM-III criteria for schizophrenia. *Am J Psychiatry* 1987;144:727–735.
28. McGlashan TH: Selective review of recent North American follow-up studies of schizophrenia. *Schizophr Bull* 1988;14(4):515–542.
29. Angst J: European long-term follow-up studies of schizophrenia. *Schizophr Bull* 1988;14(4):501–514.
30. Huber G, Gross C, Schuttler R: A long-term follow-up study of schizophrenia: psychiatric course of illness and prognosis. *Acta Psychiatrica Scand* 1975;52:49–57.
31. Huber G, Gross C, Schuttler R, et al: Longitudinal studies of schizophrenic patients. *Schizophr Bull* 1980;6(4):592–605.
32. Bleuler M: A 23-year longitudinal study of 208 schizophrenics and impressions in regard to the nature of schizophrenia, in Rosenthal D, Kety SS (eds): *The Transmission of Schizophrenia*. New York, Pergamon Press, 1968, pp 3–12.
33. Bleuler M: *The Schizophrenic Disorders*, Clemens SM (trans). New Haven, Yale University Press, 1978.
34. Ciompi L: Catamnestic long-term study of the course of life and aging of schizophrenics. *Schizophr Bull* 1980;6:606–618.
35. Ciompi L: Three lectures on schizophrenia. *Br J Psychiatry* 1980;136:413–420.
36. Carpenter WT, Kirkpatrick B: The heterogeneity of long-term course of schizophrenia: implications for future research. *Schizophr Bull* 1988;14(4):645–652.

37. Shelton RC, Weinberger DR: X-ray computed tomography studies in schizophrenia: a review and synthesis, in Nasrallah HA, Weinberger DR (eds): *Handbook of Schizophrenia,* vol 1. New York, Elsevier Science Publishers, 1986, pp 207–250.

38. Vaillant GE: The prediction of recovery in schizophrenia. *J Nerv Ment Dis* 1962;35:534–543.

39. Stephens JH: Long-term prognosis and follow-up in schizophrenia. *Schizophr Bull* 1978;4:25–47.

40. Strauss JS, Carpenter WT: The prognosis of schizophrenia, in Bellak L (ed): *Disorders of the Schizophrenic Syndrome.* New York, Basic Books, 1979, pp 472–491.

41. Lewine RJ, Watt NF, Prentky RA, et al: Childhood social competence in functionally disordered psychiatric patients and in normals. *J Abn Psychiatry* 1980;89:132–138.

42. Watt N, Stolorow R, Lubensky A, et al: School adjustment and behavior of children hospitalized for schizophrenia as adults. *Am J Orthopsychiatry* 1970;40:637–657.

43. Parnas J, Schulsinger F, Schulsinger H, et al: Behavioral precursors of schizophrenia spectrum. *Arch Gen Psychiatry* 1982;39:658–664.

44. Kendler KS, Gruenberg AM, Strauss JS: An independent analysis of the Copenhagen sample of the Danish adoption study of schizophrenia: V. The relationship between childhood social withdrawal and adult schizophrenia. *Arch Gen Psychiatry* 1982;39:1257–1261.

45. Kendler KS, Hays P: Schizophrenia with premorbid inferiority feelings. *Arch Gen Psychiatry* 1982;39:643–647.

46. McGlashan TH: Late onset improvement in schizophrenia and aging, in Miller NE, Cohen GD (eds): *Chronic Schizophrenia: Characteristics and Prediction.* New York, Guilford Publications, 1987, pp 61–73.

47. Andreasen NC: The diagnosis of schizophrenia. *Schizophr Bull* 1987;13:9–22.

48. Gottesman II, McGuffin P, Farmer AE: Clinical genetics as clues to the "real" genetics of schizophrenia (A decade of modest gains while playing for time). *Schizophr Bull* 1987;13:23–47.

49. Kety SS, Rosenthal D, Wender PH, et al: The types and prevalence of mental illness in the biological and adoptive families of adopted schizophrenics. *J Psychiatric Res* 1968;6:345–362.

50. Wagman AMI, Heinrichs DW, Carpenter WT: Deficit and nondeficit forms of schizophrenia: neuropsychological evaluation. *Psychiatry Res* 1987;22:319–330.

51. Heston LL: Psychiatric disorders in foster home reared children of schizophrenic mothers. *Br J Psychiatry* 1966;112:819–825.

52. Leonhard K: The question of prognosis in schizophrenia. *Internat J Psychiatry* 1966;2:633–635.

53. Langfeldt G: Schizophrenia: diagnosis and prognosis. *Behav Sci* 1969;14:173–182.

54. Kleist K: Schizophrenic symptoms and cerebral pathology. *J Ment Sci* 1960;106:246–253.

55. Hawk AB, Carpenter WT, Strauss JS: Diagnostic criteria and 5-year outcome in schizophrenia: a report from the International Pilot Study of Schizophrenia. *Arch Gen Psychiatry* 1975;32:343–347.

56. Brockington IF, Kendell RE, Leff JP: Definition of schizophrenia: concordance and prediction of outcome. *Psychol Med* 1978;8:387–398.
57. Kendell RE, Brockington IF, Leff JP: Prognostic implications of six alternative definitions of schizophrenia. *Arch Gen Psychiatry* 1979;35:25–31.
58. Flekkoy K, Lund I, Astrup C: Prolonged clinical and experimental follow-up of hospitalized schizophrenics. *Neuropsychobiology* 1975;1:47–58.
59. Lin K, Kleinman AM: Psychopathology and clinical course of schizophrenia: a cross-cultural perspective. *Schizophr Bull* 1988;14(4):555–568.
60. McGlashan TH: The Chestnut Lodge follow-up study: II. Long-term outcome of schizophrenia and the affective disorders. *Arch Gen Psychiatry* 1984;41:586–601.
61. Kane JM: Low dose medication strategies in the maintenance treatment of schizophrenia. *Schizophr Bull* 1983;9:528–532.
62. Kane JM, Rifkin A, Woerner M, et al: Low-dose neuroleptic treatment of outpatient schizophrenics: I. Preliminary results for relapse rates. *Arch Gen Psychiatry* 1983;40:893–896.
63. Marder SR, Van Putten T, Mintz J, et al: Low- and conventional-dose maintenance therapy with fluphenazine decanoate. *Arch Gen Psychiatry* 1987;44:518–521.
64. Schooler NR: Symptoms of psychopathology as predictors of relapse in schizophrenia, in Lieberman JA, Kane JM (eds): *Predictors of Relapse in Schizophrenia.* Washington, American Psychiatric Press, Inc, 1986, pp 33–45.
65. Heinrichs DW, Carpenter WT: Experiences with a drug-free month in schizophrenic outpatients. *Psychopharmacol Bull* 1985;21:117–119.
66. Prien RF, Cole JO, Belkin NF: Relapse in chronic schizophrenics following abrupt withdrawal of tranquillizing medication. *Br J Psychiatry* 1968;115:679–686.
67. Prien RF, Levine J, Switkalski RW: Discontinuation of chemotherapy for chronic schizophrenics. *HCP* 1971;January:20–23.
68. Andrews P, Hall JN, Smith RP: A controlled trial of phenothiazine withdrawal in chronic schizophrenic patients. *Br J Psychiatry* 1976;128:451–455.
69. Chouinard G, Jones BD, Annable L: Neuroleptic-induced supersensitivity psychosis: clinical and pharmacologic characteristics. *Am J Psychiatry* 1980;137:16–21.
70. Koenigsberg HW, Handley R: Expressed emotion: from predictive index to clinical construct. *Am J Psychiatry* 1986;143:1361–1373.
71. Parker G, Johnston P, Hayward L: Parental 'Expressed Emotion' as a predictor of schizophrenic relapse. *Arch Gen Psychiatry* 1988;45:806–813.
72. Kanter J, Lamb HR, Loeper C: Expressed emotion in families: a critical review. *HCP* 1987;38:374–380.
73. Hogarty GE, McEvoy JP, Munetz M, et al: Dose of fluphenazine, familial expressed emotion, and outcome in schizophrenia. *Arch Gen Psychiatry* 1988;45:797–805.
74. Lieberman JA, Kane JM, Galdaleta D, et al: Methylphenidate challenge as a predictor of relapse in schizophrenia. *Am J Psychiatry* 1984;141:633–638.
75. Van Kammen DP, Docherty JP, Bunney WE Jr: Prediction of early relapse after pimozide discontinuation by response to d-amphetamine during pimozide treatment. *Biol Psychiatry* 1982;17:233–242.

76. Lieberman JA, Kane JM, Sarantakos S, et al: Prediction of relapse in schizophrenia. *Arch Gen Psychiatry* 1987;44:597–603.

77. Angrist B, Peselow E, Rotrosen J, et al: Relationship between responses to dopamine agonists, psychopathology, neuroleptic maintenance in schizophrenic subjects, in Angrist B, Burrows G, Lader M, et al (eds): *Recent Advances in Neuropsychopharmacology*, vol. 31. New York, Pergamon Press, 1981. pp 49–54.

78. Zander K, Fischer B, Zimmer R, et al: Long-term neuroleptic treatment of chronic schizophrenic patients: clinical and biochemical effects of withdrawal. *Psychopharmacology* 1981;73:43–47.

79. Brown W, Laughren T: Low serum prolactin and early relapse following neuroleptic withdrawal. *Am J Psychiatry* 1981;138:237–239.

80. Lieberman JA, Kane JM, Gadaletta D, et al: Methylphenidate challenge tests and course of schizophrenia. *Psychopharmacol Bull* 1985;21:123–129.

81. Faraone SV, Curran JP, Laughren T, et al: Neuroleptic bioavailability, psychosocial factors, and clinical status: a 1-year study of schizophrenic outpatients after dose reduction. *Psychiatry Res* 1986;19:311–322.

82. Faraone SV, Brown WA, Laughren T: Neuroleptic bioavailability and clinical status: a two-year study of schizophrenic outpatients. *J Clin Psychiatry* 1987;48:151–154.

83. Wilkins JN, Marder SR, Van Putten T, et al: Circulating prolactin predicts risk of exacerbation in patients on depot fluphenazine. *Psychopharmacol Bull* 1987;23:522–525.

84. Brown GM, Cleghorn JM, Kaplan RD, et al: Longitudinal growth hormone studies in schizophrenia. *Psychiatry Res* 1988;24:123–136.

85. Carpenter WT. Early targeted pharmacotherapeutic intervention in schizophrenia. *J Clin Psychiatry* 1986;47(suppl):23–29.

86. Baldessarini RJ, Cole JO, Davis JM, et al: Clinical indications for prolonged neuroleptic treatment. American Psychiatric Association Task Force on Tardive Dyskinesia. Washington, DC, American Psychiatric Association, 1980, pp 98–136.

87. Baldessarini RJ, Davis JM: What is the best maintenance dose of neuroleptics in schizophrenia? *Psychiatry Res* 1980;3:115–122.

88. Hogarty GE, Goldberg SC, Schooler NR, et al: Drug and sociotherapy in the aftercare of schizophrenic patients: II. Two year relapse rates. *Arch Gen Psychiatry* 1974;31:603–608.

89. Davis J: Overview: maintenance therapy in psychiatry: 1. Schizophrenia. *Am J Psychiatry* 1975;132:1237–1245.

90. Falloon IRH, Liberman RP: Interactions between drug and psychosocial therapy in schizophrenia. *Schizophr Bull* 1983;9:543–554.

91. Goldstein MJ: Psychosocial issues. *Schizophr Bull* 1987;13:157–171.

92. Marder SR, Van Putten T, Mintz J, et al: Maintenance therapy in schizophrenia: new findings, in Kane JM (ed): *Drug Maintenance Strategies in Schizophrenia*. Washington, DC, American Psychiatric Press, 1984, pp 32–49.

93. Lehmann HE, Wilson WH, Deutsch M: Minimal maintenance medication: effects of three dose schedule on relapse rates and symptoms in chronic schizophrenic outpatients. *Comp Psychiatry* 1983;24:293–303.

94. Faraone SV, Cirelli V, Curran JP, et al: Neuroleptic dose reduction for schizophrenic outpatients: a three-year follow-up study. *HCP* 1988;39:1207–1208.

95. Herz MI, Szymanski HV, Simon JC: Intermittent medication for stable schizophrenic outpatients: an alternative to maintenance medication. *Am J Psychiatry* 1982;139:918–922.
96. Carpenter WT, Heinrichs DW: Early intervention, time-limited, targeted pharmacotherapy of schizophrenia. *Schizophr Bull* 1983;9:533–542.
97. Herz MI, Glazer W: Intermittent medication in schizophrenia—preliminary results. *Schizophr Res* 1988;1(2–3):224–225.
98. Carpenter WT, Heinrichs DW, Hanlon T, et al: Continuous targeted medication in schizophrenia outpatients: outcome results. *Schizophr Res* 1988;1(2–3):223–224.
99. Carpenter WT, Stephens JH, Rey AC, et al: Early intervention *vs* continuous pharmacotherapy of schizophrenia. *Psychopharm Bull* 1982;18:21–23.
100. Carpenter WT, Heinrichs DW, Hanlon TE: A comparative trial of pharmacologic strategies in schizophrenia. *Am J Psychiatry* 1987;144:1466–1470.

Part II
Recent Advances in the Diagnosis and Treatment of Schizophrenia

6
Risk Factors in Schizophrenia: Interaction Between Genetic Liability and Environmental Factors

FINI SCHULSINGER AND JOSEF PARNAS

This chapter does not focus strictly on the genetic liability for schizophrenia[1] or the effects of environment in producing schizophrenia,[2,3] but rather mainly on the interaction of genetic liabilities with experiential factors. This nature–nurture approach focuses on the degree of genetic risk and interactions with and effects of various environmental stressors.[4] This is a relatively new field with few studies on these interactions.

Historical Perspectives of Genetic Studies

The German geneticist, Bruno Schulz, published in 1932 a study of the influence of mental trauma, somatic illnesses, and accidents on the distribution of schizophrenic subclasses (hebephrenia, catatonia, etc).[5] In a sample of 660 schizophrenic patients, he found an especially high prevalence of catatonic cases with somatic factors as definite precipitants. The prognosis was best in cases with pure or mixed catatonic symptomatology, but poor in cases with somatic factors as precipitants. This was the beginning of interaction studies of genetic liability and environmental factors.

Manfred Bleuler reported in 1941 on the family characteristics of 89 schizophrenic probands who improved or recovered under treatment with electroconvulsive therapy (ECT) as compared with the relatives of an unselected schizophrenic sample.[6] Bleuler found that for the schizophrenic siblings of the probands who improved with ECT, the disorder had a more benign course than it had in the probands themselves. Further, relatives of the ECT-responsive probands were less likely to have pathological personalities and were less frequently found to be schizoid or psychopathic premorbidly than were the relatives of the unselected schizophrenic patients who did not receive ECT. Moreover, the described differences were further strengthened if those probands whose ECT remissions were only seeming and not reliable were excluded from the analysis.

A more potent method was the study of differences in experiential factors between monozygotic twins who were discordant for schizophrenia. The classical investigation of a series of these twins was published in the late 1960s by Pollin and Stabenau.[7] Eventually, other methods were found to be effective for the study of genetic factors in schizophrenia, such as the studies initiated by Seymour Kety and co-workers in 1963.[8-10] These American–Danish studies were conducted in Denmark because of the country's advantages including size, homogeneity, stability of population, and well-kept records both for population and for psychiatric admissions. These studies evaluated the biological and adoptive relatives of schizophrenic patients who were adopted away in their early childhood to nonbiologically related adoptive families. They clearly demonstrated the presence of a genetic liability for schizophrenia. The role of genetic factors was emphasized by the finding of a high prevalence of schizophrenia in biological paternal half-siblings of the schizophrenic probands with whom they shared only a degree of genetic overlap and not in utero or neonatal experiences.

Longitudinal Prospective Research: The Copenhagen High Risk Study

The research of my colleagues and myself has centered on the longitudinal prospective study of individuals at high risk.[4,11-17] In 1962 the American psychologist Sarnoff Mednick and I began the so-called 1962 Copenhagen High Risk Study by assessing 207 children between 10 and 20 years old at high risk for schizophrenia, and 104 matched low-risk controls.[11] The index children all had severely schizophrenic mothers. The theory behind this study was Mednick's learning theory on schizophrenia, which assumed a special vulnerability of the autonomic nervous system; if people with this vulnerability were exposed to chronic anxiety-provoking living conditions in childhood, they might develop tangential thinking and eventually become schizophrenic. The goal of these studies was to make possible the early identification of future schizophrenics and to develop strategies for preventing such a course.

The initial assessment of these children in 1962 to 1964 consisted of psychophysiological measures, learning experiments, school information, birth records, psychiatric interviews, and extensive psychological testing. In 1967, the subjects were all visited at home by social workers who described their life course since the first assessment and gave a detailed account of how they appeared mentally, physically, and culturally at that time.

Ten years after the first assessment, in 1972 and 1974, the subjects were reassessed using the same type of measures as those used in the original evaluation. In addition, they were given thorough clinical diagnostic assessment using several of the then modern interview instruments.[13] These

TABLE 6.1. Design of the project.*

1962	1967	1972	1980
Initial assessment	5-year follow-up	10-year diagnostic follow-up	subsample follow-up

This table shows the major assessment years in our study. In addition, we received information on the subjects from various sources.
*Modified from Schulsinger et al. with permission.[4]

instruments provided computer-derived diagnoses. These included the Present State Examination and the Current and Past Psychopathology Scale, which was a predecessor of the Schedule for Affective Disorders and Schizophrenia. Also, the evaluation included other more impressionistic interviewing using various scales and making ICD-8 diagnoses.

In 1980 we examined, with a renewed interview and this time with a CT scan, a subgroup that consisted of 10 schizophrenics, 10 patients with schizotypal personality disorders, and 10 high-risk children with no psychopathology whatsoever. Separately, we did a personal study of all the fathers.[18] After this we subsequently obtained an update on the mothers from one of our co-workers who has been analyzing the mothers' hospital records from the very beginning, before 1962, when we selected them as severely schizophrenic models. Thus, our study design is extremely complex with varied data sets obtained over time (Table 6.1).

Our original child subjects now average about 40 years of age and currently are completing the final follow-up which includes interviews assessing psychopathology and personality, eye tracking, and CT scanning. We are now virtually completed with this final follow-up. Presented here are our preliminary findings in a number of areas including: behavioral precursors of the schizophrenic spectrum; effects of early institutional vs family rearing; the role of pregnancy and birth complications; and relation of brain morphology to schizophrenia.

There are a number of ways in which one can analyze such longitudinal data in the psychopathological framework. One can compare those who become schizophrenic with those high-risk children who have no mental illness, or one can compare those schizophrenic high-risk children with those high-risk children who became schizotypal. We did both and it turned out to be fruitful to use such paradigms.

Premorbid Behavior Correlates of the Schizophrenia Spectrum

Table 6.2 summarizes the data on premorbid behavior precursors of the schizophrenia spectrum. In general, the behavioral precursors pertaining to schizophrenia spectrum disorders are similar for those who are schizophrenic and those who have schizotypal personality disorders.[15] The one

TABLE 6.2. Behavioral precursors of schizophrenia spectrum.*

Early childhood	Passivity, short attention span
School behavior	Isolated (rejected by others), poor affect control†
Clinical assessment	Subtle formal thought disorder, defective emotional rapport (mean age 15 yrs)

*Modified from Schulsinger et al. with permission.[4]
†This item significantly discriminated between preschizophrenics and preschizotypes, being characteristic for the former.

exception relates to school behavior and, in particular, poor affect control. This was the only one of the behavioral measures that discriminated between the patients who became schizophrenic and those who eventually developed schizotypal personality disorders (or, before DSM-III, termed borderline disorders). For those who became schizophrenic, their school behavior was characterized by more interpersonal difficulties, rejection by others, uneasiness about criticism, and isolation. Most striking was their poor affect control. This means that premorbidly when these children became upset, it took them a very long time, not minutes but the rest of the day, before they calmed down. In contrast, most of the other children were relaxed in just a few minutes after having been upset.

Early Institutional Versus Family Rearing

Figure 6.1 illustrates the number of months of institutionalization during the first 5 years of life of the children of schizophrenic mothers. These data are distributed over the children's diagnostic outcome 10 years after the first assessment in four categories: schizophrenic, schizotypal, other diagnoses, and no mental illness. In analyzing these data we adjusted for the age of the mother at the time of first hospitalization and the amount of contact with the mother during the first 5 years of life. This analysis showed that institutionalization had a strong effect on diagnostic outcome. Such effects from deprivation are not surprising.[19] Further statistical analysis showed that children who spent time in an institution were apt to have mothers with more severe illness of earlier onset; also, they spent less time with these mothers. Thus, children with the genetic liability for schizophrenia have a more favorable outcome if reared in a family setting, even when the mother is severely disturbed, than if reared in an institution during the first years of life when the chances of having personal attachments are more limited. In general, these data support a diathesis-stress model for the development of psychopathology.

Pregnancy and Birth Complications

In our prospective study, we also evaluated, by detailed midwife reports, the presence or absence of pregnancy and birth complications as well as the pre- and postnatal condition of both the mother and infant.[14] Two

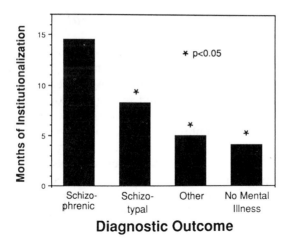

FIGURE 6.1. Institutionalization during the first five years of life adjusted for age of maternal schizophrenia and contact with parents.

thirds of the schizophrenic patients experienced some form of obstetrical complication. It was found that those high-risk children who had a history of the most pregnancy–birth complications were those who became schizophrenic (Fig 6.2). Other groups studied were those who had no mental illness, and those with other psychiatric diagnoses. The group in which almost no obstetrical complications were reported were those diagnosed as schizotypal personality disorders in 1972 to 1974. Again, these findings were interpreted as supporting the diathesis-stress model for schizophrenia.

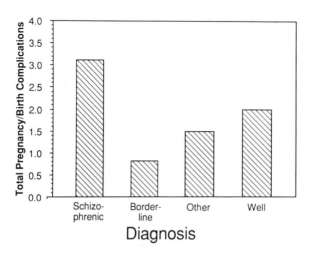

FIGURE 6.2. Pregnancy and birth complications in high-risk group. Reprinted with permission from Parnas et al.[14]

Brain Morphology and Schizophrenia: Ventricular Size

In a small substudy done in 1980 assessing ventricular size in the children of schizophrenic mothers, we selected a small subgroup instead of using the whole sample.[16] We sampled from among those who lived not too far from our institute, which is located in central Copenhagen. Thus, our sample was not especially psychopathologically selective. However, those who became schizophrenic had the largest ventricle-to-brain ratio, and those who were found schizotypal exhibited the smallest ventricle-to-brain ratio. The same distribution occurs as is seen (Fig 6.2) for the obstetrical complications when they are distributed over the diagnostic outcomes. Also, the ventricle-to-brain ratio is statistically significantly correlated with a score of obstetrical complications. Although it is not a very large correlation, it nevertheless is significant, and it offers possibilities for additional explanations.

What can we conclude from this small subset of results? Those with schizophrenia have been most damaged obstetrically, and they also have the highest degree of cerebral atrophy. From other studies derived from the American–Danish Adoption Studies we know that schizotypal personality disorder and schizophrenia occur in the same biological families. Before we did the CT scan study, the assumption was that perhaps schizotypal personality disorder is closer to the genotype than schizophrenia itself. It is possible that schizophrenia is a neurologically complicated form of schizotypal personality disorder. Based on this assumption, we have found two factors as giving a poor prognosis for those who have a genetic liability for schizophrenia: the obstetrical factors and the early institutional rearing factors. To have a genetic liability is of course the same as having an increased risk. If the individual in addition suffers from obstetrical complications or institutional rearing, his risk increases. There is a great need to replicate some of these findings, for instance, the schizotypal–schizophrenia dichotomy in relation to cerebral ventricular size, and so on. Eventually, the at-risk individuals might be selected to be targeted for attempts at offering individual prevention to the pregnant women. That might be a small step toward the goal of preventing some cases of schizophrenia.

Interaction Between High Risk and Stress: Prospective Study Design

In our study of persons at high risk, and a comparison low-risk group, it appears that if the low-risk group is exposed to stressors, it does not change their level of psychopathology considerably. But if they belong to the group at risk, for instance genetically at risk, then stressors are found to interact, with the result of an increased level of psychopathology. By using this paradigm of design for research, it is possible to examine different degrees of the same type of stress on one level of genetic risk, or the effect of one kind or degree of stress can be examined in different levels of genetic risks. This prospective study design, which I recommend, has had a very good potential. It has also kept several of us busy for 25 years.

Some other observations have grown out of this research. For instance, obstetrical complications cannot explain everything about schizophrenia; it is not the only contributing factor and it is not the only reason for ventricular enlargement. There have been numerous theories about viral infections as contributing factors. The coinvestigator, Mednick, has just completed a study in Helsinki where there was a neurotoxic A2 influenza epidemic in 1957.[20] This world-wide epidemic was very virulent in Helsinki. Mednick subsequently examined the offspring of infected pregnant mothers. He and Finnish co-workers went through mental hospital records in Helsinki and surroundings to determine the number of schizophrenics whose mothers were pregnant during the influenza epidemic. As a control group he used the offspring of mothers from the 5 preceding years when there had been no neurotoxic influenza epidemic in Finland. The researchers found that when the offspring had an excess of schizophrenia, the whole excess came from those whose mothers were in the second trimester of pregnancy during the peak epidemic period. These results are statistically strong. They offer support also for the viral etiology theory proposed by Timothy Crow along with other British investigators,[21] and for the second trimester as the crucial period of pregnancy.[20] There is a whole group of researchers who think that the second trimester is a critical period for brain development, which may have importance for the vulnerability to schizophrenia. We now intend to collect fetal brains from the second trimester to subject them to neuropathological and histochemical studies.

High Risk Research and Development of Classical Schizophrenia Concept

The last part of this discussion considers the Kraepelinian–Bleulerian concept of schizophrenia,[22–24] which more or less has been the joint heritage of many European psychiatrists. We will examine if it stands up to our present knowledge and, in particular, what we have learned about this old concept of schizophrenia from our risk studies and some related research.

Diagnosis and Changing Criteria

The first question to examine is that of schizophrenia diagnosis *vs* changing criteria for the disorder over time. What did we learn from our studies? In 1962 we had the opportunity to select 129 severely schizophrenic mothers of the 207 children who were our index children. They were selected through a review of their hospital records. The selection was done before the DSM-II, in the era of DSM-I, which was absolutely unknown in Denmark. It was also before we had the ICD, and we used some prototypical descriptions of diseases from a diagnostic list issued by the Danish Psychiatric Society. More recently, a co-worker reexamined all of these mothers' records for various purposes, and also assigned them DSM-III-R diagnoses. Of these 129 mothers, all but 11 met the DSM-III-R diagnostic criteria for schizophrenia. The remaining 11 met the criteria for disorders such as schizophreniform psychosis and delusional disorder. The old Bleulerian schizophrenia concept,[24] in which we had been trained and which was used in Denmark, seems to have held up on the whole.

Unitary Psychosis

Another question, which is a little more provocative, is that of unitary psychosis. Unitary psychosis means that it is doubtful whether there is a dichotomy between manic-depressive psychosis and schizophrenia.[25-27] Thus, Kraepelin's distinction is considered as spurious. This issue comes up periodically. Possibly it is due to nosological frustration or to unsophisticated use of advanced statistics on poor data. Also, in the emotional search for justification of polygenetic theories of the mode of transmission of schizophrenia some may feel tempted to regress to the unitary psychosis concept. The idea of unitary psychosis is understandable in light of our former lack of diagnostic sophistication. Also, it is a well-established fact that depression is prevalent over long periods in the life of many schizophrenic patients. There are many explanations for the unitary psychosis concept. However, in our project we have not found affectively ill offspring among the children of severely schizophrenic mothers, not even in the two families where the fathers suffered from bipolar affective illness. This makes us somewhat doubtful about the unitary psychosis concept.

Heterogeneity

The third question is the question of heterogeneity. This phenomenon concerns the question of whether schizophrenia is one nosological entity or is actually a set of different disorders. The discussion goes back to the title of Bleuler's famous book from 1911 titled *Dementia Praecox or the Group of Schizophrenias*.[24] If you look closely at his classic monograph and at the book of his contemporary (Karl Jasper)[28] on general psychopathology, it is quite obvious that they conceived of schizophrenia as one entity, but with different constellations of the fundamental and auxillary symptoms. No evidence confirms the existence of phenocopies of schizophrenia. Researchers who have studied epileptic psychosis, amphetamine psychosis, and other organic schizophrenic-like psychosis, do not find those conditions as being real or certain phenocopies; there are too many differences. A lot of modern twin studies, such as those of Gottesman and Shields[29] and the American–Danish Adoption Data,[8-10] show that various manifestations of schizophrenia occur in the same families. In our high risk study we learned that many schizotypals had certain premorbid behavior features, but had no pregnancy and birth complications, and had small cerebral ventricles. The actual schizophrenics had many birth complications and large cerebral ventricles.

We believe that schizophrenia is a nosological entity, which can manifest itself due to various stressors or experiential factors. This also pertains to the dichotomy between negative-symptom schizophrenia and positive-symptom schizophrenia. Some psychiatrists hold the view that negative-symptom schizophrenia is a schizophrenia represented by patients with no remissions, poor response to neuroleptic drugs, and poor prognosis. The intriguing fact is that these are the same patients who are characterized by having many Schneiderian first-rank symptoms. All Schneiderian first-rank symptoms are positive schizophrenia symptoms, so what is described is a confused picture which makes us doubt the validity of the positive–negative concept.

Many old time schizophrenia researchers described the peculiarities, the oddness, the eccentricity, the smell, and many other nonunderstandable features in schizophrenic patients. The lack of understanding is not based on the impossibility of perceiving the patient's feelings and thoughts, but on the impossibility of attunement with these thoughts and feelings. There are examples of the attempts to clarify the Bleulerian postulate of what he called "peculiar stamp only observable in schizophrenic conditions." Many investigators interpret these findings as a reflection of a lack of congruence among several relatively intact mental functions. Stransky[30] called it "intrapsychic ataxia," and there are other people who used terminology based on this concept. Numerous authors ascribe the formation of primary delusions, this Schneiderian first-rank symptom, which is an auxilliary symptom in the Bleulerian scheme, to disturbances in elementary cognitive-affective processes of the integration of mental activities.

It is currently of paramount importance to address the issue of which symptoms most adequately demarcate a schizotype, because schizotypal disorders may constitute a relatively environmentally uncontaminated expression of the schizophrenic genotype. This issue was repeatedly raised in the literature by Meehl[31] in the early 60s, and later by Shields and co-workers.[32] In one study, John Gunderson[33] used data from the Danish adoption sample which adequately deals with this question. This study showed that social isolation and anxiety, emotional detachment, suspiciousness, eccentricity, and odd communication are all characteristic of genetically defined schizotypes. Similar results emerge from other studies, including a Norwegian twin study[34] where social isolation, suspiciousness, eccentricity, peculiar communication, and social dysfunction characterized the schizotypes. In our own study, as I showed, we examined behavioral precursors of schizophrenia and schizotypal personality disorders and found that there was little difference in the premorbid characteristics of the two groups. There were more commonalities than uncommonalities from a psychopathological view.[15]

In general, there emerges an agreement that the so-called negative symptoms best characterized a schizotype rather than sub-psychotic phenomena, such as perceptual distortions. Researchers are sometimes at pain with respect to the stages of formal thought disorder. We believe that common deemphasis of the uniqueness of formal thought disorder is partly due to a failure to distinguish formal aspects of disordered thinking from the disorder of thought content (ie, delusions and disorders of perception, hallucinations). We are liable to consider formal thought disorder as a trait common both for schizophrenia and for schizotype. It has been shown predictive of subsequent schizophrenia and schizotype, exhibiting continuity from childhood to adulthood. It also has been shown to be a good indicator of a genetically defined schizotype, it seems specific for schizophrenic psychosis and tends to persist during neuroleptic-induced remissions of schizophrenia.

We hope this discussion has illustrated the longitudinal prospective study of persons at risk for schizophrenia and the potential powerfulness of this method. Also in the context of such studies, it may be fruitful to reconsider the old prophets.

Summary

From a historical standpoint, the interaction between hereditary and environmental factors in the pathogenesis of diseases has been studied only rarely in psychiatry before the 1960s. During the 1960s, the role of genetics in psychiatric disorders developed strongly due to methodological sophistication of study design as well as improved psychopathological systematization.

A special type of research design, the longitudinal prospective study of individuals at high risk, is a powerful methodology with regard to disentangling the environmental and genetic factors that contribute to mental illness. In a longitudinal prospective study begun in Denmark, The 1962 Copenhagen High Risk Study, 207 school children having schizophrenic mothers were followed along with 104 control children. In 1967, there was a 5-year follow-up, and a 10-year follow-up was completed between 1972 and 1974. A subsample was followed up in 1980, and a diagnostic study of the fathers was carried out between 1980 and 1983.

The premorbid behavioral precursors of the schizophrenia spectrum in early childhood were noted to be passivity and short attention span.

School behavior included isolation and poor affect control. Clinical assessments showed subtle, formal thought disorder and defective emotional rapport premorbidly. Also, the specific interaction between genetic liability on one hand, and perinatal complications or institutional rearing on the other, have been shown to be important. These latter factors may even be considered as possible targets for preventive intervention. Those who developed schizophrenia at follow-up had a high rate of institutionalization early in life and a high rate of pregnancy and birth complications. Furthermore, schizophrenic patients showed the highest ventricle-to-brain ratio.

With an increased level of stress, psychopathology increased in the high-risk group, but hardly so in the low-risk group. Viral infections are suspected as a possible contributing factor toward schizophrenia. An excess of schizophrenia occurred in individuals whose mothers were pregnant during the 1957 viral influenza epidemic, particularly in mothers with influenza in the second trimester of pregnancy.

The development of the classical schizophrenia concept of Kraepelin and Bleuler is examined in light of the results of high risk research and other contemporary studies. The stability of diagnostic criteria over time has implications for long-term prospective studies. In 1962, which was pre-DSM-II, 129 mothers were diagnosed as being severely schizophrenic using a chart review. When these charts were re-reviewed using DSM-III-R criteria, 118 of this group of 129 still met the new criteria.

Phenomena, such as the unitary psychosis, heterogeneity, and the positive–negative symptom schizophrenia dichotomy, are discussed. The concept of unitary psychosis negates a real dichotomy between affective and schizophrenic psychoses. However, the unitary psychosis concept is severely questioned, based on results of a study of children with bipolar as well as schizophrenic parents.

The validity of the concept of negative and positive symptoms for schizophrenia is also questioned. From a genetic viewpoint, schizotypal disorders may represent the environmentally uncontaminated expression of the schizophrenic genotype. This includes the social isolation and anxiety, suspicion, and peculiar communication which are similar to the negative symptoms of schizophrenia. Thus, schizotypal disorders represent disorder in the form of thought, and schizophrenic disorders represent disorder in the content of thought, characterized by hallucinations or delusions. These phenomena, however, are present in many conditions other than schizophrenia.

References

1. Gottesman II, Shields J: *Schizophrenia and Genetics: a Twin Study Vantage Point.* New York, Academic Press, 1972.
2. Gottesman II, Shields J: Rejoinder: toward optimal arousal and away from original din. *Schiz Bull* 1976;2:447–453.

3. Lidz T, Fleck S, Cornelison A: *Schizophrenia and the Family*. New York, International University Press, 1965.
4. Schulsinger F, Parnas J, Schulsinger H, et al: Recent trends from nature–nurture research in schizophrenia, in Stefanis CN, Rabavilas AD (eds): *Schizophrenia: Recent Biosocial Developments*. New York, Human Sciences Press, Inc., 1988.
5. Schulz B: Zur Erbpathologic der Schizophrenen. *Zeitschr ges Neurol und Psychiatr* 1932;143:175–293.
6. Bleuler M: Das Wesen der Schizophrenie nach Schockbehandlung. *Zeitschr ges Neurol und Psychiatr* 1941;173:553–597.
7. Pollin W, Stabenau JR: Biological, psychological, and historical differences in a series of monozygotic twins discordant for schizophrenia. *J Psychiat Res* 1968;6(suppl)(1):317–332.
8. Kety SS, Rosenthal D, Wender PH, et al: The types and prevalence of mental illness in the biological and adoptive families of adopted schizophrenics, in Rosenthan D, Kety SS (eds): *The Transmission of Schizophrenia*. Oxford, Pergamon, 1968, pp 345–362.
9. Kety SS, Rosenthal D, Wender PH, et al: Mental illness in the biological and adoptive relatives of adopted individuals who became schizophrenic, in Fieve R, Rosenthal D, Brill H (eds): *Genetic Research in Psychiatry*. Baltimore, MD, Johns Hopkins University Press, 1975.
10. Rosenthal D, Wender PH, Kety SS, et al: Schizophrenics' offspring reared in adoptive homes, in Rosenthan D, Kety SS (eds): *The Transmission of Schizophrenia*. Oxford, Pergamon, 1968, pp 377–391.
11. Mednick SA, Schulsinger F: A longitudinal study of children with a high risk for schizophrenia: a preliminary report, in Vnderberg S, (ed): *Methods and Goals in Human Behavior Genetics*. New York, Academic Press, 1965.
12. Mednick SA, Schulsinger F: Studies of children at high risk for schizophrenia, in MSS Information Service (eds): *Schizophrenia: The First Ten Dean Award Lectures*. New York, MSS Information Service, 1973, pp 245–293.
13. Schulsinger H: A ten-year follow-up of children of schizophrenic mothers: clinical assessment. *Acta Psychiatr Scand* 1976;53:371.
14. Parnas J, Schulsinger F, Teasdale TW, et al: Perinatal complications and clinical outcome within the schizophrenia spectrum. *Br J Psychiatry* 1982;140:416–420.
15. Parnas J, Schulsinger F, Schulsinger H, et al: Behavioral precursors of schizophrenia spectrum. *Arch Gen Psychiatry* 1982;39:658–664.
16. Schulsinger F, Parnas J, Petersen ET, et al: Cerebral ventricular size in the offspring of schizophrenic mothers: a preliminary study. *Arch Gen Psychiatry* 1984;41:602–606.
17. Parnas J, Teasdale TW, Schulsinger H: Institutional rearing and diagnostic outcome in children of schizophrenic mothers. *Arch Gen Psychiatry* 1985;42:762–769.
18. Parnas J: Mates of schizophrenic mothers: a study of associative reacting from the American–Danish High Risk Project. *Br J Psychiatry* 1985;140:490–497.
19. Rutter M: *Maternal Deprivation Reassessed*. Hammondworths, Penguin Books Ltd., 1981.
20. Mednick SA, Machon RA, Huttunen MO, et al: Adult schizophrenia following prenatal exposure to an influenza epidemic. *Arch Gen Psychiatry* 1988;45:189–192.

21. Crow TJ: A re-evaluation of the viral hypothesis: is psychosis the result of retroviral integration at a site close to the cerebral dominance gene? *Br J Psychiatry* 1984;145:243–253.
22. Kraepelin E: *Psychiatrie,* ed 4. Leipzig, JA Barth, 1896.
23. Kraepelin E: *Psychiatrie,* ed 8. Leipzig, JA Barth, 1915.
24. Bleuler E: *Dementia Praecox or the Group of Schizophrenias.* New York, International University Press, 1911/1950.
25. Crow TJ: The continuum of psychosis and its implications for the structure of the gene. *Br J Psychiatry* 1986;149:419–429.
26. Claridge GS: The schizophrenia as nervous types revisited. *Br J Psychiatry* 1987;151:735–743.
27. *Lancet:* A continuum of psychosis? 1987;October:889–890.
28. Jaspers K: *General Psychopathology.* Chicago, University of Chicago Press, 1963.
29. Gottesman II, Shields J: *Schizophrenia and Genetics: A Twin Study Vantage Point.* New York, Academic Press, 1972.
30. Stransky E: Zur Kenntnis gewisser ervorbener Bloedsinnsformen. *Neurologisches Zentralblatt* 1903;24:1–149.
31. Meehl PE: Schizotaxia, schizotypy, schizophrenia. *Am Psychol* 1962;17:827–838.
32. Shields J, Heston LL, Gottesman II: Schizophrenia and the schizoid: the problem for genetic analysis, in Fieve RR, Rosenthal D, Brill H (eds): *Genetic Research in Psychiatry.* Baltimore, Johns Hopkins University Press, 1975, pp 167–198.
33. Gunderson JG, Siever LJ, Spaulding E: The search for a schizotype. *Arch Gen Psychiatry* 1983;40:15–22.
34. Torgersen S: Relationship of schizotypal personality disorder to schizophrenia: Genetics. *Schizophr Bull* 1985;11:554–563.

7
The Role of Molecular Genetics in Psychiatry: Unraveling the Etiology for Schizophrenia

Lynn E. DeLisi and Michael Lovett

This chapter reviews the evidence for a genetic basis to schizophrenia. It also discusses attempts that have been made to discover some biological correlate that might be used as a marker for the disease, from the peripheral biochemical measurements to the protein and chromosomal marker studies, and finally the more recent application of systematic molecular genetic techniques to the study of this problem. This latter approach, which is the first step in what is now called "reverse genetics," promises to yield great insights into the genetics, etiology, pathogenesis, and diagnostic boundaries of this disease.

Evidence for a Genetic Cause for Psychosis

Kraepelin in his textbook of psychiatry[1] upon discussing the etiology of dementia praecox wrote that ". . . defective heredity is a very prominent factor . . . and appears in about 70% of cases. . . ." This, of course, was a conclusion drawn from his personal clinical experience, and not a systematic survey of families. Since his time and the beginnings of attempts to characterize schizophrenia, several family, twin, and adoption studies have clearly established a genetic influence on the development of schizophrenia in a significant portion of cases (reviewed by Gottesman and Shields[2]).

Family studies on schizophrenia can be divided into the older European (pre-DSM-III era) studies and the few American surveys published after 1980. Gottesman and Shields,[2] in a summary of the pooled European family data, estimated the risk for schizophrenia in relatives of schizophrenic probands to be 10.1% in siblings, 5.6% in parents, and 12.8% in children. The risk to second-degree relatives varies from 2.4 to 4.2% and to third-degree relatives is approximately 2.4%. The risks are generally equal for males and females, although pairs of first-degree relatives with psychosis are more likely to be the same than opposite sex,[3] and in parent–child pairs, it is more likely that the mother will be affected than the father.[2] All the above risks are significantly higher than would be expected in the unrelated general population (.1 to 1%), although these studies have generally not surveyed a specific control group for comparison. The more recent American studies are separately notable for their more structured diagnostic design and use of carefully examined controls. Taken together these also define a significant excess of schizophrenia in first degree relatives of schizophrenic probands using DSM-III criteria, ranging to approximately 8%.[4–7]

There are approximately 12 major studies of schizophrenic twin pairs comparing monozygotic (MZ) with same-sex dizygotic (DZ) concordance rates. Although the rates vary from study to study, it is clear that significantly higher concordance rates are found among monozygotic compared with dizygotic twins in all studies. Proponents of environmental causes for psychoses, however, emphasize that in no study does the monozygotic concordance rate reach 100%.[2] Nevertheless, using twin concordance rates or family study data, several investigators have calculated the heritability, or extent to which the variance in liability for schizophrenia is due to genetic factors, to be between 60 and 70%.[8–13] To distinguish the relative importance of the genetic *vs* environmental component to the development of schizophrenia, Rosenthal and Kety and their colleagues[14,15] embarked on a landmark series of studies that strongly suggest that children removed from biological parents at birth are still significantly at greater risk for schizophrenia if there is schizophrenia among their biological relatives, but not their adoptive relatives. A more recent adoption study completed in Finland has independently confirmed this finding.[16]

Another piece of evidence against an environmental cause for at least the onset of psychosis comes from a series of studies examining the age of onset of illness in pairs of siblings, both of whom were diagnosed as schizophrenic. In a recent review of this literature, Crow and Done[17] combined all studied pairs and calculated whether or not onset of illness in one member of a pair influenced the time of onset of illness in the second member. They found, however, that age of onset among siblings was significantly correlated, whereas the actual time of onset was not, suggesting a prenatal determination, possibly genetic, on the timing of onset of illness within families with no significant effect of a postnatal "contagious" environmental factor.

Finally, although rarer than the family prevalence statistics may suggest, families are occasionally found with clusters of members with schizophrenia spanning multiple generations. Given that the illness is only present in less than 1% of the general population, it is unlikely that this could happen by chance, and implies that genetic transmission must be occurring in some proportion of cases.

The Mode of Inheritance

Despite numerous clinical studies based on large populations, a specific pattern of inheritance has not as yet been established and the literature in this area remains inconsistent. Using morbid risk figures, or segregation analysis, several mechanisms have been proposed, but none definitively determined. These include a single major locus, a large number of genes, each with small additive effects (polygenic), or a combination of a number of underlying genetic and environmental liability factors such that if a person reaches a quantitative threshold of these factors, he develops schizophrenia. Single locus and polygenic inheritance can be differentiated on the basis that they predict different patterns of inheritance in relatives of patients and can be modeled mathematically. Rao and colleagues,[10] using morbid risk figures from an aggregate of family data from European studies, showed that a multifactorial threshold model could most adequately explain transmission. Other studies using segregation analysis, which take into account pedigree structure, however, are contradictory. Some provide evidence for dominant single major locus transmission, others are consistent with polygenes,[9] and, in one, the investigators conclude that a pure polygenic model could not be distinguished from a model including a major recessive locus and polygenic component.[13] Taken together these analyses appear to suggest a mode of transmission consistent with polygenes; however, most do not rule out that a single major locus could be responsible for schizophrenia in at least some families.

All these models have been limited in their power to identify a mode of transmission for several reasons: (1) Many of the family studies on which analyses are based have relied on family history diagnoses that may not meet present-day criteria for the disorder and also have not had the sensitivity to include the broader spectrum disorders. In fact, the extent of the clinical boundaries that define the genetic factor or factors are unknown.[18] There may actually be considerable genetic overlap between schizophrenia and affective disorder,[4,7] a previously dismissed finding. (2) The analyses to date have not considered the role played by unknown environmental variables in the expression of the disorder, and they do not deal adequately with incomplete gene penetrance. Simulation studies have shown that a single major locus is often not detectable by segregation analysis when the heterozygote penetrance is low (5 to 20%) or when there are substantial numbers of nongenetic phenocopies in the population. However, under these conditions, a major locus can be detected if there is a closely linked marker locus.[19,20] (3) Perhaps most important, the above inconsistencies may have resulted from considering schizophrenia as a single etiologic entity. It is possible that significant subgroups may emerge with different, but clear patterns of inheritance, and that in at least these subgroups, schizophrenia may be caused by one or more major genetic loci.

Given the above limitations in our research designs and the fact that no biological factor has been found to be abnormal in schizophrenic patients and to segregate with the illness within high-density families (reviewed in references 21 and 22) it is not surprising that, at present, there are no obvious clues for determining what is inherited and which gene is the most likely one to pursue. Nevertheless, as will be seen below, some potential candidate genes have been described that might have some (frequently rather tenuous) biological correlation with the schizophrenic phenotype.

Biological Marker and Heritability Studies

During the past few decades numerous studies have been published comparing samples of unrelated schizophrenic patients with control groups quantifying different biochemical substances in urine, plasma, cerebrospinal fluid (CSF), and postmortem brain.[21,22] Interpretation of these studies has been complicated by the unclear influences of environmental variables even though some abnormalities have been consistently replicated in several independent populations.

The most extensively studied substance in schizophrenic patients, an enzyme of major importance in monoamine metabolism, is monoamine oxidase (MAO). The B form of the enzyme is easily assayed in platelets and thought to be representative of the B form in human brain. The hypothesis that abnormalities in MAO may be associated with schizophrenia is supported by the known major role of MAO in the metabolism of dopamine. Low MAO activity could explain elevated dopaminergic activity and would be consistent with the dopamine hypothesis of schizophrenia. Numerous studies of platelet MAO activity in the 1970s resulted in reports of reduced activity of this enzyme in populations of chronic schizophrenic patients, individuals with other major psychiatric disease, as well as miscellaneous other conditions (reviewed by DeLisi et al[23]). The level of MAO activity was found to be highly heritable and having a pattern of inheritance consistent with X linkage.[24] Two studies of monozygotic twins discordant for schizophrenia show lower platelet MAO activity in twins with one schizophrenic member than in control twin pairs, although the ill twins tend to have lower enzyme activity than their well twin pairs despite having identical genes.[25,26] This work, although interpreted as an indication of a genetic vulnerability toward decreased MAO activity in schizophrenia, also suggests an environmental effect on enzyme activity. Neuroleptics were subsequently found to lower platelet MAO activity to the degree seen in populations of schizophrenic patients,[27,28] and thus interest was lost in the use of this measurement as a biological marker of illness.

Examples also exist of other enzymes crucial to monoamine metabolism that have been examined in tissue studies, but for which significant differences have generally not emerged. These enzymes include dopamine beta-hydroxylase and catechol-O-methyl transferase, both of which also have been found to have highly heritable measurable peripheral activity.[29,30] Although peripheral enzymes themselves may no longer be valid markers for studying brain metabolism, newer approaches, focusing directly on the structural genes for these enzymes, may be warranted.

The metabolites of monoamine neurotransmitters (dopamine, norepinephrine, and serotonin) have been studied in the CSF by Sedvall and colleagues[31,32] using the family history dichotomy for detection of inheritance of differences in the metabolism of these transmitters as markers for illness. Patients with positive family history were found to have higher CSF 5-HIAA and HVA than patients with negative family history, indicating increased turnover of both dopamine and serotonin in the familial subgroup of patients. Normal individuals with a family history of psychosis also tend to have higher CSF 5-HIAA and HVA then those with negative family histories, although the numbers of individuals in these studies are small. The same investigators also examined the heritability of these markers using MZ and DZ comparisons.[33] Although a familial influence was found for both HVA and 5-HIAA, cultural heritability (familial environment) appeared larger than the genetic effect. Further studies to determine whether altered catechol or indolamine metabolism is related to the genetics of schizophrenia, and thus whether these can be useful as biological markers of illness, have not been done.

An increased amount of functionally available dopamine receptors also may be another important marker of psychosis. Previous evidence from postmortem studies finding significantly increased D-2 dopamine receptors in the striatum of schizophrenic patients has been controversial due to the unclear influence of neuroleptic treatment.[34] The more recent in vivo positron-emission tomography (PET) spiperone binding studies, unfortunately, have only added to the controversy.[35,36] The peripheral lymphocyte spiperone binding results of Bondy and Ackenheil,[37] although confirming the postmortem studies and further demonstrating a familial aggregation of increased binding, have remained unreplicated, although several unpublished attempts have been made.

Another possibility is that subtle brain morphological abnormalities (often of inherited origin) can be an early marker of illness in some patients, although it has not yet been clearly shown that they proceed, rather than result, from the chronic deterioration characteristic of the illness. Despite the apparent demonstrated heritability of variations in brain ventricular size,[38,39] additional nongenetic factors also appear to contribute to the enlargement associated with schizophrenia.[39,40]

Whereas physiological traits appear the most removed from the basic defect, they also may serve as easily measurable markers of an illness if consistently present. The most interesting trait associated with schizophrenia is the presence of deviant smooth pursuit eye movements (SPEM), or "tracking" (the ability of the eye to follow a moving target). More than 60% of schizophrenics have been found to have abnormal SPEM in several studies.[41,42] This trait has also been shown to be heritable in twin and family studies and unaffected by neuroleptic medication.[43,44] The family studies of schizophrenic probands, however, do not show that abnormal SPEM segregates with schizophrenic illness, and schizophrenics with normal eye tracking are found to have well relatives with abnormal tracking. Nevertheless, abnormal SPEM has been found in excess among well first-degree relatives of schizophrenics. To provide an explanation for these findings, Matthysse and colleagues[45] have speculated that the gene (or genes) involved with genetic vulnerability for psychosis are expressed in variable ways; although some individuals with these genes may develop a psychosis, others may only have the presence of abnormal eye tracking. Perhaps the delineation of the mechanism for abnormal eye tracking will clarify the significance of these findings.

Genetic Marker Studies

Protein Polymorphisms as Genetic Markers

Before the advent of techniques to systematically derive genetic maps of human chromosomes using polymorphic deoxyribonucleic acid (DNA) probes, and to correlate the inheritance of these markers with the incidence of a specific disease, protein polymorphisms were the only direct genetic markers available. These primarily consisted of blood group and human leukocyte antigens (HLA) because of their highly variable expression. They were used to detect higher frequencies of specific variants occurring in association with a specific disorder ("association" studies), or to "mark" the inherited pattern to a specific gene and those portions of the same chromosome closely linked to it within families (linkage studies). Linkage of the HLA region on chromosome 6 to schizophrenia was reported by Turner in 1979,[46] but subsequently rejected in two other more recent independent studies that were, unlike the Turner study, based on systematic diagnoses of family members.[47,48] ABO blood types have been studied in schizophrenic populations, with no consistent deviations from normal control distributions noted.[49] Human leukocyte antigen typing of lymphocytes has also been extensively compared. Many studies finding significant associations have been reported, but no specific HLA type has consistently been associated with schizophrenia.[49,50] Other genetic marker loci have been reported to be associated with schizophrenia in single studies (e.g., Gc, Gm, Km, complement C4B, and C3), although they remain unconfirmed[49,51,–53].

Cytogenetic Abnormalities as Genetic Markers

Previous chromosomal studies of schizophrenic patients, although based on large populations, remain inconclusive. Most are extensive surveys of all psychiatric hospital patients and do not use systematically defined diagnostic criteria. In addition, in the majority of studies complete karyotypes of patients were not performed; rather, only the X chromosome number was assessed by examining buccal smears.

A summary of these data (Table 7.1) suggests that there is a modest excess of XXY males and XXX females among psychiatric hospital patients, although these aberrations in no way account for the vast majority of major psychiatric illness. Case reports also exist of schizophrenic-like symptoms in patients with known Klinefelter (XXY) and triple X syndromes;[70-72] no study to date, however, has reported the prevalence of psychosis in these patients. There also is no existing hypothesis which has been put forth to explain why the presence of an extra dose of genes on the X chromosome could lead to psychosis, particularly if inactivation of the extra X chromosomes occurs at the cellular level. Although the location of a psychosis gene could be deduced from these data to be within the pseudoautosomal region of the X chromosome, where inactivation does not take place, there are still no clues to the nature of the gene.

Another genetic condition linked to an X chromosome abnormality which has gained recent attention in psychiatry is the fragile site mapped to the X_{q27} region (end of the long arm). The presence of the fragile site is now known to be associated with approximately 30 to 50% of all X-linked mental retardation in males[73] and 4 to 5% of all mental retardation in males.[74,75] This form of mental retardation, named the Martin-Bell syndrome after its first describers[76] is clinically characterized by mild dysmorphic facial features (long narrow facies, large ears) and other physical anomalies, including macroorchidism and joint hyperextensibility. Fragile X males and females also have been reported to show autistic and psychotic symptoms. An excess of fragile X has also been reported among children diagnosed with autism.[77] Systematic family diagnostic studies[78,79] suggest that the female carriers of the fragile X site may have an increased prevalence of schizoaffective disorder and schizophrenia spectrum personality disorders.

Another possibility that has recently been proposed to account for apparently variable X linkage for psychoses and the frequent associations of X chromosome anomalies to schizophrenia is that the locus may be situated within the pseudoautosomal region[80-82] of the sex chromosomes. This is a region at the distal end of the short arms of the X and Y chromosomes with a gradient of completely autosomal-like recombinational events between both chromosomes at the distal end, to almost no crossing over at the proximal end, thus enabling defects on the X chromosome to be transmitted by the Y chromosome in a "pseudoautosomal" fashion

TABLE 7.1. XXY (Klinefelter's syndrome) and XXX in psychiatric hospital patients.

Study	# of male pts with XXY	# of female pts with XXX	Diagnosis
Cowie et al, 1960[54]	0/22	0/20	Schizophrenia
Tedeschi & Freeman, 1962[55]	3/248		Schizophrenia
Raphael & Shaw, 1963[56]	1/105	1/105	Schizophrenia
Nielsen & Fischer, 1965[57]	3/14 hypogonadal		Not schizophrenia
Asaka et al, 1967[58]		2/424	Schizophrenia
Judd & Brandkamp, 1967[59]	1/22	0/18	Schizophrenia
Anders et al, 1968[60]	6/529	1/445	Chronic psychosis
MacLean et al, 1968[61]	30/6000	7/6241	13 males = schizophrenia All females = schizophrenia
Kaplan, 1970[62]		4/1061	Schizophrenia
Vartanian & Gendelis, 1972[63]		9/2431	Schizophrenia
Dasgupta et al, 1973[64]	2/500		Schizophrenia
Tsuang, 1974*		2/614	Chronic psychosis
Trixler et al, 1976[65]	2/310		Not schizophrenia
Axelsson & Wahlstrom, 1984[66]	2/134		Paranoid psychosis
DeLisi et al, 1988[67]	0/46		RDC schizophrenia
Total	50/7930 (.63%)	36/11,359 (.32%)	

XXY = .09–.15% live male births[68,69]; XXX = .07–.11% live female births.[68,69]
* Tsuang MT: Sex chromatin anomaly in Chinese females: psychiatric characteristics of XXX. *Br. J Psychiatry* 1974;124:299–305.

or as partially X linked.[83-85] This is also the only region of the X chromosome that does not undergo the usual inactivation process that takes place in individuals with more than one X chromosome. Thus, in the case of Klinefelter (XXY) males and triple X (XXX) females, the pseudoautosomal region of the X chromosome specifically is functionally in excess and may explain the association of psychosis with these syndromes. Clinical information on the pattern of inheritance in pairs of schizophrenic siblings recently has been shown to be consistent with inheritance in the pseudoautosomal region.[82] Whereas several previous studies of sibling pairs showed significantly greater same-sex than opposite-sex concordance for schizophrenia,[86-90] a further analysis found that this same-sex concordance rate was specifically relevant when inheritance of illness was from the paternal, but not the maternal, side of the family.[82] This particular pattern could be specific to inheritance of a gene within the pseudoautosomal region, because when carried on the X chromosome from the father it must be transmitted only to daughters unless recombination occurs in meiosis. Similarly, when on the Y it will most likely be transmitted only to sons. In the case of maternal transmission, however, opposite-sex siblings with illness are just as likely as same sex, as mothers can transmit the same X equally to sons and daughters. Thus, polymorphic probes for this region (already available[83-85]) will enable the testing of this hypothesis.

Other miscellaneous chromosomal anomalies have been described in several isolated unconfirmed reports (Table 7.2). One study[66] describes an unusually high percentage of aberrations (approximately 30%) among patients with paranoid psychoses. These include long Y chromosomes, duplications in the heterochromatin regions of several chromosomes, inversion of a region on chromosome 9, and fragile sites on chromosome 17 and 9. Another report found an association between a fragile site on the long arm of chromosome 3 and schizophrenia,[91] and another fragile site on chromosome 19 was seen in schizophrenic members within one family.[92] Both trisomy 8[93] and trisomy of a portion (q11–q13) of the long arm of chromosome 5[94], as well as a balanced translocation of the distal long arm of 2,[95] also have been associated with schizophrenia. Thus, no consistent pattern of chromosomal abnormalities have emerged. Nevertheless, some investigators assume that these abnormalities may each be markers of regions of the genome to further investigate in the search for the putative psychosis gene. In the case of trisomy of part of the long arm of chromosome 5, this observation led to several molecular genetic linkage studies of this region, culminating most recently in the detection of apparent linkage between this region and schizophrenia in one set of pedigrees.[107] It is unclear at present whether this observation is of any functional relevance in the original trisomic pedigree, or whether the correlation is fortuitous in that family. The counterargument to pursuing obser-

TABLE 7.2. Other associations of chromosomal deviations with schizophrenia.

Study	Chromosomal aberration	Clinical descriptions
Reiss et al, 1986; 1988[78,79]	Fragile site X_{q27}	35 female obligate carriers of fragile X had increase in schizophrenia spectrum disorders
Bassett et al, 1988[94]	Translocation (5.1) (ql3.3q11.2;q32.3)	Case report of schizophrenia segregating with the unbalanced translocation in one family
Chodirker et al, 1987[92]	Fragile site 19_{p13}	4 brothers (2 with schizophrenia, 1 autism, and 1 mental retardation)
Rudduck & Franzen, 1983[91]	Fragile site 3_{p21}	2 siblings with schizophrenia
Genest et al, 1976[95]	Translocation (2;18) (q21;q23)	Father with schizophrenia and daughter with undiagnosed behavioral problems
Sperber, 1975[93]	Trisomy 8	1 case with schizophrenia

vations of cytogenetic abnormalities is that although it may be successful in some cases, it is unlikely to be productive; many diverse diseases have been correlated (through observations of chromosomal abnormalities) to specific chromosomal regions, that upon further investigation, have been discovered not to be the correct locations. Perhaps, however, these reports will at least initiate searches for a gene that, although only defective in rare cases of schizophrenia, is part of a common pathway underlying the pathogenesis of the disorder. Other genes influencing this pathway also may be found on other chromosomes.

DNA Polymorphisms as Genetic Markers

Using cloned DNA probes that reveal sequence polymorphisms, the human genome can now be scanned for disease markers. This methodology, reviewed in several publications,[96-98] enables large regions of DNA to be examined. Using multiple probes for loci on different chromosomes, it is possible to identify a specific region that is linked to a disease locus before identifying the defective gene itself. This recombinant DNA approach is based on the existence of DNA sequence variations in different individuals which can be detected because they may alter the recognition site of type II restriction endonucleases, which catalyze sequence-specific breaks in double-stranded DNA.

Deoxyribonucleic acid is generally prepared from whole blood or lymphocytes of individuals, and, commonly, the lymphocytes are transformed in culture with Epstein-Barr virus, which ensures continuous karyotypically normal growth of the cells. Thus, established lines can be stored and grown indefinitely to replenish supplies of DNA for multiple studies. The DNA is then isolated from these cells in a series of routine extraction procedures. The DNA is cut into fragments by restriction enzymes, and separated by gel electrophoresis. The fragments are then fixed by transfer to a nylon or nitrocellulose filter (Southern blot) and hybridized with a radiolabelled cloned DNA, which marks a specific locus. Autoradiograms of these fragments can then be visualized and scored for each individual (specific procedures are outlined in Maniatis et al[99]). It should be noted that this approach does not require a gene or a gene product as the probe, but rather depends on detecting a DNA sequence alteration that is sufficiently frequent in the population to have a high chance of being informative in any pedigree. Frequently, the probe used is an anonymous noncoding piece of genomic DNA, and it is the degree of cosegregation of the sequence alteration recognized by this probe and the disease gene that is subsequently measured (see below). These diverse patterns of restriction fragments are heritable and referred to as restriction fragment length polymorphisms (RFLPs).

Many inherited disorders already have been linked to specific genes using this methodology. Of particular interest to neuropsychiatry is the linkage of a locus on the distal short arm of chromosome 4 to Huntington's disease,[100] a linkage that has subsequently resulted in the development and availability of presymptomatic diagnostic markers for this disorder. A linkage of manic-depressive illness in a large Amish family to a region of chromosome 11 near the Harvey-Ras 1 (HRAS1), insulin, and tyrosine hydroxylase genes,[101] as well as in other pedigrees to the long arm of the X chromosome,[102] and finally the linkage of Alzheimer's disease to a linked marker on chromosome 21[103] are also of great interest.

Feder and colleagues[104] were the first to publish any RFLP examinations of psychiatric patients with their attempt to test the hypothesis that endogenous opiate production was abnormal in psychotic disorders. They failed to find any associations of RFLPs of the opiate precursor, the propiomelanocortin gene, with schizophrenia or bipolar illness. During the past few years other preliminary studies using some cell lines from patients with schizophrenia described in DeLisi et al[86] were similarly performed. These studies made use of identified polymorphisms for several other neuropeptides and related substances[105,106] (published and unpublished data). Groups of unrelated schizophrenic patients were compared with screened controls to look for rare polymorphisms that were more frequent among schizophrenics. No such associations were found when using cloned probes for neuropeptide Y, somatostatin, substance P, gastrin-releasing peptide, vasoactive intestinal polypeptide (VIP), insulin, HRAS1, tyrosine hydroxylase, and phenylalanine hydroxylase. Only a polymorphism in the adenosine deaminase gene was significantly more frequent in schizophrenics compared with controls (Chi square 4.09; $P <$ .05), but has yet to be examined in a larger population, probably because little clinical relevance seems apparent in this chance finding.

There has recently been a report by Sherrington and co-workers[107] of a linkage of schizophrenia in seven families from Iceland and the United Kingdom to a region on the proximal small arm of chromosome 5. However, in the same issue of *Nature,* there appeared a second independent study[108] failing to find a similar linkage in a large pedigree from a genetic isolate in northern Sweden. One possible conclusion that has been drawn from these observations is that genetic heterogeneity is present in familial schizophrenia. Thus, the significance of the reported chromosome 5 linkage will be unclear until further investigations of this region in other collections of pedigrees have been made. In this regard it is of interest that linkage studies have also been performed in four extended schizophrenia pedigrees from the United States (Detera-Wadleigh and colleagues, NIMH, as presented by Gershon[109]) using a probe for the glucocorticoid receptor mapped to the distal portion of the long arm of chromosome 5 and several polymorphic markers in the region more proximal reported to be associated with the translocation (resulting in partial trisomy) previously described in one family with schizophrenia.[94] These studies have thus far not resulted in a positive linkage of schizophrenia to this region,[109] and neither have several recent studies by other investigators. In addition, linkage to the short arm of chromosome 11 using HRAS-1 and insulin polymorphisms has been ruled out in the same families (Detera-Wadleigh et al, unpublished data). Most recently, a suggestion of possible linkage to an area of chromosome 2 in four families with schizophrenia was described using a DNA probe that detects a highly polymorphic locus mapped to a region of unknown function or clinical relevance (Cloninger et al, unpublished data). This is particularly interesting in view of the one report of an association of schizophrenia with a translocation from the same general area of chromosome 2.[95]

Thus, with the exception of the Huntington's disease finding, none of these several recent reports of neuropsychiatric disorders have been confirmed in a wide sample of families with the same illness. They remain isolated suggestions that have yet to be generalizable to other samples of families and thus considered as definitive locations for the gene. Several laboratories are therefore pursuing systematic searches for linked markers in various pedigrees using RFLP markers that cover the entire genome. Nevertheless, there are still several candidate regions of the genome that are worth pursuing in schizophrenia. These include the areas mentioned above and several others based on hypotheses generated about the pathogenesis of the disorder.

The "Candidate Gene" Approach

As has already been mentioned, little information exists on which particular metabolic pathway(s), physiological functions, or phenotypic parameters are involved in the susceptibility to schizophrenia. The candidate gene approach seeks to test linkage hypotheses based on the candidate gene encoding products that might have some (frequently quite tenuous) functional connection with the disease. Such substances may be related to brain metabolism or brain growth and development. Other candidate "regions" have already been mentioned, namely regions based on cytogenetic observations and the pseudoautosomal region of the X and Y chromosomes. Summarized below are potential candidate genes (also, see Table 7.3). Although in many cases there is really no compelling reason to favor one of these candidate genes over another, their investigation has the added possibility that such candidate genes may be located in close proximity to genes of similar tissue specificity and/or function. Thus, while the candidate gene itself might not be the mutant locus, it may lead to identification of a linked but distinct disease gene.

Enzymes

Both catecholamine and indolamine neurotransmitters and related substances have been found to be abnormally concentrated in blood, CSF, and brain in schizophrenia. These findings have been reviewed extensively elsewhere.[110,112] Metabolites of dopamine (eg, HVA) have been found to be increased. Studies of indoleamines in schizophrenia have suggested that circulating serotonin is increased in some schizophrenics, and that some endogenous indoleamine hallucinogenic substances (ie, bufotenine, dimethyltryptamine) may sometimes be present.[111,112] These findings could be explained by defects in enzymes catalyzing their synthesis or metabolism. These issues raised by past studies showing reduced peripheral measures of both monoamine oxidase and dopamine beta-hydroxylase in schizophrenic patients have not been resolved. Catechol-O-methyl transferase is another major enzyme involved in the metabolism of dopamine and norepinephrine, both neurotransmitters hypothesized to be in excess in some forms of schizophrenia. Tyrosine hydroxylase is the enzyme involved in the rate-limiting step in dopamine synthesis. In addition, phenylalanine hydroxylase, the enzyme deficient in patients with phenylketonuria, has been hypothesized to play a role in schizophrenia based on several studies of serum phenylalanine and phenylethylamine concentrations in patients with schizophrenia, particularly

TABLE 7.3. Proposed candidate genes and their locations, as established by the Human Gene Mapping Collaborative Workshops.*

Candidate factors	Chromosome location	Probe	Enzymes for known RFLPs
Enzymes			
Monoamine oxidase (MAO)	X		No
Catecholamine-O-methyl transferase (COMT)	22		No
Dopamine β-hydroxylase (DBH)	9		No
Tyrosine hydroxylase (TH)	11p15.5	HTH TY	PstI, EcoRI
Phenylalanine hydroxylase (PAH)	12p22–q24.2	PH72	MspI, SphI, HindIII, BglII, PvuII, XmnI, EcoRV
Neuropeptides			
CCK	3		No
VIP	6		No
NPY	7pter–q22	NPY	TaqI
Neurotensin			SacI
Somatostatin	3q28	HS7	EcoRI, BamHI
Receptors:			
Dopamine			
Serotonin			
Alpha-adrenergic			
Beta-2-adrenergic	5q31–q32	TF	BanI
Nerve growth factor receptor	17q22	E51	XmnI, HincII
Miscellaneous:			
Huntington's Dis. linked probe	4		
Probes on proximal portion of long arm (q11.2–q13)	5		Several
Nerve growth factor (beta)	1p22.1	NBC6	BglII HincII TaqI XbaI
Growth factors/oncogenes	several		
Fragile site	Xq27		several
Pseudoautosomal region	Xp telomeric	several	several

*Information obtained from Howard Hughes Medical Institute, The New Haven Gene Mapping Library, Chromosome Plots, Book 4, 1988.

of the paranoid type. The above hypotheses are reviewed in DeLisi and Wyatt.[113]

Both A and B forms of monoamine oxidase (MAO) have been mapped in humans to the proximal short arm of the X chromosome and recently cloned.[114,115] Tyrosine hydroxylase has been mapped to the distal short arm of chromosome 11, whereas phenylalanine hydroxylase has been similarly mapped to the short arm of chromosome 12, cloned and used in some of the first reported human RFLP studies.[116] Phenylketonuria (PKU), which has long been known to be due to a deficiency in phenylalanine hydroxylase activity, is now detectable prenatally using polymorphisms identified with probes for this gene.[117]

Neuropeptides

Several of the neuropeptides have been found to co-exist with catecholamines intraneuronally and have modulating effects on their activity.[118] Some [cholecystokinin (CCK), somatostatin (SOM)] also have been found to be in abnormal concentrations in regions of postmortem brain of schizophrenic patients.[119]

Receptors

Numerous studies (pharmacologic, physiologic, clinical, and postmortem, and most recently, in vivo positron emission tomography) have implicated abnormalities of dopamine receptors in schizophrenia.[120] Other receptors, such as the noradrenergic and the serotonergic receptor types may also be worth examination.

Growth Factors

It has been suggested that psychosis may be associated with abnormal regulation or production of a cellular growth factor that determines the asymmetries in human brain, as disturbances of normal brain laterality have been noted in schizophrenia.[121] For this reason, growth factors could also be considered as potential candidate genes.

Miscellaneous

Patients with Huntington's disease may, as part of their clinical spectrum of symptoms, exhibit psychotic symptoms sometimes misdiagnosed as schizophrenia, as well as major affective disorder. Although schizophrenia and Huntington's disease obviously do not result from the same mutation, it is still possible that they might be allelic or that their loci may be linked on the same chromosome.

Thus, at present, although there are several somewhat promising candidate genes to pursue, the relative lack of definitive knowledge about the nature of the gene, its location, and mode of inheritance suggest that a more systematic genomic search for linkage may be necessary. Using a large panel of evenly spaced highly polymorphic probes that span all chromosomes may prove more productive than preferentially pursuing the above candidate loci. The first step in this "reverse genetic" approach is the isolation of a linked genetic marker using RFLP analysis. The next step is the further refinement of the genetic map of the chromosomal subregion and the isolation of markers on both sides of the gene. These markers can usually be used as reasonably accurate diagnostic tools. The final stage in this scheme is the movement inwards to eventually isolate the specific coding sequences of the disease locus. However, there are several methodological problems in this approach to be aware of, and these are described below.

Methodologic Problems

I. Informativeness of Probe

Many DNA probes are not very informative because they vary little in the general population. The ideal marker should have a high level of heterozygosity among individuals within families to exhibit a high degree of informativeness for linkage analysis.

The most commonly used RFLP to date is one caused by the mutation of a single base pair so that a cleavage site for the restriction enzyme is destroyed or a new one is created. Such polymorphisms are detected by single-copy cloned DNAs and frequently occur at the highly mutable dinucleotide CpG. This is part of the recognition sequence of several restriction enzymes, such as MspI (CCGG) and TaqI (TCGA), which are frequently used to detect RFLPs. Most RFLPs result in the presence or absence of a cleavage site and are thus dimorphic (two alleles with a frequency of heterozygosity that can never exceed 50%, and is usually much less).

This type of genetic analysis would be greatly simplified if a series of marker loci with multiallelic variation and high heterozygosity were found distributed on many chromosomes. The first of such hypervariable regions was isolated by chance;[122] several others have subsequently been discovered. Deoxyribonucleic acid sequencing has revealed that the basis for the variation in restriction fragment lengths is variation within the fragment in the number of short tandem oligonucleotide repeats. These repeats, which are shorter than 50 base pairs, are known as "minisatellites," and the type of RFLP generated by them has been called a variable number of tandem repeat (VNTR) marker.

When DNA from an individual is digested with a restriction enzyme that cuts outside the repeats and is probed with a short oligonucleotide corresponding to the repeat "core" sequence, a very complex pattern of restriction fragments is detected. Specific oligonucleotide probes can recognize as many as 200 VNTR loci, and more than 10 alleles have been found at many of these loci. If this type of experiment is repeated with other oligonucleotide probes known to be contained within minisatellites, then more than 1,000 hypervariable loci in the human genome can be detected. The net effect of all this variability is that no two people share every minisatellite marker allele.

All the VNTR loci corresponding to a particular oligonucleotide repeat can be isolated as molecular clones and these provide a series of dispersed loci of high heterozygosity.[123] A cloned VNTR locus, when used at high hybridization stringencies, can be used to detect just its own homolog within various individuals. In this way, these repeated loci can be mapped and used as hypervariable RFLP markers that frequently yield linkage information with disease loci in a pedigree analysis.

II. Procedural Errors

Procedural errors can lead to totally erroneous conclusions. Rigorous "quality control" must be introduced when typing large numbers of samples with multiple probes. The most common errors are introduced by mislabelling of samples, because many serial steps are involved. Occasionally these can be detected through visualization of a pattern of DNA fragments that are totally inconsistent with other members of the particular pedigree. Of course, this latter problem could be the result of nonpaternity, which will be revealed when the sample preparation is repeated. It could also be the result of partial digestion (see below). However, in most cases mislabelling or poor data handling and storage are difficult to detect and can lead to misassignments of alleles and to incorrect exclusion of linkage.

Partial digestion products also can lead to incorrect typing. Incomplete digestion of a genomic DNA sample can lead to the visualization of a lower number of fragments than are actually present in a sample. In the case of a probe that recognizes two alleles, this can lead to assigning a homozygous designation to a sample that is in fact heterozygous. In cases where multiple fragments are detected by one probe, partial digestion can lead to great confusion in assigning alleles. Occasionally this problem can be detected as an inconsistent fragment pattern within a pedigree.

Cross-hybridization can occasionally be a problem. Some probes may, under certain hybridization conditions, cross-hybridize with regions of the genome other than the one that is being searched for linkage. With the usual two allele type of RFLP this is immediately obvious. With probes that detect multiple bands, probes from a different species, or probes that are members of multigene families, care must be taken in designing the stringency of hybridization to minimize this possibility. In dubious cases, a relatively simple method to determine whether or not only one chromosomal location is being detected is to conduct a control hybridization to a Southern blot of a pulsed field gel. As mentioned below, this type of gel system separates very large DNA fragments; detecting only one large fragment with a particular probe would indicate that only one chromosomal location is being detected.

Nevertheless, although care in adequate sample handling and vigilance for some of the most obvious pitfalls must be observed, the derivation of Southern blot data from genomic DNAs is fairly straightforward. Detecting a linked marker is only the first (and probably technically the easiest) step in the path to isolating a disease gene. However, it is time consuming and laborious.

New Approaches in the Laboratory

One type of technique currently under development that promises to greatly accelerate the speed with which linkage analysis can be conducted is "multiplexing" ordinary RFLP methodology (C. Cantor and C. Smith, personal communication). "Multiplexing" means designing methods to combine several serial steps into one, and then resolving the identity of the product at as near the final stage of analysis as possible. In DNA sequencing by multiplexing, one can mix different DNA samples and use specific probes to examine the sequence of one component of the mixture at a time.[124] In RFLP multiplexing, which has yet to be fully developed for human disease application, a single sample could be hybridized in solution to many probes at once. Restriction enzymatic digestion after the hybridization will detect the presence or absence of particular sites in the probes, and the resulting pattern of probe lengths can be analyzed by an automated DNA sequencer. Other strategies for multiplexing will also be possible with the application of multiple fluorescent dyes for probe labelling. These newer approaches still under development should accelerate the search for genetic vulnerability factors for all human diseases, particularly those (eg, schizophrenia) in which family material is fragmented and no clear candidate genes have been identified.

Another new approach that should add to the efficiency of the above searches is pulsed field gel electrophoresis (PFGE). A recently developed technique, PFGE allows the separation of very large (up to several million base pairs) DNA molecules. Such large fragments are generated by digesting specially prepared DNAs with rare cutting restriction enzymes. Most of these enzymes recognize sites that contain one or more CpG dinucleotides, sites that are very rare in human genomic DNA and which can in some cases delineate the ends of actively transcribed genes.[125] This method already has produced macrorestriction maps of several megabase regions of the human genome as well as a complete restriction map of *Escherichia coli*.[126–129] They are particularly valuable whenever the routinely used DNA marker probes show evidence of possible linkage. The probe can then be used to make a restriction map of the surrounding region. The map may quickly identify any major DNA rearrangements in the region which could eventually be found to actually represent specific disease alleles.

In addition, it is here that cytogenetic abnormalities have a potentially valuable role in the localization of the disease gene. Translocations, deletions, insertions, and inversions will all result in alterations to a long-range restriction map. They can provide valuable "anchors" on which to base the map and may represent the exact location of the mutant locus. The availability of such physical markers can greatly simplify the interpretation and time course of this type of analysis.

It is also possible to use large DNA methods for direct linkage analysis. Some moderately repetitive DNA probes show extreme degrees of polymorphism, reminiscent of that of the hypervariable minisatellites, using large DNA techniques. However, the size scale of PFGE means that one can analyze 10 megabases of DNA, or more, in a single gel lane by using such a probe to detect 10 to 20 fragments at once. Although such a repetitive probe makes identifying the exact genomic region of linkage more complicated, the power of screening such a large amount of DNA at once has obvious advantages (C. Cantor and C. Smith, personal communication).

Another strategy would be to use the specific techniques of genomic DNA sequencing[130] or Polymerase Chain Reaction (PRC) amplification,[131] plus sequencing,[132] on the DNA from schizophrenic families once linkage information is available on which chromosomal region to focus upon. This might possibly be derived by initially screening DNAs from both affected and unaffected individuals for conserved RFLPs. Such sequence alterations might reflect the presence of a specific mutation, and their sequence can be identified by these methods.

However, the proper interpretation of genetic linkage data and the movement from an apparent linkage to the immediate vicinity of the gene itself, require more extensive expertise than just Southern blotting. Before discussing some of the future possibilities in moving from linked marker to gene we shall first briefly describe the process of statistical linkage analysis by which a likelihood of linkage is calculated.

Statistical Analyses of Genetic Data

Loci that are situated close to each other on the same chromosome do not assort independently and are said to be linked. However, rearrangement of alleles between pairs of homologous chromosomes by crossing-over (recombination) occurs during meiosis, so that alleles at linked loci are not always transmitted together. The further apart two loci are situated, the more chances they have to recombine. When recombination occurs less than 50% of the time, the two loci are considered linked, and the distance is expressed as percentage recombination between them. Two different methods of linkage analysis can be used, the regular likelihood or Lod score method (developed by Morton[133] in 1956), and the affected sib-pair method developed by a number of investigators (reviewed in Goldin and Gershon[50]).

Methods of Linkage Analysis

Lod Score Method

With linkage analyses by the Lod score method, the detection of linkage is more powerful with a small number of large family pedigrees than a larger number of small families,[134] because the more relatives and generations of relatives available, the more likely that the exact alleles for parents can be established with certainty. In addition, for relatively uncommon diseases, it is likely that the illness is homogeneous within the same family pedigree, thus increasing its informativeness for linkage analysis, and bypassing the issue of illness heterogeneity.

With the Lod score method, one tests linkage by assuming the mode of transmission of each locus (ie, dominant or recessive) and all parameters (ie, degree of penetrance) are known. One then compares the probability of observing the pattern of segregation of the two loci in a family (given a specific pattern of inheritance) if there is linkage, to the probability of observing the pattern if there is no linkage as follows:
The Lod score of the probability of the odds for linkage versus nonlinkage is:

$$\log_{10} \frac{\text{Probability of observing a family configuration assuming linkage (eg, the recombination fraction is less than } \frac{1}{2})}{\text{Probability of observing a family configuration assuming no linkage (eg, the recombination fraction } = \frac{1}{2})}$$

The Lod score for a sample of families is obtained by adding the scores for separate families. A Lod score of 1.0 means that linkage is 10 times more likely than no linkage. A Lod score of 3.0 is the accepted cutoff for acceptance of the linkage hypothesis, and indicates that the odds of linkage to no linkage is 1,000:1. Computer programs, such as LIPED,[135] enable relatively easy calculation of these likelihood ratios using multiple parameters and multiple estimations of the frequency of recombination. However, when the questions of heterogeneity, penetrance, and problems in diagnostic boundaries are factored into these calculations, the complexity of the analysis demands considerable statistical talent. For data containing alleles for multiple closely linked genetic markers, "multipoint analysis" can then be used.[136] Although the Lod score method requires that the mode of inheritance for the schizophrenia susceptibility gene be specified, at least in the initial stages in the search for a gene, linkages are being tested assuming a few different models and parameters.

It is always possible that after a few years of systematically searching the genome, no clearly established linkage to schizophrenia will be found, that a few will be found not clearly defining any specific etiological subtypes, or even that more than one will be found linked to illness in the same families. New methods for mathematical analysis of linkage might then reveal the involvement of more than one gene locus for the causation of illness and distinguish between the alternative possibilities.

The presence of heterogeneity may also decrease the power of linkage detection. Whereas a sample of 5 to 10 families may not be enough to confirm linkage between a schizophrenia locus and a genetic marker, it may be sufficient to determine suggestive linkages that can stimulate independent testing in new samples. Gershon and Goldin[137] have estimated the number of families necessary to confirm linkage given varying degrees of heterogeneity with both major dominant and recessive loci. This number ranges from less than 10 to more than 50. Computer models for calculating linkage can also detect the statistical likelihood of heterogeneity, given specific data sets.[134] That is, with respect to a given marker, one assumes a mixture of two family types, a type that is linked and a type that is unlinked to the marker. It is then tested whether one can significantly discriminate between these two components.

Affected Sib-Pair Method

As the nature of the clinical syndrome corresponding to a particular gene defect is not certain, particularly for the clinical syndrome we call "schizophrenia," linkage studies that depend on the delineation of ill and well family members may use erroneous assumptions to calculate likelihood scores for linkage. With schizophrenia genetic studies it may be more reliable to concentrate on analyzing pairs of ill siblings with clearly defined symptoms of nuclear schizophrenia and not attempt to define the clinical boundaries of the illness. Linkage studies making use of ill sibling pairs are also particularly valuable because they do not depend on knowledge of the mode of inheritance, as does the Lod score method. In addition ill sib-pairs are valuable in determining the extent of generalization of a linkage result that has been observed in a smaller set of one or a few large families. Moreover, sib-pair analyses may be the only practical alternative for genetic studies of schizophrenia, because large families with multiple ill members are rarely available.

The sib-pair method is based on the assumption that if a marker locus is linked to a disease locus, then affected pairs of siblings will have the same phenotype at the marker locus more often than would be expected by chance (originally proposed by Penrose[138,139]). This technique has been applied extensively to detect linkage of disease to the HLA loci.[140,141] It is determined whether affected sib-pairs share two, one, or no parental haplotypes identical by descent (IBD). Having cell lines from at least one parent, while not necessary for analysis, is useful for establishing definite parental haplotypes. If there is no linkage, this distribution among pairs of siblings would be 1/4, 1/2, and 1/4, respectively. If linkage is present, then this distribution is skewed so that more than 25% of affected sib-pairs have identical haplotypes. Thus, linkage is tested by comparing observed vs expected IBD distributions. This method has been extended to make inferences about the mode of inheritance,[141] and also to account for families with more than two affected siblings.[142] The method, however, is most useful when the loci examined are highly polymorphic (ie, numerous alleles exist; thus, parental alleles are likely to be heterozygous and different from each other). When the number of alleles is reduced, the likelihood of two siblings sharing both alleles increases, and thus the ability of this technique to detect linkage is reduced.

It has been calculated that with a sample size of 20 affected sib-pairs, if schizophrenia is genetically homogeneous, linkage will be detected to a disease susceptibility gene with a population frequency of less than 45% if it is recessive, and a frequency of less than 5% if it is dominant.[143] Because schizophrenia may well be genetically heterogeneous, more pairs of siblings will be needed. Gershon and Goldin[137] have calculated the number of sib-pairs needed as a function of the degree of heterogeneity. With a gene locus that is linked to the illness in at least 50% of cases, approximately 40 pairs of siblings would be the minimum needed, assuming the marker loci are highly polymorphic.

The Reverse Genetic Approach Once Linkage is Established

The identification of a genetic linkage is only the first step in the process of isolating and characterizing the actual gene that causes a disease. The detection of linked markers that are on both sides of the disease locus is the first step in defining the exact location of the gene. Multipoint linkage analysis of several markers in the region is used for this purpose. Once flanking markers are identified, then a physical map of the region between these markers would be constructed by pulsed field gel electrophoresis, and on overlapping map of the entire region could then be produced. Assuming that a 2-cm region could be defined by genetic mapping, this would on average comprise about 2 million base pairs of DNA, which would have to be mapped and traversed to isolate the disease gene. Ideally, if the transcription units within this long-range physical map can be defined, particularly those expressed in brain, whole areas could then be eliminated as possible loci. At present the large DNA technologies that could be used in such an analysis include: "jumping libraries"[144,145] to move rapidly over large regions and to isolate closer markers for genetic analysis, yeast artificial chromosome cloning[146] to isolate an entire large fragment for further analysis, and "chromosome walking" to isolate overlapping clones of sequences within the region of interest. Molecular clones isolated in these ways could then be screened by hybridizing to "zoo blots" (southern blots of genomic DNAs from several species) to detect evolutionarily conserved sequences that might reflect functional genes. Interesting clones could then be hybridized to blots of brain mRNA from both normal and schizophrenic postmortem specimens in the search for the candidate gene.

It is during these later stages of trying to identify the exact gene that causes the disease that the absence of more defined information on the biology, biochemistry, and physiology of schizophrenia will hamper efforts. For example, if a defined sublocalized region of the brain were known to be the site of action of the mutant allele, then cDNA libraries from that specific region would be screened for candidate genes. Likewise, the absence of a defined in vitro assay for the defect means that definitively proving that a candidate gene is the real disease gene will be difficult. Nevertheless, several current technologies are available, and many are under development, that should allow the rapid identification of mutant alleles. Among these are strategies to use denaturing gradient gels to identify altered coding sequences, various schemes using the polymerase chain reaction,[131] and the use of genomic DNA sequencing[130,132] to identify regions that might be part of the disease locus.

Summary

A genetic vulnerability for major psychiatric illness, including schizophrenia, seems likely, although the details of the underlying mechanisms remain unknown. Evidence is derived from European and American family studies that show the risk for schizophrenia in relatives of affected probands to be significantly higher than in the general population. Because monozygotic concordance rates do not reach 100%, the issue of environmental factors has been raised. However, the importance of genetic factors is shown by the higher rates of schizophrenia in adopted children having biological relatives with schizophrenia. In sibling pairs diagnosed as schizophrenic, the similar age of onset suggests a genetically predetermined time of onset of illness rather than environmental contagion.

Several mechanisms for a mode of inheritance have been proposed but not definitively determined. These mechanisms include: single major locus, polygenic loci, and a combination of genetic and environmental factors. During the past few decades the role of various biochemical substances has been evaluated in a search for biological markers for schizophrenia, but not yet clearly established to be associated with the genetics of schizophrenia.

With the availability of new technology to examine the human genome, the search for putative genes has accelerated. In fact, a few suggestions of chromosomal regions for linkage have already emerged. These include regions of 5, 11 and X chromosomes. Many psychiatric researchers remain skeptical about this approach due to the knowledge that the majority of individuals with psychosis have no family history of a similar disorder. However, they are missing the essence of the reason to focus on molecular genetics in the quest for the cause of the disorder. It is the realization that the tools provided by molecular genetics can be used for the detection of specific causes of abnormal psychopathology, whether ultimately genetic or nongenetic, that makes this the single most promising area for future focus. Finding a gene that can cause psychosis, uncovering its biochemical characteristics, and charting its subsequent array of dysfunction and pathology, may lead to the elucidation of a clear generalizable model for the development of abnormal behavior.

Acknowledgments. The following individuals, as collaborators in our search for a "gene for schizophrenia" contributed substantially to the formation of this review of the field. The information contributed forms the basis of our multicenter collaborative project. They are: C. Cantor, F. Collins, T. Crow, K. Davies, J. Ott, C. Smith, and S. Weissman. One of us (LED) would also like to acknowledge Dr. E. Gershon, who taught her the importance of linkage analysis and study designs using multiplex families with schizophrenia, as well as guiding her entry into this field.

References

1. Kraepelin E: *Lehrbuich der Psychiatrie,* Diefendorf AR (trans). New York, MacMillan Company, 1907.
2. Gottesman II, Shields J: *Schizophrenia: The Epigenetic Puzzle.* New York, Cambridge University Press, 1982.
3. Rosenthal D: Familial concordance by sex with respect to schizophrenia. *Psychol Bull* 1962;59:401–421.
4. Tsuang MT, Winokur G, Crowe RR: Morbidity risks of schizophrenia and affective disorders among first-degree relatives of patients with schizophrenia, mania, depression, and surgical conditions. *Br J Psych* 1980;137:497–504.
5. Guze SB, Cloninger CR, Martin RL, et al: A follow-up and family study of schizophrenia. *Arch Gen Psychiatry* 1983;40:1273–1276.
6. Baron M, Gruen R, Rainer JD, et al: A family study of schizophrenia and normal control probands: implications for the spectrum concept of schizophrenia. *Am J Psychiatry* 1985;142:447–454.
7. Gershon ES, DeLisi LE, Maxwell ME, et al: A controlled family study of psychosis. *Arch Gen Psychiatry* 1988;45:328–337.
8. Kendler KS: Overview: a current perspective on twin studies of schizophrenia. *Am J Psychiatry* 1983;140:1413–1425.
9. Carter CL, Chung CS: Segregation analysis of schizophrenia under a mixed genetic model. *Human Heredity* 1980;30:350–356.
10. Rao DC, Morton NE, Gottesman II, et al: Path analysis of quantitative data on pairs of relatives: application to schizophrenia. *Human Heredity* 1981;31:325–333.
11. McGue M, Gottesman II, Rao DC: The transmission of schizophrenia under a multifactorial threshold model. *Am J Human Genetics* 1983;35:1161–1178.
12. McGue M, Gottesman II, Rao, DC: Resolving genetic models for the transmission of schizophrenia. *Genetic Epidemiol* 1985;2:99–110.
13. Risch N, Baron M: Segregation analysis of schizophrenia and related disorders. *Am J Human Genetics* 1984;36:1039–1059.
14. Rosenthal D, Wender PH, Kety SS, et al: The adopted away offspring of schizophrenics. *Am J Psychiatry* 1971;128:397–411.
15. Kety SS, Rosenthal D, Wender PH, et al: Mental illness in the biologic and adoptive families of adopted individuals who become schizophrenic: a preliminary report based on psychiatric interviews, in Fieve RR, Rosenthal D, Brill H (eds): *Genetic Research in Psychiatry.* Johns Hopkins University Press, Baltimore, 1975, pp 147–165.

16. Tienari P, Sorri A, Lahti I, et al: The Finnish adoptive family study of schizophrenia. *Yale J Biol Med* 1985;58:227–237.
17. Crow TJ, Done DJ: Age of onset of schizophrenia in siblings: a test of the contagion hypothesis. *Psych Res* 1986;18:107–117.
18. Crow TJ: The continuum of psychosis and its implication for the structure of the gene. *Br J Psychiatry* 1986;149:419–428.
19. Goldin IR, Kidd KK, Matthysse S, et al: The power of pedigree segregation analysis for traits with incomplete penetrance, in Gershon ES, Matthysse S, Ciaranello RD, Breakefield XO (eds): *Genetic Strategies in Psychobiology and Psychiatry*. Pacific Grove, CA, Boxwood Press, 1981, pp 305–317.
20. Goldwin IR, Cox NJ, Pauls DL, et al: The detection of major loci by segregation and linkage analysis: a stimulation study. *Genetic Epidemiol* 1984;1:285–296.
21. DeLisi LE, Goldin LR, Gershon ES: Studies of biological factors associated with the inheritance of schizophrenia: a selective review. *J Psychiatric Res* 1987;21:507–513.
22. Erlenmeyer-Kimling L: Biological markers for the liability to schizophrenia, in Helmchen H, Henn FA (eds): *Biological Perspectives in Schizophrenia: Dahlem Workshop Reports LS 40*. Cambridge, Wiley and Sons, 1987, pp 33–56.
23. DeLisi LE, Wise CD, Bridge TP, et al: Monoamine oxidase and schizophrenia, in Usdin E, Hamin I (eds): *Biological Markers in Psychiatry and Neurology*. Oxford, Pergamon Press, 1982, pp 89–96.
24. Nies A, Robinson DS, Lamborn KR, et al: Genetic control of platelet and plasma monoamine oxidase activity. *Arch Gen Psychol*. 1971;28:834–838.
25. Wyatt RJ, Murphy DL, Belmaker R, et al: Reduced monoamine oxidase in platelets: a possible marker for vulnerability to schizophrenia. *Science* 1973;179:916–918.
26. Reveley MA, Reveley AM, Clifford CA, et al: Genetics of platelet MAO activity in discordant schizophrenic and normal twins. *Br J Psychiatry* 1983;142:89–93.
27. DeLisi LE, Wise CD, Bridge TP, et al: A probable neuroleptic effect on platelet monoamine oxidase activity. *Psychiatry Res* 1981;4:95–107.
28. Owen F, Bourne RC, Crow TJ, et al: Platelet monoamine oxidase activity in acute schizophrenia: relationship to symptomatology and neuroleptic medication. *Br J Psychiatry* 1981;139:16–22.
29. Weinshilbaum RM, Schrott HG, Raymond FA, et al: Inheritance of very low serum dopamine-beta-hydroxlase activity. *Am J Human Genetics* 1975;27:573–585.
30. Weinshilbaum RM, Raymond FA: Inheritance of low erythrocyte catechol-O-methyltransferase activity in man. *Am J Human Genetics* 1977;29:125–135.
31. Sedvall GC, Wode-Helgodt B: Aberrant monoamine metabolite levels in CSF and family history of schizophrenia. *Arch Gen Psychiatry* 1980;37:1113–1116.
32. Sedvall GC, Fyro B, Gullberg B, et al: Relationships in healthy volunteers between concentrations of monoamine metabolites in cerebrospinal fluid and family history of psychiatric morbidity. *Br J Psychiatry* 1980;136:366–374.

33. Oxenstierna G, Edman G, Iselius L, et al: Concentrations of monoamine metabolites in the cerebrospinal fluid of twins and unrelated individuals—a genetic study. *J Psychiatr Res* 1986;20:19–29.
34. Kornhuber J, Riederer P, Reynolds GP, et al: ^{3}H-spiperone binding sites in postmortem brains from schizophrenic patients: relationship to neuroleptic drug treatment, abnormal movements, and positive symptoms. *J Neural Transmission* 1989;75:1–10.
35. Wong DF, Wagner HN, Tune LE, et al: Positron emission tomography reveals elevated brain D-2 dopamine receptors in schizophrenia. *Science* 1986;234:1558–1563.
36. Farde L, Wiesel F-A, Hall H, et al: No D_2 receptor increase in PET study of schizophrenia. *Arch Gen Psychiatry* 1987;44:671–672.
37. Bondy B, Ackenheil M: ^{3}H-spiperone binding sites in lymphocytes as possible vulnerability marker in schizophrenia. *J Psychiatr Res* 1987;21:521–529.
38. Reveley AM, Reveley MA, Clifford CA, et al: Cerebral ventricular size in twins discordant for schizophrenia. *Lancet* 1982;i:540–541.
39. DeLisi LE, Goldin LR, Hamovit JR, et al: A family study of the association of increased ventricular size with schizophrenia. *Arch Gen Psychiatry* 1986;43:148–153.
40. Reveley AM, Reveley MA, Murray RM: Cerebral ventricular enlargement in nongenetic schizophrenia: a controlled twin study. *Br J Psych* 1984;144:89–93.
41. Lipton RB, Levy DL, Holzman PS, et al: Eye movement dysfunctions in psychiatric patients: a review. *Schizophrenia Bulletin* 1983;9:13–22.
42. Holzman PS: Eye movement dysfunction and psychosis. *Int Rev Neurobiol* 1985;27:179–205.
43. Holzman PS, Proctor LR, Levy DL, et al: Eye-tracking dysfunctions in schizophrenic patients and their relatives. *Arch Gen Psychiatry* 1974;31:143–151.
44. Holzman PS, Kringlen E, Levy DL, et al: Deviant eye tracking in twins discordant for psychosis: a replication. *Arch Gen Psychiatry* 1980;32:627–631.
45. Matthysse S, Holzman PS, Lange K: The genetic transmission of schizophrenia: application of Mendelian latent structure analysis to eye-tracking dysfunction in schizophrenia and affective disorder. *J Psychiatric Res* 1986;20:57–67.
46. Turner WD: Genetic markers for schizotaxia. *Biol Psychol.* 1979;14:177–205.
47. McGuffin P, Festenstein H, Murray R: A family study of HLA antigens and other genetic markers in schizophrenia. *Psychological Medicine* 1983;13:31–43.
48. Goldin LR, DeLisi LE, Gershon ES: The relation of HLA to schizophrenia in 10 nuclear families. *Psychiatry Res* 1987;20:69–77.
49. McGuffin P, Sturt E: Genetic markers in schizophrenia. *Human Heredity* 1986;36:65–88.
50. Goldin LR, Gershon ES: Association and linkage studies of genetic marker loci in major psychiatric disorders. *Psychiatric Devel* 1983;4:387–418.
51. Book JA, Wetterberg L, Modrzewska K: Schizophrenia in a north Swedish geographical isolate, 1900–1917. Epidemiology, genetics, and biochemistry. *Clin Genetics* 1978;14:373–394.

52. Ruddick C, Granzen G, Hanson A, et al: G serum groups in schizophrenia. *Human Heredity* 1985;35:11–14.
53. Ruddick C, Beckman L, Franzen G, et al: C3 and C6 complement types in schizophrenia. *Human Heredity* 1985;35:255–258.
54. Cowie V, Coppen A, Norman P: Nuclear sex and body build in schizophrenia. *Br Med J* 1960;ii:431–433.
55. Tedeschi L, Freeman D: Sex chromosomes in male schizophrenics. *Arch Gen Psychiatry* 1962;6:17–19.
56. Raphael T, Shaw MW: Chromosome studies in schizophrenia. *JAMA* 1963;183:1022–1028.
57. Nielsen J, Fisher M: Sex chromatin and sex chromosome abnormalities in male hypogonadal mental patients. *Br J Psychiatry* 1965;111:641–647.
58. Asaka A, Tsuboit T, Inove E, et al: Schizophrenic psychosis in triple-X females. *Folia Psychiatr Neurol Jap* 1967;21:271–81.
59. Judd LL, Brandkamp WW: Chromosome analyses of adult schizophrenics. *Arch Gen Psychiatry* 1967;16:316–324.
60. Anders JM, Jagiello G, Polani PE, et al: Chromosome findings in chronic psychotic patients. *Br J Psychiatry* 1968;114:1167–1174.
61. MacLean, N, Court-Brown WM, Jacobs PA, et al: A survey of sex chromatin abnormalities in mental hospitals. *J. Medical Genetics* 1968;5:165–172.
62. Kaplan AR: Chromosomal mosaicisms and occasional acentric chromosomal fragments in schizophrenic patients. *Biological Psychiatry* 1970;2:89–94.
63. Vartanian ME, Gendelis VM: The role of chromosomal aberrations in the clinical polymorphism of schizophrenia. *Int J Ment Health* 1972;1:93–106.
64. Dasgupta J, Dasgupta D, Balasubrahmanyan M: XXY syndrome XY/XO mosaicism and acentric chromosomal fragments in male schizophrenics. *Indian J Med Res* 1973;61:62–70.
65. Trixler M, Kosztolani G, Mehes K: Sex chromosome aberration screening among male psychiatric patients. *Arch Psychiat Nervenkr* 1976;221:273–282.
66. Axelsson R, Wahlstrom J: Chromosome aberrations in patients with paranoid psychosis. *Hereditas* 1984;100:19–31.
67. DeLisi LE, Reiss AL, White BJ, et al: Cytogenetic studies of males with schizophrenia: screening for the fragile X chromosome and other chromosomal abnormalities. *Schizophrenia Res* 1988;1:277–281.
68. Hamerton JL, Canning N, Ray M, et al: A cytogentic survey of 14,069 newborn infants I. Incidence of chromosomal abnormalities. *Clin Genetics* 1975;8:223–243.
69. Ratcliffe SG, Murray L, Teague P: Edinburgh study of growth and development of children with sex chromosome abnormalities III. *Birth Defects* 1986;22:73–118.
70. Money J, Hirsch SR: Chromosome anomalies, mental deficiency, and schizophrenia. *Arch Gen Psychol* 1963;8:54–63.
71. Polani PE: Abnormal sex chromosomes and mental disorder. *Nature* 1969;223:680–686.
72. Forssman H: The mental implications of sex chromosome aberrations. *Br J Psychiatry* 1970;117:353–63.
73. Turner G, Gill R, Daniel A: Marker X chromosomes, mental retardation, and macroorchidism. *N Engl J Med* 1978;299:1472.

158   Lynn E. DeLisi and Michael Lovett

74. Rogers RC, Simensen RJ: Fragile X syndrome: a common etiology of mental retardation. *Am J Mental Defic* 1987;91(5):445–449.
75. Webb TP, Thake AI, Bundey SE, et al: A cytogenetic survey of a mentally retarded school age population with special reference to fragile sites. *J Mental Defic Res* 1987;31(part 1):61–71.
76. Martin JB, Bell J: A pedigree of mental defect showing sex linkage. *J Neurol Psychiatry* 1943;6:154–157.
77. Brown WT, Jenkins EC, Cohen IL, et al: Fragile X and autism: a multicenter survey. *Am J Med Genetics* 1986;23:341–52.
78. Reiss AL, Feinstein C, Toomey KE, et al: Psychiatric disability associated with the fragile X chromosome. *Am J Med Genetics* 1986;23:393–402.
79. Reiss AL, Hagerman RJ, Vinogradov S, et al: Psychiatric disability in female carriers of the fragile X chromosome. *Arch Gen Psychiatry* 1988;45:25–30.
80. Crow TJ: Pseudoautosomal locus for psychoses? *Lancet* 1987;ii:1532.
81. Crow TJ: Sex chromosomes and psychosis: the case for a pseudoautosomal locus. *Br J Psychiatry* 1988;153:675–683.
82. Crow TJ, DeLisi LE, Johnstone EC: Clues to the nature and location of the psychosis gene: is schizophrenia due to an anomaly of the cerebral dominance gene located in the pseudoautosomal region of the sex chromosomes? in Wetterberg L (ed): *Genetics of Neuropsychiatric Diseases*. Wenner-Gren Center International Symposium No. 51. New York, McMillan Press, 1989.
83. Rouyer F, Simmler M-C, Johnsson C, et al: A gradient of sex linkage in the pseudoautosomal region of the human sex chromosomes. *Nature* 1986;319:291–295.
84. Rouyer, F, Simmler M-C, Vergnaud G, et al: The pseudoautosomal region of the human sex chromosomes. *Cold Spring Harbor Symposia on Quantitative Biology* 1986;LI:221–228.
85. Page DC, Bieker K, Brown LG, et al: Linkage, physical mapping, and DNA sequence analysis of pseudoautosomal loci on the human X and Y chromosomes. *Genomics* 1987;1:243–256.
86. DeLisi LE, Goldin LR, Maxwell ME, et al: Clinical features of illness in siblings with schizophrenia or schizoaffective disorder. *Arch General Psychiatry* 1987;44:891–896.
87. Schulz B: Zur Erbpathologie der schizophrenie. *Zeitschrift Gesammie Neurologie und Psychiatrie* 1932;143:175–293.
88. Zehnder M: Uber Krankheitsbild und Krankheitsverlauf bei schizophrenen Geschwistern. *Monatschrift fur Psychiatrie und Neurologie* 1941;103:231–277.
89. Penrose LS: Survey of cases of familiar mental illness. *Digest Neurology Psychiatry* 1945;13:644.
90. Tsuang MT: A study of pairs of sibs both hospitalized for mental disorder. *Br J Psychiatry* 1967;113:283–300.
91. Rudduck C, Franzen G: Brief report: a new heritable fragile site on human chromosome 3. *Hereditas* 1983;98:297–299.
92. Chodirker BN, Chudley AE, Ray M, et al: Fragile 19p13 in a family with mental illness. *Clinical Genetics* 1987;31:1–6.
93. Sperber MA: Schizophrenia and organic brain syndrome with trisomy 8 (group C trisomy 8 [47,XX,8 +]). *Biol Psychiatry* 1975;10:27–43.
94. Bassett AS, McGillivray BC, Jones BD, et al: Partial trisomy chromosome 5 cosegregating with schizophrenia. *Lancet* 1988;i:799–801.

95. Genest, P, Dumas L, Genest FB: Translocation chromosomique t (2;18) (q21;q23) chez un individual schizophrene et sa fille. *L'Union Medicale Du Canada TOME* 1976;105:1617–1681.
96. White RL: DNA in medicine: human genetics. *Lancet* 1984;ii:1257–1262.
97. Gershon ES, Merrill CR, Goldin LR, et al: The role of molecular genetics in psychiatry. *Biol Psychiatry* 1987;22:1388–1405.
98. Baron M, Rainer JD: Molecular genetics and human disease: implications for modern psychiatric research and practice. *Br J Psychol* 1988;152:741–753.
99. Maniatis T, Fritsch EF, Sambrook J: *Molecular Cloning: A Laboratory Manual.* New York, Cold Spring Harbor Laboratory, 1982.
100. Gusella JF, Wexler NS, Conneally PM, et al: A polymorphic DNA marker genetically linked to Huntington's disease. *Nature* 1983;306:234–238.
101. Egeland JR, Gerrhard DS, Pauls DL, et al: Bipolar affective disorders linked to DNA markers on chromosome 11. *Nature* 1987;325:783–787.
102. Mendlewicz J, Sevy S, Brocas H, et al: Polymorphic DNA marker on X chromosome and manic depression. *Lancet* 1987;i:1230–1232.
103. Tanzi RE, Gusella FF, Watkins PC, et al: Amyloid beta-protein gene: cDNA, mRNA distribution, and genetic linkage near the Alzheimer locus. *Science* 1987;235:880–884.
104. Feder J, Gurling HMD, Darby J, et al: DNA restriction fragment analysis of the proopiomelanocortin gene in schizophrenia and bipolar disorders. *Am J Human Genetics* 1985;37:286–294.
105. Detera-Wadleigh, S, DeLisi LE, Berrettini WH, et al: DNA polymorphisms in schizophrenia and affective disorders, in Shagass C, et al (eds): *Proceedings of the IVth World Congress of Biological Psychiatry.* New York, Elsevier Publishing Co., 1986.
106. Detera-Wadleigh SD, deMiguel C, Berrettini WH, et al: Neuropeptide gene polymorphisms in affective disorder and schizophrenia. *J Psychiatric Res* 1987;21(4):581–587.
107. Sherrington R, Brynjolfsson J, Petersson, H, et al: Localization of a susceptibility locus for schizophrenia on chromosome 5. *Nature* 1988;336:164–167.
108. Kennedy JL, Gluffrat LA, Moises HW, et al: Evidence against linkage of schizophrenia to markers on chromosome 5 in a northern Swedish pedigree. *Nature* 1988;336:167–170.
109. Gershon ES: Presented at the 27th Annual Meeting of the American College of Neuropsychopharmacology, San Juan, Puerto Rico, Dec 12–16, 1988.
110. Crow TJ: Two syndromes of schizophrenia as one pole of the continuum of psychosis: a concept of the nature of the pathogen and its genetic locus, in Henn FA, DeLisi LE (eds): *Neurochemistry and Neuropharmacology of Schizophrenia.* Amsterdam, Elsevier, 1987, pp 17–48.
111. DeLisi LE, Wyatt RJ: Endogenous hallucinogens and other behavior modifying factors in schizophrenia, in Henn FA, DeLisi LE (eds): *Neurochemistry and Neuropharmacology of Schizophrenia.* Amsterdam, Elsevier, 1987, pp 377–390.
112. Stahl SM, Wets K: Indoleamines and schizophrenia, in Henn FA, DeLisi LE (eds): *Neurochemistry and Neuropharmacology of Schizophrenia.* Amsterdam, Elsevier, 1987, pp 257–296.
113. DeLisi LE, Wyatt RJ: Neurochemical aspects of schizophrenia, in Lajtha JR (ed): *Handbook of Neurochemistry,* New York, Plenum Publishing Co, 1985, vol 10, pp 553–587.

114. Bach AWJ, Lan NC, Johnson DL, et al: cDNA cloning of human liver monoamie oxidase A and B: molecular basis of differences in enzymatic properties. *Proc Natl Acad Sci USA* 1988;85:4934–4938.

115. Ozelius L, Hsu Y-PP, Bruns G, et al: Human monoamine oxidase gene (MAOA): chromosome position (Xp21-p11) and DNA polymorphism, in *Genomics 198 Biochemical Basis of Neuropharmacology*, ed 4. New York, Oxford University Press, 1982, pp 295–320.

116. Woo SLC, Lidsky AS, Guttler F, et al: Cloned human phenylalanine hydroxylase gene allows prenatal diagnosis and carrier detection of classical phenylketonuria. *Nature* 1983;306,151–155.

117. Woo SLC, DiLella AG, Marvit J, et al: Molecular basis of phenylketonuria and potential somatic gene therapy. *Cold Spring Harbor Symposia on Quantitative Biology* 1986;LI,395–401.

118. Cooper JR, Bloom FE, Roth RH: Neuroactive peptides, chap 10, in *The Biochemical Basis of Neuropharmacology*, ed 4. New York, Oxford University Press, 1982, pp 295–320.

119. Roberts GW, Ferrier IN, Lee Y, et al: Peptides, the limbic lobe and schizophrenia. *Brain Research* 1983;288:199–211.

120. Crow TJ, Deakin JFW: Neurotransmitters, behavior, and metal disorder, in Shephard M (ed): *Handbook of Psychiatry*. Cambridge, Cambridge University Press, 1985, vol. 5, pp 137–182.

121. Crow TJ: A reevaluation of the viral hypothesis: is psychosis the result of retroviral integration at a site close to the cerebral dominance gene. *Br J Psychiatry* 1984;145:243–253.

122. Jeffreys AJ, Wilson V, Thein SL: Hypervariable "minisatellite" regions in human DNA. *Nature* 1985;314:67–73.

123. Nakamura Y, Leppert M, O'Connell P, et al: Variable number of tandem repeat (VNIR) markers for human gene mapping. *Science* 1987;235:1616–1622.

124. Church G, Kieffer-Higginss: Multiple DNA sequencing. *Science* 1988;240:185–188.

125. Bird AP: CpG-rich islands and the function of DNA methylation. *Nature* 1986;321:209–213.

126. Smith CL, Econome JG, Schutt A, et al: A physical map of the *Escherichia coli* K12 genome. *Science* 1987;236:1448–1453.

127. Lawrence SK, Smith CL, Srivastava R, et al: Megabase scale mapping of the HLA gene complex by pulsed field gel electrophoresis. *Science* 1987;235:1387–1390.

128. Smith CL, Cantor CR: Approaches to physical mapping of the human genome. *Cold Spring Harbor Symp Quart Biol* 1986;51:115–122.

129. Smith CL, Cantor CR: Preparation and manipulation of large DNA molecules: advances and applications. *TIBS* 1987;12(8):284–287.

130. Church GM, Gilbert W: Genomic sequencing: preliminary communication. *Proc. Natl Acad Sci USA* 1984;81:1991–1995.

131. Scharf SJ, Horn GT, Erlich HA: Direct cloning and sequence analysis of enzymatically amplified genomic sequences. *Science* 1986;233:1076–1078.

132. Engelke DR, Hoener PA, Collins FS: Direct sequencing of enzymatically amplified human genomic DNA. *Proc Natl Acad Sci USA* 1988;85:544–548.

133. Morton NE: The detection and estimation of linkage between the genes for elliptocytosis and RH blood type. *Am J Human Genetics* 1956;8:80–96.

134. Ott J: *Analysis of Human Genetic Linkage*. Baltimore and London, Johns Hopkins University Press, 1985.
135. Ott J: Estimation of the recombination fraction in human pedigrees: efficient computation of the likelihood for human linkage. *Am J Human Genetics* 1974;26:588–597.
136. Lathrop GM, Lalouel JM, Julier C, et al: Strategies for multilocus linkage analysis in humans. *PNAS* 1984;81:3443–3446.
137. Gershon ES, Goldin IR: The outlook for linkage research in psychiatric disorders. *J Psychiatric Res* 1987;21:541–550.
138. Penrose LS: The detection of autosomal linkage in data which consists of pairs of brothers and sisters of unspecificied parentage. *Ann Eugenics* 1935;6:133–138.
139. Penrose LS: The general purpose sib-pair linkage test. *Ann Eugenics* 1953;18:120–124.
140. Thomson G, Bodmer WF: The genetic analysis of HLA and disease associations, in Dausset J, Svejgaard A (eds): *HLA and Disease*. Baltimore, Williams and Wilkins, 1987, pp 84–93.
141. Suarez BIK: The affected sib-pair IBD distribution for HLA linked disease susceptibility loci. *Tissue Antigens* 1978;12:87–93.
142. Green JR, Woodrow JC: Sibling method for detecting HLA-linked genes in disease. *Tissue Antigens* 1977;9:31–35.
143. Clerget-Darpoux F, Govaerts A, Feingold N: HLA and susceptibility to multiple sclerosis. *Tissue Antigens* 1984;24:160–169.
144. Collins FS, Weissman SM: Directional cloning of DNA fragments at a large distance from an initial probe: a circulization method. *Proc Natl Acad Sci USA* 1984;81:6812–6816.
145. Poustka A, Lehrach H: Jumping libraries and linking libraries. The next generation of molecular tools in mammalian genetics. *Trends Genet* 1986;2:174–179.
146. Burke DT, Carle GF, Olson MV: Cloning of large segments of exogenous DNA into yeast by means of artificial chromosome vectors. *Science* 1987;236:806–812.

8
Diagnostic Advances in Anatomical and Functional Brain Imaging in Schizophrenia

JÖRG J. PAHL, VICTOR W. SWAYZE, AND NANCY C. ANDREASEN

The past decade has experienced an unprecedented advance in our understanding of psychiatric disorders. This has led to renewed optimism and excitement in psychiatry in general and in schizophrenia research in particular. The optimism stems primarily from developments in the basic neurosciences and computer technology as well as from refinements that have been made in established psychiatric research areas such as epidemiology and phenomenology.

It now appears possible that we will eventually be able to define the major psychotic disorders in terms of etiology, pathophysiology, and regional cerebral neurochemical alterations. It also seems likely that this goal will be achieved with laboratory tools that are currently available. These include recombinant DNA technology, neuroimaging modalities (magnetic resonance imaging [MRI], single photon emission computer tomography [SPECT], autoradiography, positron emission tomography [PET]), and improved postmortem histological methods (quantitative morphometrics and immunohistochemistry). Developments in psychiatric classification schemes and biometric techniques, which have led to a more precise definition of schizophrenia, form an integral part of these research endeavors.

Essential and ongoing postmortem pathological and biochemical investigations are now being complemented by in vivo brain imaging studies. High resolution MRI (< 2 mm in-plane) generates anatomical brain images in standard sagittal, coronal, and axial views. Software packages for MRI are being developed that will allow volumetric determinations to be performed on individual structures in addition to the linear and planimetric measurements that are routinely made. Such MRI scans can be repeated in longitudinal studies without the considerable radiation exposure of conventional x-ray computed tomography (CT). Magnetic resonance imaging also has the advantage over x-ray CT of possessing a superior gray-white matter differentiation capacity that allows improved delineation of cerebral regions.

Structural imaging techniques will undoubtedly increase our general understanding of schizophrenia. It appears evident, however, that chemical imaging modalities currently offer the greatest promise for studying pathophysiological events causing the illness. This assumption is based on present neuropathological studies in schizophrenia that have reported subtle to nonexistent alterations in a substantial number of cases. The most powerful of the available analytical techniques are autoradiography and PET.[1] It has been demonstrated that these modalities can measure picomolar concentrations of chemical species such as neuroreceptors in discrete postmortem areas in vitro (autoradiography) and defined cerebral regions in vivo (PET).

The above-mentioned brain imaging methods are currently being used to search for anatomical and biochemical substrates that underly specific schizophrenic phenomenological manifestations such as auditory hallucinations. This review will outline the diagnostic advances that have been made recently in this field of brain imaging. We will also discuss indications for the use of these techniques in everyday patient management.

Structural Brain Imaging

X-ray Computed Tomography

Pneumoencephalography was the first brain imaging technique used to study living schizophrenic subjects. As early as 1927 the European literature reported enlargement of the lateral ventricles in some, but not all, schizophrenics.[2] The unpleasantness and invasiveness of the procedure, however, precluded its widescale application to research. The studies were furthermore tainted by unreliability due to the tendency of insufflated air to increase ventricular size.[3] These drawbacks were largely overcome by the introduction of x-ray CT in 1972. Johnstone and colleagues were the first to demonstrate lateral ventricular enlargement noninvasively with the new technique in schizophrenic patients (Fig 8.1).[4]

Morphological abnormalities reported in x-ray CT studies have included enlarged lateral, third, and fourth ventricles; enlarged cortical fissures and sulci; reversed cerebral asymmetries; and apparent atrophy of the cerebellar vermis.

Lateral ventricular enlargement is not a prominent x-ray CT finding in most schizophrenics. Quantitative methods have therefore been devised to supplement qualitative evaluations of ventricular dimensions. These include linear and planimetric measurements of the ventricular spaces and, more recently, semiautomated computerized techniques to determine ventricular volumes.[5,6] The semiautomated methods use x-ray CT density numbers to determine the boundary between ventricles and surrounding brain tissue.

Lateral ventricular enlargement represents the best characterized x-ray

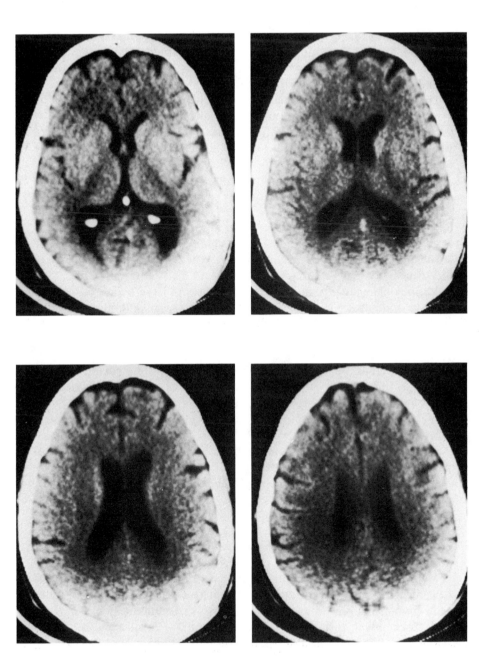

FIGURE 8.1. The figure depicts four contiguous transaxial x-ray CT scans of a 28-year- old schizophrenic (slice thickness = 10 mm). The images demonstrate typical lateral ventricular dilatation as found in a subset of schizophrenics.

CT abnormality in schizophrenia, despite the fact that it is a relatively subtle finding. Indeed, positive studies showing dilatation now outnumber negative studies by a ratio of four to one (see Fig 8. 2).[4–50] Although the cause of the dilatation remains obscure, it could be due to an early developmental abnormality or atrophic process reflecting postnatal pathological involvement of the brain.

Third ventricular enlargement has been less frequently demonstrated in schizophrenia than lateral ventricular dilatation.[48] Such a finding, if valid, could reflect a central atrophic process that would be consistent with the hypothesis of histopathological changes in the diencephalon of chronic schizophrenics as reported by Stevens in postmortem studies.[51]

X-ray CT studies also have focused on evidence of sulcal enlargement or widening because of frequent reports of cortical changes in the neuropathology literature.[52] The measurement of sulcal size has been difficult because of x-ray CT artifacts that occur at the brain–cerebrospinal fluid–skull interfaces. These include partial volume, spectral shift, and bone hardening artifacts which, when present, potentially limit the validity of linear measurement techniques and qualitative visual rating scales.

Various changes in x-ray CT density numbers have been examined in hopes of finding subtle changes reflecting pathological alterations in brain tissue. These investigations are difficult to interpret due to methodological problems that are inherent to these types of studies.[53]

A number of investigators also have used x-ray CT to scan patients suffering from tardive dyskinesia. These studies have, however, not identified specific areas in the brain that might distinguish schizophrenic patients with tardive dyskinesia from those without the disorder.[54]

A major thrust of x-ray CT schizophrenia research has been to seek morphological features that would correlate with one or more unique aspects of the schizophrenic syndrome. Naturally, then, the subgroup of patients showing lateral ventricular dilatation, third ventricle enlargement, and/or sulcal prominence might be expected to present with more prominent signs of mental illness and neuropsychological impairment than those with a normal x-ray CT.

The early investigations using x-ray CT performed clinicopathological correlations which supported the above-mentioned concept.[4,55] This resulted in a substantial number of other controlled investigations as presented. Many have examined such clinical aspects as age of onset, duration of illness, cognitive impairment, positive and negative symptoms, poor premorbid adjustment, poor response to treatment, poor outcome, and biochemical variables. Of these, cognitive impairment correlated with ventricular enlargement in several early studies,[4,14,55] but has not been found in other studies.[37,50,56] A number of investigations have supported increased negative symptoms in schizophrenia,[11,14,22,29,35,39] but an equal number have not supported this finding.[21,26,37,40,48,50] Studies of poor premorbid adjustment and poor treatment outcome have been split in the

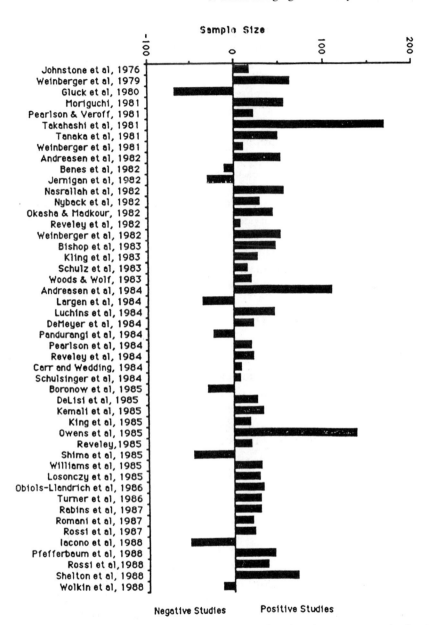

FIGURE 8.2. Lateral ventricular dilatation in schizophrenia represents the best documented morphological abnormality of the disorder. As shown, studies demonstrating increased lateral ventricular size far outnumber negative studies.

number that support or do not support a correlation with ventricular enlargement.[14,26,33,39,57] Correlations with biochemical variables such as low concentrations of homovanillic acid and 5-hydroxyindoleacetic acid in cerebrospinal fluid have suffered from mixed results as well.[58–61] Thus, x-ray CT correlations in schizophrenia still remain inconclusive. It should be noted, however, that correlation analysis on parameters that have a narrow range of variability is fraught with difficulty and may in part account for the lack of correlations in some studies when they may indeed exist.

X-ray CT brain abnormalities have not been limited to schizophrenia. Similar findings of cortical atrophy and ventricular dilatation have been noted in subgroups of patients suffering from affective illness, anorexia nervosa, and alcohol dependence.[62] The alterations may represent pseudoatrophy in the latter two conditions, as they are partly reversible in some of these patients. The limited data set presently available precludes firm conclusions from being made about the permanence of similar structural abnormalities in schizophrenia.[63,64]

Magnetic Resonance Imaging

Magnetic resonance imaging (MRI) possesses significant advantages over x-ray CT. It has vastly superior gray-white matter differentiation capability. In addition, image acquisition can occur in multiple planes, allowing detailed anatomical exploration of small limbic structures that are highly relevant to schizophrenia research. The absence of ionizing radiation represents a further appealing feature of MRI that allows it to be used for repeat studies in longitudinal investigations.

It is beyond the scope of this chapter to explain in depth the technology and complex physics of MRI. Interested readers are referred to standard texts for more thorough nonmathematical explanations.[65,66] What follows is a brief overview that is meant to help clarify the advantages of MRI over x-ray CT in anatomical imaging.

Magnetic resonance imaging is based on the physical phenomenon called nuclear magnetic resonance that was first described in the 1940s. A number of elements have at least one isotope in abundance whose nuclei have an unpaired neutron or proton. This unpaired atomic particle causes these particular elements to behave like minute bar magnets. Because each nucleus is randomly situated in relationship to other like nuclei, they cancel each other's net magnetic fields. However, if these nuclei with unpaired atomic particles are placed inside a strong, static magnetic field, the randomly spinning unpaired particle aligns either parallel or antiparallel to the direction (vector) of the external magnetic field. Parallel alignment of the particle has a slightly lower energy state than antiparallel, and so an extremely small excess (10^{-5}) of the particles are lined up in the parallel (lower energy) state. Biological substances contain several such magnetic nuclei: 1H, 13C, 31P, 15N, 23Na, 39K, 19F. The atomic particles also wobble or precess with a certain frequency, and this is "resonance." As currently used for morphometric imaging research, MRI makes use of the hydrogen atom because it is by far the most abundant element in the human body.

To create MRI images of the human body, bursts of radio frequency signals are used to tip the precessing hydrogen atoms out of the plane of the main magnetic field. Gradient magnetic fields are used to change the static magnetic field so that contiguous slices of brain tissue can be imaged simultaneously. Three parameters describe the characteristics of the signal, which produces the magnetic resonance image. These parameters are proton density and the two relaxation time constants, T1 and T2, otherwise known as transverse and longitudinal relaxation times. In quite simplistic terms these time constants refer to the chemical environment in which the protons are found, T1 relating mainly to its neighboring protons and T2 referring to neighboring molecules. It is these unique parameters that enable magnetic resonance imaging to have superior resolution and superior contrast between gray and white matter. Three imaging sequences, saturation recovery, inversion recovery, and spin echo, enable the radiologist to obtain proton density-weighted, T1-weighted, and T2-weighted images, depending on the image information sought. Use of these different imaging techniques may enable detection of subtle pathological changes in the chemical composition of tissue.

Magnetic resonance imaging has thus been shown to be quite sensitive to pathological changes in a number of neurological diseases due to the effect of the chemical environment on the hydrogen atom. Because of this effect Johnstone et al [67] conducted a MRI study based on the hypothesis that a pathologic process in the periventricular area may occur in schizophrenic subjects as a result of suffering their first acute episode of psychosis. This study examined 27 schizophrenic subjects closely matched for age to 12 control subjects. All scans were reviewed blind to diagnosis; although some of the scans did show unusual increase in signal intensity on spin echo scans at the angles of the ventricles, no significant difference between controls and the total group of schizophrenic patients was demonstrated (Fig 8.3).

Ten MRI studies of brain morphological characteristics in schizophrenia have appeared in the literature and are summarized in Table 8.1.[68–77] The utility of using multiple plane imaging to examine various anatomical regions was demonstrated in a pilot MRI study done by our research group.[71] Evaluation of the midsagittal plane revealed that the frontal lobe, cerebrum, and cranial areas were smaller in schizophrenic subjects compared with a control group consisting mainly of hospital personnel. When a slightly larger sample of schizophrenic subjects was used, this result was not replicated at our center, in part due to differences in the control group, which was educationally equivalent in this later study.[77] DeMyer, using transverse images and measuring the frontal lobes from the anterior tips of the lateral ventricles to the anterior tips of the hemispheres, noted

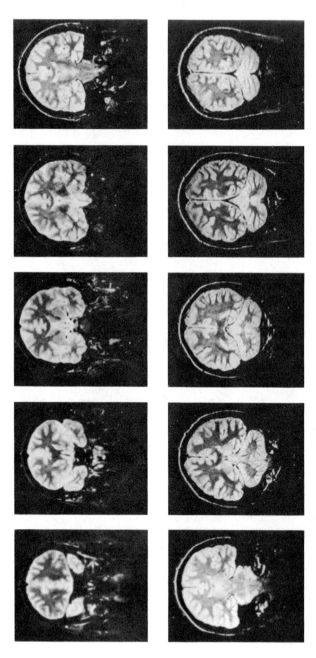

FIGURE 8.3. The MRI proton density weighted images of a normal volunteer were generated with a spin echo technique (pulse sequence TR = 3000, TE = 30) that results in superb gray-white matter differentiation. The 10 consecutive coronal scans (slice thickness = 5 mm) allow planimetric two-dimensional and volumetric three-dimensional measurements to be made. Shown with good anatomical clarity are the amygdala, hippocampi, caudate, and lenticular nuclei.

that the frontal lobes were slightly smaller in one of two slices measured in this manner.[78]

Four out of six studies to date have reported enlargement of the lateral ventricles. Only one of three studies using a planimetric ventricular brain ratio (VBR) similar to those reported in CT literature reported ventricular enlargement.[68,73,74] Two studies, one from the National Institute of Mental Health and our research center's second MRI study, used volumetric measurements of the lateral ventricles. Both used coronal slices to measure the anatomical area of the ventricles and multiplied each area by the slice thickness, adding the results to obtain total ventricular volume. Both of these studies showed ventricular enlargement in schizophrenics *vs* controls, as did the sixth study which used the midsagittal plane to measure the lateral ventricle area as it appears ventral to the corpus callosum (Fig 8.4).[70,75,77]

The two studies that used volumetric techniques to measure ventricular size also measured the size of the third ventricle. One reported that the third ventricle was significantly larger in the anterior most coronal slice

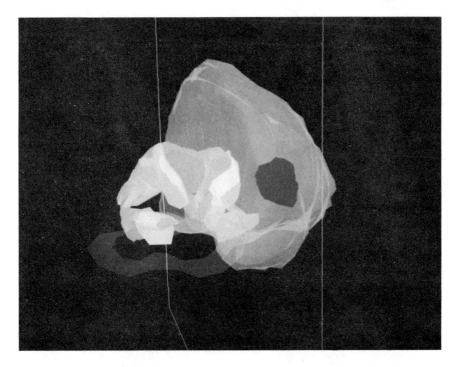

FIGURE 8.4. Semi-automated image analysis techniques developed at the University of Iowa allow three-dimensional reconstruction of two-dimensional coronal, sagittal, or transaxial MRI scans. The software enables the investigator to measure structures volumetrically and to depict single structures such as the amygdala or hippocampi individually or in combination.

TABLE 8.1. Magnetic resonance imaging studies in schizophrenia.

Source	Number of subjects controls	Imaging and measurement techniques	Regions examined	Morphological findings in schizophrenics compared with controls
Smith et al, 1984[68]	9/5	0.3-tesla scanner; spin echo, 30 ms; transverse sections; planimetry	Bifrontal ratio, bicaudate ratio, ventricular-brain ratio, corpus callosum	No difference in regions examined
Mathew and Partain, 1985[69]	12/12	0.5-tesla scanner; spin echo; 1 midsagittal section; planimetry	Cerebellar vermis, fourth ventricle	No difference in regions examined
Mathew et al, 1985[70]	18/18	0.5-tesla scanner; spin echo, 30 ms; 1 midsagittal section; planimetry	Septum pellucidum, corpus callosum anteroposterior length of corpus callosum	Increased area of septum pellucidum, increased anteroposterior length of corpus callosum
Andreasen et al, 1986[71]	38/49	0.5-tesla scanner; inversion recovery, 600 ms; 1 midsagittal section; planimetry	Frontal area, cerebral area, cranial area	Frontal area decreased, cerebral area decreased, cranial area decreased
Nasrallah et al, 1986[72]	38/41	0.5-tesla scanner; inversion recovery, 600 ms; 1 midsagittal section; planimetry	Corpus callosum	Increased callosal area, increased callosal area to midsagittal brain area ratio, increased callosal thickness
Smith et al, 1987[73]	29/21	0.3-tesla scanner; inversion recovery, 30 ms; spin echo, 30 ms; transverse, coronal and midsagittal sections; planimetry	Lateral ventricles, third ventricle, white and gray matter	No difference in lateral ventricles, no difference in third ventricle

Study	N	Methods	Measures	Results
Rossi et al, 1988[74]	12/12	0.5-tesla scanner; spin echo 30 ms, midsagittal section; spin echo 30,120 ms, transverse section; planimetry	Corpus callosum area, ventricular-brain ratio, fourth ventricle area	Decreased callosal area, increased ventricular-brain ratio, no difference in fourth ventricular area
Kelsoe et al, 1988[75]	24/14	0.5-tesla scanner; inversion recovery, 600 ms; 1 midsagittal section, multiple coronal sections; computer digitized planimetry	Lateral ventricular volume, lateral ventricular volume-to-brain volume ratio, third ventricular area, cerebral hemisphere volume, prefrontal region volume, temporal lobe volume, amygdala-hippocampal volume, caudate area, globus pallidus-putamen area, corpus callosum area, corpus callosum thickness	Increased lateral ventricular volume, increased lateral ventricular volume to brain volume ratio, increased third ventricular area, no differences in other brain regions measured
DeMyer et al, 1988[76]	24/24	0.15-tesla scanner; combined spin echo, 30 ms, and inversion recovery, 400 ms; 2 transverse slices; planimetry	Left and right hemisphere areas, frontal lobe areas	Decreased right hemisphere area on slice 1; no hemisphere differences on slice 2; decreased frontal area on slice 2; no frontal area difference on slice 1
Andreasen et al, 1989 in press[77]	55/47	0.5-tesla scanner; inversion recovery, 600/1600 ms; 1 midsagittal, multiple; coronal slices; planimetry	Frontal, parietal, occipital, cerebral, cranial, corpus callosal, and ventricular areas in midsagittal plane, lateral and third ventricular areas and volumes in the coronal planes.	Increased lateral ventricular area; no significant differences in other regions measured on midsagittal plane; increased lateral ventricular volume; no difference in third ventricular volume on coronal plane

in which it was present compared with the control group.[75] Our study found no significant difference in its volume compared with controls.[77] Smith, using transverse images, found the third ventricle to be no greater in its linear width.[73] Mathew reported that the cerebellar vermis and the fourth ventricle measured in the midsagittal plane did not differ significantly from controls.[69]

Seven studies evaluated the size of the corpus callosum.[68,70,72–75,77] One reported the callosal area to be significantly smaller in schizophrenics vs controls, [74] whereas the first study from our center reported it to be significantly larger in total midsagittal area and callosal to cerebral area ratio.[72] Two studies have shown no differences in callosal to transverse brain area ratio,[68,73] and two showed no difference in the callosal midsagittal area (no ratio reported).[70,75] Our own second MRI study agreed with the majority in reporting no significant difference in midsagittal callosal area and midsagittal callosal to cerebral area ratio.[77]

Five studies[68,73–75,78] evaluated the possibility of having T1 and T2 signal intensity parameter changes in the brain of schizophrenics vs controls. The results of these studies are quite variable, and it is at present unclear as to whether T1 and T2 have any clinical meaning and their measurement any applicability to the study of schizophrenia. Our own work has indicated significant differences between schizophrenics and controls in T2 in gray matter, a finding consistent with increased fluid in gray matter in schizophrenia.[79] Although this study has the most rigorous methodology of any to date, it clearly needs further replication.

Clinical Applications of Anatomical Imaging

The clinical indications for x-ray CT and MRI imaging in schizophrenia are well established by now. The most important indication for their use is in ruling out focal organic causes in patients presenting with schizophreniform symptoms. These include neoplasms, demyelinating disease, vasculopathies (at times associated with stimulant abuse), and various neurodegenerative conditions such as Huntington's disease and Wilson's disease. Confusion, dementia, movement disorders (all of unknown etiology), as well as prolonged catatonia and changes in personality or affect in schizophrenic patients over age 50 may all reflect such an underlying organic etiology. Age of onset, duration or severity of illness, or schizophrenia subtype do not as such indicate the need for anatomical imaging in schizophrenia.

Magnetic resonance imaging is the preferred structural imaging modality in the clinical setting because it does not use ionizing radiation and can image in multiple planes. It, rather than x-ray CT, is especially suited for identifying demyelinating disease, small primary or metastatic tumors, early lymphomas, early infarction, and early inflammation. Its use is also indicated in patients who, because of an iodine allergy, cannot tolerate iodinate contrast agents used in x-ray CT.

The use of MRI is, however, contraindicated by the presence of metal intracranial aneurysm clips or pacemakers, because the clips at times experience a significant torque, separating them from the arterial wall and leading to acute hemorrhage, and cardiac pacemakers have been shown to switch from the demand to the asynchronous mode in the magnetic field. In addition, the effect of MRI on fetal development has not been studied; thus, pregnancy remains a major contraindication for MRI studies. The primary advantages of x-ray CT over MRI lies in imaging intracranial hemorrhages and in detecting bone lesions.

Functional Brain Imaging

The foregoing review has demonstrated the usefulness of x-ray CT and MRI in schizophrenia research. The overall consensus is that brain imaging has demonstrated structural abnormalities in a subgroup of schizophrenics. It is, however, also evident that these techniques have failed to show macroscopic cortical or subcortical abnormalities in the majority (> 80%) of patients. This has led to the conclusion that phenotypic expression in schizophrenia probably primarily reflects dynamic regional biochemical abnormalities rather than local neuropathological changes. This realization has been further strengthened by the absence of pathognomonic histological changes in schizophrenic brains, despite the presence of highly psychotic manifestations or persistent negative defect states during the patient's lifetime.

The obvious need for chemical imaging in schizophrenia has led to the investigation of regional brain function with newly developed imaging devices. Initial studies were designed to detect functional regional cerebral blood flow (rCBF) and metabolic effects of such chemical alterations. More recent studies have attempted to characterize the actual chemical substrates that underlie schizophrenia.

Physiological brain imaging is based on the work of Roy and Sherrington[80] who were the first to demonstrate tight coupling of CBF and metabolism. They also showed that these parameters were directly related to brain function in healthly individuals.[80] This fundamental concept shaped the Kety and Schmidt nitrous oxide determinations of global CBF and metabolism in schizophrenia. Their initial report of normal global CBF and oxygen values in the illness has since been replicated in numerous additional studies. The authors voiced the possibility that regional rather than global CBF abnormalities might underlie the schizophrenic syndrome.[81]

Cortical Probe Blood Flow Measurement

The xenon[133] clearance technique was developed to measure rCBF using cortical probe sodium iodide detectors. This method generates two-dimensional functional images of rCBF, reflecting underlying brain activity.

Ingvar[82] studied 11 "normal" patients with this modality and demonstrated that rCBF was significantly higher (20 to 40%) in the frontal region than in the temporal, parietal, or occipital regions. The subjects were examined in a state of "resting" wakefulness. The eyes were kept occluded with a sandbag. Ingvar coined the term "hyperfrontality" to describe this "resting" rCBF pattern.[82] In 1974 Ingvar and Franzen published a CBF study of 20 chronic schizophrenics of whom the younger group (mean age 25 years; disease duration 5 years) showed a normal hyperfrontal rCBF pattern, whereas the older group (mean age 61 years; disease duration 40 years) had a relatively low frontal CBF pattern, and in most cases, high flow rates in the occipitotemporal region. Cerebral blood flow in the occipitotemporal region correlated positively with the degree of cognitive disturbance in the schizophrenic population. The appearance of relatively low frontal CBF in the patients was termed "hypofrontality" as opposed to the normal "hyperfrontality" pattern.[83] This study represents the forerunner of SPECT rCBF and PET metabolic investigations in schizophrenia.

The absence of abnormal "resting state" CBF values in acute and many chronic schizophrenics has led investigators to use cognitive activation studies in CBF measurements. The rationale for using these cognitive probes is that they may identify schizophrenics with marginally reduced resting rCBF values. Tests have been selected for their potential of preferentially activating specific brain regions. Frontal lobe activation tasks include the Wisconsin Card Sorting Test (WCST) and the Continuous Performance Test (CPT). It is hypothesized that areas of reduced frontal lobe perfusion will reflect reduced neuronal activity that one would expect to see in predominantly negative symptom schizophrenics. The WCST seems especially suited for this purpose because it challenges the ability to think abstractly and to change a cognitive set in response to a change in instructions and stimuli.

Berman et al[84] used the WCST to study activation of the dorsolateral prefrontal cortex (DLPFC) in medicated and nonmedicated schizophrenics and matched controls. During the initial resting state they found a reduction of relative, but not absolute, rCBF values with the xenon[133] technique. A simple nonprefrontal number matching task failed to activate the DLPFC. Unlike normals, both medicated and nonmedicated schizophrenics failed to show activation of the DLPFC on the WCST.[84] This finding is consistent with the general hypothesis of frontal lobe dysfunction in schizophrenia.

Single Photon Emission Computed Tomography

Single photon emission computed tomography (SPECT) has been developed recently to overcome significant disadvantages of the two-dimensional cortical probe technique.[85] These include poor visualization of central grey matter structures and poor resolution (> 25 mm for cortical structures). Xenon[133] SPECT can represent rCBF values three dimensionally and allows visualization of the basal ganglia. Gamma-cameras represent an alternative method for measuring cerebral perfusion. This technique uses a rotating detector and associated planimeter systems to collect information from different angular projections. The approach results in data acquisition from multiple planes. Gamma-cameras in combination with newly developed radiotracers such as [I[123]] iodine-labelled iodoamphetamine [I[123]-IMP) result in a significantly improved resolution (presently 12 mm full width half maximum [FWHM]). The technique is also suited for measuring radioligand uptake in specific receptor regions, including the basal ganglia.

The schizophrenia SPECT literature is still rather limited. Devous,[86] in a recent review that included his own investigations, reported a decrease in frontal CBF over resting values in schizophrenics during a special version of the WCST. This interesting finding, which may point to functional reorganization of the brain in schizophrenia, is in partial agreement with the earlier cortical probe studies.[84]

It is envisioned that SPECT will come to play an important complementary role to PET in the characterization of physiological and biochemical substrates in schizophrenia. The development of SPECT as a functional imaging modality for schizophrenia research is especially important if one considers the phenomenological heterogeneity of the condition. Extremely large patient populations may have to be sampled in schizophrenia with SPECT before it becomes possible to generate meaningful subgroups and achieve statistical (and clinical) significance in the overall data set. It may become the imaging modality of first choice in such a situation, because SPECT uses commercially available radiotracers and does not require the on site presence of a cyclotron or a team of physicists and chemists. This makes it a cost-effective alternative to PET for the relatively rapid evaluation of large samples when testing specific hypotheses about normal functional brain patterns and possible regional cerebral abnormalities in schizophrenia.

Recent advances in SPECT technology and radiotracer synthesis now enable neuroscientists to image rCBF with a resolution of 10 to 12 mm at FWHM. Newer generation SPECT cameras will achieve a resolution of 7 mm or less (ie, resolution below that of most PET cameras presently in service). This could result in the visualization of CBF and neurotransmitter changes in small limbic structures such as the parahippocampus and hippocampus.

Positron Emission Tomography

Positron emission tomography (PET) is the most powerful chemical brain imaging modality currently available for schizophrenia research. The technique allows chemical measurements to be made regionally in discrete cerebral areas in living human subjects. This in vivo analytic capability represents a phenomenal advance over conventional chemical studies that analyze body fluids (eg, cerebrospinal fluid, blood, and urine) at a considerable neurochemical distance from the cerebral region of interest (ROI). Positron emission tomography has been used to measure cerebral blood flow and metabolism. Major advances in radiotracer production and camera design have enabled neuroscientists to study an ever increasing number of chemical compounds in the brain. Advanced tracer kinetic methods allow accurate quantification of such chemical species at picomolar concentrations. Regional neurotransmitter and neuroreceptor distributions can then be displayed in two- and three-dimensional brain images. Advanced computer graphic techniques will allow us to visualize dynamic alterations in individual transmitter systems as a function of time in the future.

The generation and analysis of PET images involves the following basic steps. First a chemical compound is selected, synthesized, and tested to document that it accurately reflects the dynamic characteristics of the neurochemical process being studied. Compounds can be analogues of naturally occurring substances such as glucose and dopamine (fluorodeoxyglucose [FDG] and fluorodopa) or receptor ligands, such as raclopride and spiperone, that bind to receptors. These "cold" substances are tagged with radioisotopes to become radioactive tracers. The choice of an appropriate isotope (11-C, 18-F, 15-O) is partly dependent on the kinetics of the underlying biochemical process. Highly dynamic events are usually visualized with isotopes with a short half-life (t/2); that is, CBF using 15-O (t/2 = 2 minutes). D2 dopamine receptor studies, which typically achieve maximum binding after 20 minutes to 2 hours, require radiotracers with a longer half-life (C-11, t/2 = 20 minutes; 18-F, t/2 = 108 minutes) to allow an adequate representation of the pharmacokinetics of the neurotransmitter system studied. Positron emitters for such studies are generated on site in cyclotrons in close proximity to the PET scanner.

The precise location of the administered isotope is determined by annihilation coincidence detection (ACD). In this process a colliding positron and electron produce two 511 keV gamma rays, which are emitted 180 degrees apart. Opposing PET camera detectors are interconnected to register such photons if they strike detector pairs within 20 nanoseconds of each other. This technique of electronic collimation allows accurate three-dimensional localization of the radioisotope. The resultant PET images represent cross-sectional distributions of positron-emitting radiotracers within the brain. Further physiological modeling of the process is necessary to convert the isotope concentrations into biochemical and biophysical units (eg, micromoles of glucose per hundred gram per minute and D2 receptor density [Bmax]). This can be achieved by applying mathematical kinetic models in the form of differential equations to the data. Parameters such as rCBF can then be determined for individual cerebral structures by defining regions of interest (ROI) on the PET images.

The initial PET study of cerebral metabolism in the living human brain was performed by Reivich et al in 1979.[87] They were able to measure local cerebral glucose metabolic rates (LCMRGlc) by adapting Sokoloff's tracer kinetic autoradiographic model to PET.[88] This breakthough led to the widespread acceptance of PET as a quantitative analytical research technique for the measurement of physiological and chemical parameters in vivo.

Farkas et al[89] examined the first schizophrenic patient with 18-F fluoro-deoxyglucose (18-FDG) and PET in 1980. This study appeared to confirm Ingvar's earlier finding of hypofrontality in schizophrenia. Repeat scans of the same patient after neuroleptic medication resulted in a partial reversal of the hypofrontal pattern.[89] Subsequent PET investigators measured cerebral metabolism in acute and chronic schizophrenics on and off neuroleptics using 15-O, 11-C-glucose, and 18-FDG as radiotracers. Acute schizophrenics failed to demonstrate prominent metabolic abnormalities.[90] Some, but not all, studies in chronic schizophrenics reported reduced absolute and/or relative frontal metabolic rates.[91,92] Hemispheric asymmetry (left > right) and increased metabolic rates in the temporal lobes and basal ganglia also were found.[93] It was furthermore demonstrated that neuroleptics increased metabolism in the neostriatum and, to a lesser extent, in the cortical structures (Fig. 8.5).[94]

A substantial number of authors have failed to replicate the metabolic results of these initial PET studies.[95–100] A combination of patient- and PET-related methodological factors may account partly for the discrepant findings. Most PET studies performed in the past contained very small sample numbers ($N < 15$). Schizophrenic populations varied in mean age, disease duration, and severity of illness. Few patients were drug naive or totally drug free (ie, adequately washed out) at the time of the PET scan. The various protocols also differed in the ambient conditions that existed during isotope uptake. Lastly, the variability of metabolic PET findings may represent differences in phenotypic biochemical expression in an inherently heterogeneous schizophrenic syndrome.

It is also difficult to compare these pioneering investigations for the following PET-related methodological reasons. The various studies were performed with different tracers and camera types. The first and second generation tomographs used had a limited spatial resolution (> 15 mm in plane, full width at half maximum [FWHM]) and could only examine relatively large structures such as the caudate nucleus or entire lobes to limit partial volume effects.[101] Different anatomical localization schemes were used to delineate cerebral regions of interest.

A combination of two cardinal events has radically improved the outlook for and interest in PET schizophrenia research. First is the availability of new-generation high-resolution PET scanners. Current state-of-the-art PET cameras achieve a spatial resolution of 5.5 mm, which is close to the theoretical limit of 2 to 3 mm. They are able to acquire 15 planes

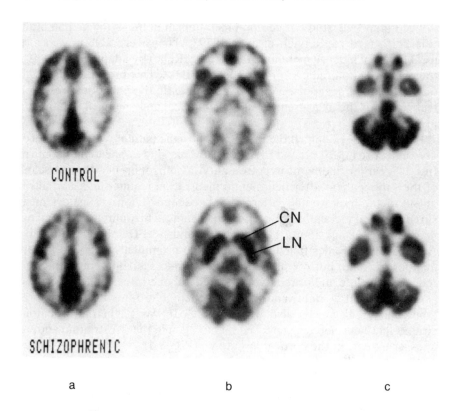

FIGURE 8.5. [¹⁸F]Fluorodeoxyglucose PET scans of a chronic schizophrenic with tardive dyskinesia (TD) and a normal control. The transaxial images reflect resting glucose metabolism of three nonconsecutive slices through the brain at the level of (a) the centrum semiovale, (b) the basal ganglia, and (c) the cerebellum. The caudate nucleus (CN) and lenticular nucleus (LN) of the TD patient appear increased in size and intensity. (Isotope uptake occurred in the eyes and ears open mode in a quiet dark room in the absence of voluntary movements.)

simultaneously in all three orthogonal planes. This major technical advance will allow us to probe small medial temporal lobe structures, such as the hippocampus, in standard axial, coronal, and sagittal views. Second, newly developed radiotracers allow us to regionally dissect component parts of individual neurochemical systems, including those that have been implicated in the pathophysiology of schizophrenia.

The decision to use PET to study the dopaminergic system in schizophrenia is primarily based on chemical lines of evidence supporting the dopaminergic hypothesis.[102] Postsynaptic D2 receptors were selected for initial PET investigation after studies of peripheral body fluids and in vitro postmortem studies failed to find presynaptic neuronal overactivity while demonstrating increases in D2 dopamine receptor density. The reasoning for this approach was further strengthened when additional neurochemical studies failed to show consistent abnormalities in other neurotransmitter systems. Lastly, PET scanning of the dopaminergic system proved eminently feasible as 85% of central dopaminergic terminals are localized in the caudate and putamen, two structures which are sufficiently large to allow accurate sampling with PET.

Two approaches have been used in the PET estimation of D2 dopamine receptor density in schizophrenia. One study using quantitative compartmental analysis was performed on haloperidol-induced inhibition of [11-C] N-methylspiperone postsynaptic binding.[103] The study showed a surprising two- to threefold elevation of D2 dopamine receptors in the basal ganglia of ten drug-naive subjects and five previously treated schizophrenic patients. The second study of Farde et al[104] used 11-C raclopride, a ligand that shows greater reversible binding than spiperone, to determine D2 dopamine receptor density. The quantitative saturation analysis method used failed to show an increase in D2 dopamine receptor numbers.[104]

The following factors could account for the inconsistent results of the above-mentioned PET examinations. Patients in the first study were older than in the second. Their disease duration was longer than that of the Farde group. Furthermore, the two ligands used, [11-C[raclopride and [11-C] N-methylspiperone, possess different receptor and serum protein binding chracteristics that necessitate radically different kinetic modeling approaches. [11-C] raclopride has a much lower affinity for the D2 dopaminergic receptor than [11-C] N-methylspiperone. Increased endogenous dopamine turnover, which is theoretically possible in a subgroup of schizophrenics, would lead to much greater displacement of [11-C] raclopride than [11-C] N-methylspiperone from the receptor. On the other hand, raclopride also has much greater specificity for the D2 receptor. Further studies of the postsynaptic D2 dopamine receptors in drug-naive schizophrenics are essential to decide whether or not elevation in receptor numbers is an inherent pathophysiological event in schizophrenia.

The focus of psychiatric research in the upcoming decade will shift even further toward the basic neurosciences. Positron emission tomography will increasingly be used as a basic neuroscience laboratory tool to determine the anatomical localization of underlying primary pathological processes and to understand the pathophysiological events resulting in schizophrenia. As a result, psychiatric diagnostic systems may become more biochemically oriented. Furthermore, PET may be used to identify subjects at high risk for developing schizophrenia. It may even become feasible to diagnose patients before they manifest their illness. It should also be possible to monitor the effects of somatic treatments by measuring their effect on selected PET variables. Lastly, new psychopharmacological agents could be developed and characterized pharmacokinetically with the aid of dynamic high-resolution PET.

Clinical Applications of Functional Imaging

This review has emphasized research findings rather than clinical applications of brain imaging in schizophrenia. Technical advances in isotope production, radiotracer synthesis, and SPECT and PET camera design may make the functional imaging modalities indispensible to clinical psychiatric practice in the near future. Psychiatrists have only recently started using structural imaging techniques to diagnose psychoses of focal organic etiology. Thus, they have used x-ray CT and MRI to identify a small percentage of subjects presenting with schizophreniform symptoms due to conditions such as Huntington's disease, temporal lobe epilepsy, or tumors.

Single photon emission computed tomography and PET may eventually come to play a central role in the everyday management of neuroleptic therapy, in routine cases and in treatment-resistant schizophrenics. Optimal neuroleptic drug doses may be related to the degree of D2 dopamine receptor occupancy in the striatum. Such occupancy studies already have been performed in the research setting.[104] Drug receptor occupancy rates may prove more relevant than serum drug levels when determining possible therapeutic windows for individual neuroleptics. Compelling evidence now exists that shows that substantial central drug occupancy remains for more than 24 hours after drug discontinuation, at a time when serum drug levels already have fallen to negligible values (Fig 8.6).[105]

Further pharmacokinetic information gained from SPECT and PET

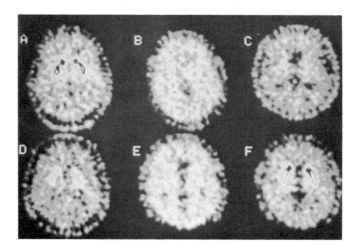

FIGURE 8.6. [¹¹-C]Raclopride PET image of a schizophrenic before and after neuroleptic treatment. As shown, [¹¹-C]raclopride binds specifically to the D2 receptor. Prior occupancy of the receptor with "cold" haloperidol reduces radioligand binding. Images were acquired by the research group at the Karolinska Institute, Stockholm. (Modified and reproduced with permission from Farde et al.[105] Copyright © 1988, American Medical Association.)

studies will also help to determine minimal efficacious antipsychotic doses for individual schizophrenics. This approach hopefully will lead to a reduction in neuroleptic cognitive and extrapyramidal side effects including akathisia, parkinsonism, and tardive dyskinesia.

Single photon emission computed tomography and PET are presently undergoing further technical refinements that will allow them to be implemented in routine psychiatric patient management. Both radioisotope production and chemical tracer synthesis can now be performed on a semiautomatic basis, thus substantially reducing the expense of PET studies. However, SPECT, which uses commercially available noncyclotron based radiotracers, will probably become the functional imaging modality of choice due to the ease of operation and cost-effectiveness of this imaging technique.

Summary

Psychiatric neuroscientists are currently focusing their research efforts on identifying anatomical and neurochemical substrates for the schizophrenic syndrome. Structural and functional brain imaging studies in living human beings complement post-mortem histologic and autoradiographic investigations in this endeavor.

Studies have focused mainly on the ventricles, the frontal and temporal lobes, and the dopaminergic neurotransmitter system. Thus, pathological investigations have shown a reduction in the size of medial temporal lobe structures and compensatory dilatation of the adjacent temporal horn of the lateral ventricle. Histologic examinations have detected malalignment of hippocampal pyramidal cells. Autoradiographic studies have demonstrated increased D2 dopamine receptor numbers in the putamen of both drug naive and neuroleptically treated schizophrenics.

X-ray CT and MRI have replicated post-mortem structural findings. They have shown lateral ventricular enlargement in a subset (20%) of schizophrenics. The majority of patients and most female patients, however, fail to demonstrate ventricular dilitation. Thus, schizophrenia researchers must also focus their research efforts on the in vivo neurochemistry and metabolic function of the brain.

Functional brain imaging modalities such as positron emission tomography (PET) and single photon emission computed tomography (SPECT) have become powerful new tools in these research endeavors. Initial PET studies in schizophrenia have shown hypometabolism of the frontal lobes in chronic schizophrenics, and one study has reported increased numbers of D2 dopaminergic receptors in drug-naive schizophrenics. These results have not been consistently replicated, however. Further studies are underway using new ligands and PET cameras of improved design and resolution capability. Thus, it would seem that neuroscientists have entered into a new phase of biological psychiatric research.

References

1. Phelps ME, Mazziotta JC: Positron emission tomography: human brain function and biochemistry. *Science* 1985;228:799–809.
2. Jacobi W, Winkler H: Encephalographische studien an chronischen schizophrenen. *Arch Psychiatr Nervenkr* 1927;81:299–332.
3. LeMay M: Changes in ventricular size during and after pneumoencephalography. *Radiology* 1967;88:57–63.
4. Johnstone EC, Frith CD, Crow TJ, et al: Cerebral ventricular size and cognitive impairment in chronic schizophrenia. *Lancet* 1976;ii:924–926.
5. Jernigan TL, Zatz LM, Moses JA, et al: Computed tomography in schizophrenics and normal volunteers: I. Fluid volume. *Arch Gen Psychiatry* 1982;39:765–770.
6. Reveley MA: Ventricular enlargement in schizophrenia: the validity of computerised tomographic findings. *Br J Psychiatr* 1985;147:233–240.
7. Weinberger DR, Torrey EF, Neophytides AN, et al: Lateral cerebral ventricular enlargement in chronic schizophrenia. *Arch Gen Psychiatry* 1979;36:735–739.
8. Glück E, Radu EW, Mundt C, et al: A computed tomographic protective trohoc study of chronic schizophrenics. *Neuroradiology* 1980;20:167–171.
9. Moriguchi I: A study of schizophrenic brains by computerized tomography scans. *Folia Psychiatrica et Neurologica Japonica* 1981;35:55–72.
10. Pearlson GD, Veroff AE: Computerised tomographic scan changes in manic-depressive illiness. *Lancet* 1981;ii:470.
11. Takahashi R, Inaba Y, Inanaga K, et al: CT scanning and the investigation of schizophrenia. *Biol Psychiatry* 1981;9:259–268.
12. Tanaka Y, Hazama H, Kawahara R, et al: Computerized tomography of the brain in schizophrenic patients. *Acta Psychiatr Scand* 1981;63:191–197.
13. Weinberger DR, DeLisi LE, Neophytides AN, et al: Familial aspects of CT scan abnormalities in chronic schizophrenic patients. *Psychiatry Res* 1981;4:65–71.
14. Andreasen NC, Smith MR, Jacoby CG, et al: Ventricular enlargement in schizophrenia: definition and prevalence. *Am J Psychiatry* 1982;139:292–296.
15. Benes F, Sunderland P, Jones BD, et al: Normal ventricles in young schizophrenics. *Br J Psychol* 1982;141:90–93.
16. Nasrallah HA, Jacoby CG, McCalley-Whitters M, et al: Cerebral ventricular enlargement in subtypes of chronic schizophrenia. *Arch Gen Psychiatry* 1982;39:774–777.
17. Nyback H, Wiesel F-A, Berggren B-M, et al: Computed tomography of the brain in patients with acute psychosis and in healthy volunteers. *Acta Psychiatr Scand* 1982;65:403–414.
18. Okasha A, Madkour O: Cortical and central atrophy in chronic schizophrenia: a controlled study. *Acta Psychiatr Scand* 1982;65:29–34.
19. Reveley AM, Clifford CA, Reveley MA, et al: Cerebral ventricular size in twins discordant for schizophrenia. *Lancet* 1982;i:540–541.
20. Weinberger DR, DeLisi LE, Perman GP, et al: Computed tomography in schizophreniform disorder and other acute psychiatric disorders. *Arch Gen Psychiatry* 1982;39:778–783.
21. Bishop RJ, Golden CJ, MacInnes WD, et al: The BPRS in assessing symp-

tom correlates of cerebral ventricular enlargement in acute and chronic schizophrenia. *Psychiatry Res* 1983;9:225–231.

22. Kling AS, Kurtz N, Tachiki K, et al: CT scans in sub-groups of chronic schizophrenics. *J Psychiatr Res* 1983;17:375–384.

23. Schulz SC, Koller MM, Kishore PR, et al: Ventricular enlargement in teenage patients with schizophrenia spectrum disorder. *Am J Psychiatry* 1983;140:1592–1595.

24. Woods BT, Wolf J: A reconsideration of the relation of ventricular enlargement to duration of illness in schizophrenia. *Am J Psychiatry* 1983;140:1564–1570.

25. Largen JW, Smith RC, Calderon M, et al: Abnormalities of brain structure and density in schizophrenia. *Biol Psychiatry* 1984;19:991–1013.

26. Luchins DJ, Lewine RRJ, Meltzer HY: Lateral ventricular size, psychopathology, and medication response in the psychoses. *Biol Psychiatry* 1984;19:29–44.

27. DeMeyer MK, Gilmore R, DeMeyer WE, et al: Third ventricle size and ventricular brain ratio in treatment-resistant psychiatric patients. J *Operational Psychiatry* 1984;15:2–8.

28. Pandurangi AK, Dewan MJ, Lee SH, et al: The ventricular system in chronic schizophrenic patients: a controlled computed tomography study. *Br J Psychiatr* 1984;144:172–176.

29. Pearlson GD, Garbacz DJ, Breakey WR, et al: Lateral ventricular enlargement associated with persistent unemployment and negative symptoms in both schizophrenia and bipolar disorder. *Psychiatry Res* 1984;12:1–9.

30. Andreasen NC: CT scan data in male and female schizophrenics. Abstracts, American Psychiatric Association Annual Meeting, 1984.

31. Carr EG, Wedding D: Neuropsychological assessment of cerebral ventricular size in chronic schizophrenics. *Int J Clin Neuropsychol* 1984;6:106–111.

32. Schulsinger F, Parnas J, Petersen ET, et al: Cerebral ventricular size in the offspring of schizophrenic mothers. *Arch Gen Psychiatry* 1984;41:602–606.

33. Boronow J, Pickar D, Ninan PT, et al: Atrophy limited to the third ventricle in chronic schizophrenic patients. *Arch Gen Psychiatry* 1985;42:266–271.

34. DeLisi LE, Goldin LR, Hamovit JR, et al: Cerebral ventricular enlargement as a possible genetic marker for schizophrenia. *Psychopharmacol Bull* 1985;21:365–367.

35. Kemali D, Maj M, Galderisi S, et al: Clinical and neuropsychological correlates of cerebral ventricular enlargement in schizophrenia. *J Psychiatr Res* 1985;19:587–596.

36. King DJ, Cooper SJ, Earle JAP, et al: Serum and CSF antibody titres to seven common viruses in schizophrenic patients. *Br J Psychiatr* 1985;147:145–149.

37. Owens DGC, Johnstone EC, Crow TJ, et al: Lateral ventricular size in schzophrenia: relationship to the disease process and its clinical manifestations. *Psychol Med* 1985;15:27–41.

38. Shima S, Kanba S, Masuda Y, et al: Normal ventricles in chronic schizophrenics. *Acta Psychiatr Scand* 1985;71:25–29.

39. Williams AO, Reveley MA, Kolakowska T, et al: Schizophrenia with good and poor outcome. II: Cerebral ventricular size and its clinical significance. *Br J Psychiatr* 1985;146:239–246.

40. Losonczy MF, Song IS, Mohs RC, et al: Correlates of lateral ventricular size in chronic schizophrenia, I: Behavioral and treatment response measures. *Am J Psychiatry* 1986;143:976–981.
41. Obiols-Llandrich JE, Ruscalleda J, Masferrer M: Ventricular enlargement in young chronic schizophrenics. *Acta Psychiatr Scand* 1986;73:42–44.
42. Turner SW, Toone BK, Brett-Jones JR: Computerized tomographic scan changes in early schizophrenia—preliminary findings. *Psychol Med* 1986;16:219–225.
43. Rabins P, Pearlson G, Jayaram G, et al: Increased ventricle-to-brain ratio in late-onset schizophrenia. *Am J Psychiatry* 1987;144:1215–1218.
44. Romani A, Merello S, Gozzoli L, et al: P300 and CT scan patients with chronic schizophrenia. *Br J Psychiatr* 1987;151:506–513.
45. Rossi A, de Cataldo S, Stratta P, et al: Cerebral atrophy and neuropsychological correlates in schizophrenia. *Acta Psychiat Belg* 1987;87:670–675.
46. Iacono WG, Smith GN, Moreau M, et al: Ventricular and sulcal size at the onset of psychosis. *Am J Psychiatry* 1988;145:820–824.
47. Rossi A, Stratta P, de Cataldo S, et al: Cortical and subcortical computed tomographic study in schizophrenia. *J Psychiat Res* 1988;22:99–105.
48. Shelton RC, Karson CN, Doran AR, et al: Cerebral structural pathology in schizophrenia: evidence for a selective prefrontal cortical defect. *Am J Psychiatry* 1988;145:154–163.
49. Wolkin A, Angrist B, Wolf A, et al: Low frontal glucose utilization in chronic schizophrenia: a replication study. *Am J Psychiatry* 1988;145:251–253.
50. Pfefferbaum A, Zipursky RB, Lim KO, et al: Computed tomographic evidence for generalized sulcal and ventricular enlargement in schizophrenia. *Arch Gen Psychiatry* 1988;45:633–640.
51. Stevens JR: Neuropathology of schizophrenia. *Arch Gen Psychiatry* 1982;39:1131–1139.
52. Benes FM, Davidson J, Bird ED: Quantitative cytoarchitectural studies of the cerebral cortex of schizophrenics. *Arch Gen Psychiatry* 1986;43:31–35.
53. Jacobson RR, Turner SW, Baldy RD, et al: Densitometric analysis of scans: important sources of artefact. *Psychol Med* 1985;15:879–889.
54. Swayze II VW, Yates WR, Andreasen NC, et al: CT abnormalities in tardive dyskinesia. *Psychiatry Res* 1988;26:51–58.
55. Donnelly EF, Weinberger DR, Waldman IN, et al: Cognitive impairment associated with morphological brain abnormalities on computed tomography in chronic schizophrenic patients. *J Nerv Ment Dis* 1980;168:305–308.
56. Kolakowska T, Williams AO, Jambor K, et al: Schizophrenia with good and poor outcome, III: Neurological 'soft' signs, cognitive impairment and their clinical significance. *Br J Psychiatr* 1985;146:348–357.
57. Weinberger DR, Cannon-Spoor E, Potkin SG, et al: Poor premorbid adjustment and CT scan abnormalities in chronic schizophrenia. *Am J Psychiatry* 1980;137:1410–1413.
58. van Kammen DP, Mann LS, Sternberg DE, et al: Dopamine-β-hydroxylase activity and homovanillic acid in spinal fluid of schizophrenics with brain atrophy. *Science* 1983;220:974–977.
59. van Kammen DP, Mann LS, Scheinin M, et al: Spinal fluid monoamine metabolites and anticytomegalovirus antibodies and brain scan evaluation in schizophrenia. *Psychopharmacol Bull* 1984;20:519–522.
60. Potkin SG, Weinberger DR, Linnoila M, et al: Low CSF 5-hydroxyindole-

acetic acid in schizophrenic patients with enlarged cerebral ventricles. *Am J Psychiatry* 1983;140:21–25.

61. Nyback H, Berggren B-M, Hindmarsh T, et al: Cerebroventricular size and cerebrospinal fluid monoamine metabolites in schizophrenic patients and healthy volunteers. *Psychiatry Res* 1983;9:301–308.

62. Jaskiw GE, Andreasen NC, Weinberger DR: X-ray computed tomography and magnetic resonance imaging in psychiatry, in Hales RE, Frances AJ (eds): *American Psychiatric Association Annual Review*, vol. 6. Washington, DC, American Psychiatric Press, Inc., 1987, pp 260–299.

63. Nasrallah HA, Olson SC, McCalley-Whitters M, et al: Cerebral ventricular enlargement in schizophrenia. *Arch Gen Psychiatry* 1986;43:157–159.

64. Illowsky BP, Juliano DM, Bigelow LB, et al: Stability of CT scan findings in schizophrenia: results of an 8-year follow-up study. *J Neurol Neurosurg Psychiatry* 1988;51:209–213.

65. Brant-Zawadski M, Norman D (eds): *Magnetic Resonance Imaging of the Central Nervous System*. New York, Raven Press, 1987.

66. Oldendorf W, Oldendorf Jr W: Basics of magnetic resonance imaging. Hingham, MA, Martinus Nijhoff, 1988, pp 1–180.

67. Johnstone EC, Crow TJ, Macmillan JF, et al: A magnetic resonance study of early schizophrenia. *J Neurol Neurosurg Psychiatry* 1986;49:136–139.

68. Smith RC, Calderon M, Ravichandran GK, et al: Nuclear magnetic resonance in schizophrenia: a preliminary study. *Psychiatry Res* 1984;12:137–147.

69. Mathew RJ, Partain CL: Midsagittal sections of the cerebellar vermis and fourth ventricle obtained with magnetic resonance imaging of schizophrenic patients. *Am J Psychiatry* 1985;142:970–971.

70. Mathew RJ, Partain CL, Prakash R, et al: A study of the septum pellucidum and corpus callosum in schizophrenia with MR imaging. *Acta Psychiatr Scand* 1985;72:414–421.

71. Andreasen NC, Nasrallah HA, Dunn VD, et al: Structural abnormalities in the frontal system in schizophrenia: a magnetic resonance imaging study. *Arch Gen Psychiatry* 1986;43:136–144.

72. Nasrallah HA, Andreasen NC, Coffman JA, et al: A controlled magnetic resonance imaging study of corpus callosum thickness in schizophrenia. *Biol Psychiatry* 1986;21:274–282.

73. Smith RC, Baumgartner R, Calderon M: Magnetic resonance imaging studies of the brains of schizophrenic patients. *Psychiatry Res* 1987;20:33–46.

74. Rossi A, Stratta P, Gallucci M, et al: Standardized magnetic resonance image intensity study in schizophrenia. *Psychiatry Res* 1988;25:223–231.

75. Kelsoe JR, Cadet JL, Pickar D, et al: Quantitative neuroanatomy in schizophrenia. *Arch Gen Psychiatry* 1988;45:533–541.

76. DeMyer MK, Gilmor RL, Hendrie HC, et al: Magnetic resonance brain images in schizophrenic and normal subjects: influence of diagnosis and education. *Schizophr Bull* 1988;14:21–37.

77. Andreasen NC, Ehrhardt JC, Swayze VW, et al: Magnetic resonance imaging of the brain in schizophrenia: pathophysiological significance of structural abnormalities. *Arch Gen Psychiatry* 1989, in press.

78. Besson JAO, Corrigan FM, Cherryman GR, et al: Nuclear magnetic resonance brain imaging in chronic schizophrenia *Br J Psychiatr* 1987;150:161–163.

188   Jörg J. Pahl, Victor W. Swayze, and Nancy C. Andreasen

79. Andreasen NC, Ehrhardt JC, Swayze VW, et al: T1 and T2 relaxation times in schizophrenia as measured with magnetic resonance imaging. *Arch Gen Psychiatry* 1989, in press.
80. Roy CS, Sherrington CS: The regulation of the blood supply of the brain. *J Physiol* 1890;11:85–121.
81. Kety SS, Woodford RB, Harmel MH, et al: Cerebral blood flow and metabolism in schizophrenia: the effects of barbiturate seminarcosis, insulin coma and electroshock. *Am J Psychiatry* 1948;104:765–770.
82. Ingvar DH: "Hyperfrontal" distribution of the cerebral grey matter flow in resting wakefulness; on the functional anatomy of the conscious state. *Acta Neurol Scandinav* 1979;50:425–462.
83. Ingvar DH, Franzen G: Abnormalities of cerebral blood flow distribution in patients with chronic schizophrenia. *Acta Psychiatr Scand* 1974;50:425–462.
84. Berman KF, Zec RF, Weinberger DR: Physiologic dysfunction of dorsolateral prefrontal cortex in schizophrenia. II. Role of neuroleptic treatment, attention, and mental effort. *Arch Gen Psychiatry* 1986;43:126–135.
85. Shirahata N, Henriksen L, Vorstrup S, et al: Regional cerebral blood flow assessed by ^{133}Xe inhalation and emission tomography: normal values. *J Comput Assist Tomogr* 1985;9:861–866.
86. Devous MD: Imaging brain function by single photon emission computer tomography in Andreasen NC (ed): *Brain Imaging: Applications in Psychiatry*. American Psychiatric Press, Inc., 1989.
87. Reivich M, Kuhl D, Wolf A: The [18F]fluorodeoxyglucose method for the measurement of local cerebral glucose utilization in man. *Circ Res* 1979;44:127–137.
88. Sokoloff L, Reivich M, Kennedy C: The [14C]deoxyglucose method for the measurement of local cerebral glucose utilization theory, procedure, and moral values in the conscious and anesthetized albino rat. *J Neurochem* 1977;28:897–916.
89. Farkas T, Reivich M, Alavi A, et al: [18F]2-deoxy-2-fluoro-D-glucose and positron emission tomography in the study of psychiatric conditions, in Passonneau JV, Hawkins RA, Lust WD, Welsh FA (eds): *Cerebral Metabolism and Neural Function*. Baltimore/London, Williams & Wilkins, 1980, pp. 403–408.
90. Sheppard G, Gruyzelier J, Manchanda R, et al: 150 positron emission tomographic scanning in predominantly never-treated acute schizophrenic patients. *Lancet* 1983;24/31:1448–1452.
91. Buchsbaum MS, Ingvar DH, Kessler R, et al: Cerebral glucography with positron tomography. Use in normal subjects and in patients with schizophrenia. *Arch Gen Psychiatry* 1982;39:251–259.
92. Farkas T, Wolf AP, Jaeger J, et al: Regional brain glucose metabolism in chronic schizophrenia: a positron emission transaxial tomographic study. *Arch Gen Psychiatry* 1984;41:293–300.
93. Widen L, Blomqvist G, Greitz T, et al: PET studies of glucose metabolism in patients with schizophrenia. *AJNR* 1983;4:550–552.
94. Wolkin A, Jaeger J, Brodie JD, et al: Persistence of cerebral metabolic abnormalities in chronic schizophrenia as determined by positron emission tomography. *Am J Psychiatry* 1985;142:564–571.
95. Jernigan TL, Sargent T, Pfefferbaum A, et al: 18Fluorodeoxyglucose PET in schizophrenia. *Psychiatry Res* 1985;16:317–329.

96. Gur RE, Resnick SM, Alavi A, et al: Regional brain function in schizophrenia. I. A positron emission tomography study. *Arch Gen Psychol* 1987;44:119–125.
97. Gur RE, Resnick SM, Gur RC, et al: Regional brain function in schizophrenia. II. Repeated evaluation with positron emission tomography. *Arch Gen Psychiatry* 1987;44:126–129.
98. Kling AS, Metter EJ, Riege WH, et al: Comparison of PET measurement of local brain glucose metabolism and CAT measurement of brain atrophy in chronic schizophrenia and depression. *Am J Psychiatry* 1986;143:175–180.
99. Volkow ND, Brodie JD, Wolf AP, et al: Brain organization in schizophrenia. *J Cereb Blood Flow Metab* 1986;6:441–446.
100. Williamson P: Hypofrontality in schizophrenia: a review of the evidence. *Can J Psychiatry* 1987;32:399–404.
101. Mazziotta JC, Phelps ME, Kuhl DE: Quantitation in positron emission computed tomography. 5. Physical-anatomical effects. *J Comput Assist Tomogr* 1981;5:734–43.
102. Seeman P: Dopamine receptors and the dopamine hypothesis of schizophrenia. *Synapse* 1987;1:133–152.
103. Wong DF, Wagner HN, Tune LE, et al: Positron emission tomography reveals elevated D2 dopamine receptors in drug-naive schizophrenics. *Science* 1986;234:1558–1563.
104. Farde L, Hall H, Ehrin E, et al: Quantitative analysis of D2 dopamine receptor binding in the living human brain by PET. *Science* 1986;231:258–261.
105. Farde L, Wiesel FA, Halldin C, et al: Central D2-dopamine receptor occupancy in schizophrenic patients treated with antipsychotic drugs. *Arch Gen Psychiatry* 1988;45:71–76.

9
Risk Factors and Prevention in Schizophrenia

MICHAEL J. GOLDSTEIN

Current thinking concerning the prevention of schizophrenia focuses on two issues, whether or not the initial onset of the disorder is preventable and whether recurrence can be prevented or delayed substantially once the initial episode has occurred. To answer these questions it is necessary to establish risk factors either within the individual or his or her social environment whose modification can alter the probability of the initial onset or recurrence of a schizophrenic disorder. The purpose of the present chapter is to review the current state of evidence regarding the establishment of risk factors within the domain of psychosocial variables (including those usually termed neurobehavioral), as well as to review any attempts to use these risk factors in intervention studies. The emerging data from studies of high-risk populations (see Goldstein and Asarnow[1] and Goldstein and Tuma[2] for a summary of some of these studies) have not generated as yet controlled clinical trials designed to prevent the initial episode of schizophrenia. Most intervention studies have focused on the important but more modest goal of preventing recurrence.

Vulnerability Stress Model

Psychosocial issues refer to psychological attributes of individuals or their social environment that play a contributory role to the onset, course, or treatment of a schizophrenic disorder. Most contemporary researchers investigate psychosocial variables within the context of a vulnerability stress model[3] in which behavioral markers of personal vulnerability are studied within the context of environmental stressors, both intra- and extrafamilial.

Whereas the vulnerability stress model is intuitively appealing, to be useful it requires greater specification of potential vulnerability markers and stressor conditions likely to relate to the onset and course of schizophrenia. Figure 9.1 presents one model developed by Nuechterlein and Liberman designed to specify the variables likely to relate to the onset

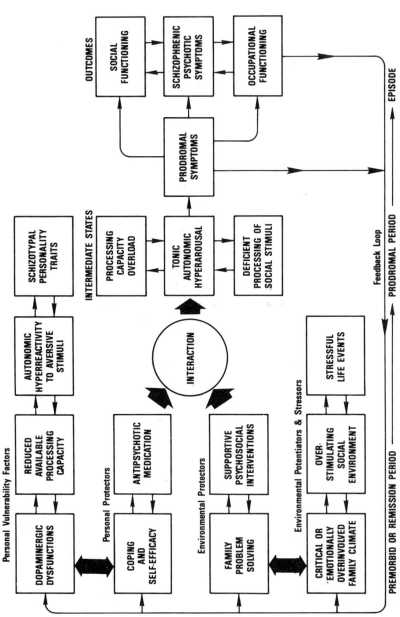

FIGURE 9.1. A schematic articulation of the vulnerability-stress model which specifies the complex interactions among hypothetical personal vulnerability and stressor conditions involved in the onset and course of schizophrenia. For both vulnerability and stress conditions, factors potentially protective of their impact are suggested as well. (Reprinted with permission from Nuechterlein.[4])

and course of schizophrenia.[4] Note that the scheme proposed is an iterative one in which similar variables, hypothesized to be present in the premorbid phase of development, are also relevant factors after an episode of the disorder has occurred. The scheme in Figure 9.1 also distinguishes between factors that increase the risk for the onset of relapse of the disorder and those deemed protective against these events.

There is some question as to the conceptual independence of risk and protective factors, as it has been noted that frequently one is simply the inverse of the other. Ideally, a protective factor should be identified by its ability to modify the outcome for an individual previously identified as being at risk for a disorder. At the present time, there are no clear biological or behavioral markers of the risk for schizophrenia applicable to individuals that permit a clear analysis of modification of life course by protective factors. However, there are some suggestions from the high-risk studies summarized below that research of this sort will be possible in the near future.

In the review that follows, we first examine the nature of the evidence for personal vulnerability markers for schizophrenia. Following this, we examine the evidence regarding stressors that may interact with these personal vulnerability factors to increase the probability of an initial episode of a schizophrenic disorder. In the remaining sections of the chapter we evaluate the role of vulnerability and stress factors in determining the course of schizophrenia and the implications of these findings for intervention programs.

Childhood and Adolescent Markers of Vulnerability High-Risk Studies

Most of the evidence regarding early behavioral signs of a vulnerability to schizophrenia have come from what have been termed high-risk studies, in which samples of individuals hypothesized to be at greater than the population risk for schizophrenia are studied prospectively from a developmental period that antedates the onset of schizophrenia or its prodromal phases. Most high-risk projects have examined children considered to be at risk by virtue of having a biological parent with schizophrenia. Ultimately it will be necessary to test the value of these vulnerability markers in samples lacking parents with schizophrenia to determine whether they can be used in large scale screening or preventive intervention trials.

High-risk studies are designed to answer three important questions: (1) Are there behavioral indicators that discriminate the offspring of schizophrenics likely to develop the disorder from those who will not? (2) Are these discriminating attributes unique to schizophrenia or are they merely nonspecific signs of maladaptation indicative of a vulnerability to psychiatric disorder in general? (3) Are these attributes observed in the children of nonpsychiatrically affected parents and do they have any prognostic significance in this context?

It is important to recognize that analogous questions are applicable to the identification of stressor conditions likely to increase the risk for schizophrenia in vulnerable persons, namely do these stressor conditions have a specific connection to schizophrenia or are they nonspecific stressors likely to increase the risk for psychiatric disorders in general? Are they generalizable to samples where parental schizophrenia was not present?

To provide a developmental perspective of potential vulnerability markers for schizophrenia, we consider the results of studies separately for four age periods: (1) conception to infancy, (2) early childhood, (3) middle childhood, and (4) adolescence. The potential vulnerability markers fall into three broad categories: (1) neurointegrative functioning, a general term that refers to neuromotor, attentional, autonomic nervous system reactivity, and cognitive processes; (2) social behavior; and (3) early symptoms of maladjustment.

It should be noted that different high-risk studies have used different kinds of comparison groups. Generally when high-risk subjects were compared with children of parents with other forms of psychiatric disorder, differences were not as pronounced as when they were compared with children of normal controls. This section of this chapter is based on a previous review of the high-risk literature by Asarnow and Goldstein.[5]

Conception to Infancy

Much of the data on the general status and neurointegrative functioning of the infant are contradictory. Walker and Emory[6] conclude that the bulk of the evidence on fetal neonatal death and birth weight for surviving infants indicate no significant differences between children of schizophrenics and controls. The exception is McNeil et al,[7] who found that children of schizophrenics were small for gestational age, relative to offspring of controls, but not different in length, head circumference, or shoulder circumference. This may relate to reports from other studies of children of schizophrenics of erratic growth and deviations in musculoskeletal development[8,9]. As Walker and Emory[6] point out, being small for gestational age may reflect intrauterine growth retardation, which when extreme has been linked to later learning and attentional problems.

Three studies[8,10-14] have identified subgroups of infant children of schizophrenic mothers who showed deviant development and were the subgroup most likely to develop schizophrenia or related disorders in adulthood. However, the type of deviant development identified was not consistent across studies. Fish's[8] deviant sample showed pandysmaturation or periods when gross motor, visual motor, and physical development were transiently disorganized. Preschizophrenic and preschizotypal infants in the Danish sample[13] were described as passive, unenergetic, and having a short attention span, whereas Marcus et al[11] described 13 infants of schizophrenic mothers who showed poor motor and sensorimotor performance during their first year. Although these findings are intriguing, as they suggest the emergence of signs of vulnerability to schizophrenia in infancy, they must be interpreted with caution as there is little evidence that these patterns are consistent across studies or that they are specific markers for subsequent schizophrenia.

It has frequently been hypothesized that certain patterns of social behavior in infancy might serve as vulnerability markers for schizophrenia. According to a recent review,[5] infants of schizophrenic mothers were found to have: more difficult temperaments; show a lower threshold to stimulation; be more inhibited, apathetic, or withdrawn; be less responsive to verbal commands; and be less spontaneous and initiative. Recent findings[15] indicate that offspring of psychotic parents are less likely to show a fear of strangers during the first year of life. One-year-old infants of schizophrenics, but not infants of mothers with other psychotic conditions, also were found to show significantly increased rates of anxious attachment as defined by Ainsworth and Wittig's[16] classification system. This finding should be viewed with caution however, as Sameroff et al[17] did not find deviant attachment patterns in infants of schizophrenic mothers.

Early Childhood (Ages Two to Four)

Two studies support observations of neurointegrative problems in early childhood. Sameroff et al[17] found lower reactivity in 2.5-year-old children of schizophrenics than in controls, and Hanson et al[18] reported poorer gross and fine motor performance in children of schizophrenics when compared with children of nonschizophrenic psychiatric controls.

With regard to signs of deviance in social behavior in early childhood, Sameroff et al[17] found more parental reports of depression in children of schizophrenics than in children of well controls. Goodman[19] found that children of schizophrenic mothers were more likely to receive diagnoses of developmental disorders than were children of depressed or well mothers. Hanson et al[18] reported that children of schizophrenics were more often described as schizoid (ie, emotionally flat, withdrawn, distractable, passive, irritable, and negativistic).

Middle Childhood (Ages Five to Twelve)

Reports of the various high-risk studies that have assessed neuropsychological functioning during this period have consistently indicated some impairment in certain high-risk children.[8,11,20–22] Impaired fine motor coordination is the single sign reported by all investigators.[20] Several studies also reported delays in motor development similar to those reported in infancy and early childhood. Marcus et al[11,12] in their follow-up of the Israeli High-Risk Study, showed that 5 of 6 children who later showed "schizophrenia spectrum psychoses" showed earlier difficulties in neuropsychological functioning.

In the analyses of attention and information processing (AIP) tasks in children of schizophrenics in middle childhood, three of five studies[20,23] found some impairment in children of schizophrenics. With one exception,[24] studies have found that children of schizophrenics tend to show cognitive impairment on more complex tasks that assess impairment under stimulus overload conditions.[20,25–27]

Further, when subgroups of children of schizophrenics who manifest these AIP deficits in middle childhood are followed up into late adolescence these children, in contrast to nonimpaired offspring of schizophrenics, are more likely to require some form of psychiatric treatment.[25] However, although the sensitivity and composite index of multiple measures of AIP in middle childhood for predicting later psychopathology was excellent, the specificity was only moderate.

Consistent with the data from earlier age periods, data from middle childhood indicate that a subset of children of schizophrenics show disturbed social functioning relative to children of normal controls.[26,28–30] However, in these studies impaired social role functioning in the child relates to the severity of parental psychopathology in general rather than to the existence of parental schizophrenia per se, as children of severely disturbed affective disorder parents show social dysfunctions comparable to those of offspring of severely disturbed schizophrenics.

Although psychological disturbance has been observed in children of schizophrenics, it does not typically reach the level found in children referred for clinical levels of psychopathology.[26,30] Despite previous theories that emphasize social withdrawal as a vulnerability marker for schizophrenia, no specific pattern of disturbance in social relations has been identified across studies. As with many samples of clinically disturbed children, some children of schizophrenics have been negatively evaluated variously by their peers and teachers as aggressive, disruptive, low in social and cognitive competence, emotionally flat, withdrawn, distractable, passive, irritable, negativistic, hyperactive, emotionally labile, and immature.[10,18,21,26,30–33]

Adolescence

Several studies point to the continued existence of neurointegrative problems in children of schizophrenics studied as adolescents. Marcuse and Cornblatt[34] found deficits in motor coordination, balance, and sensory perceptual signs in adolescent children of schizophrenics. When the subjects from the Erlenmeyer-Kimling and Cornblatt project[35] were re-evaluated as teenagers, it was found that comparable patterns to those observed earlier were found on AIP measures. Further, the middle childhood AIP measures were strongly related to adolescent clinical status.

Early reports from the Danish high-risk study[36] indicated that, when tested in adolescence, offspring of schizophrenics, who subsequently developed schizophrenia, showed unusual patterns of autonomic nervous system reactivity to a series of loud tones, particularly in skin conductance reactivity and recovery pattern. However, recent studies[37] have not supported these findings to date.

Studies that have included or started with adolescent samples have, without exception, shown some evidence of social dysfunction of offspring of schizophrenics. Similar to findings in middle childhood, many of the deviant social patterns are also found in other clinical and high-risk populations.

In the Danish high-risk project,[13] teacher's reports of poor affective control and difficulty in making friends, were found to discriminate those offspring of schizophrenics who developed schizophrenia in early adulthood from those with healthier outcomes.

In summary, children of schizophrenic parents show a number of early signs and dysfunctions that discriminate them from their peers. Typically, however, only a subsample of the offspring show these signs and dysfunction, and it appears that it is those offspring who are at greater risk for the disorder. The most promising markers are signs of neurointegrative and social dysfunction in middle childhood and attention and information processing deficits in middle childhood and adolescence. The specificity of these markers to schizophrenia remains to be demonstrated.

Family Environmental Stressors

As indicated previously in this chapter, the second part of the vulnerability stress model outlined schematically in Figure 9.1, attempts to specify the nature of stressful life events that interact with indices of personal vulnerability. We can see in Figure 9.1 that heavy emphasis is placed on the family environment as a source of chronic stress. The attempt to identify patterns of family relationships that may play a contributory role in the development of schizophrenia goes back to the mid-1950s when clinical investigators, working with families with adult schizophrenic offspring, hypothesized that unique patterns of family organization and relationships existed in the families of schizophrenics. These investigators[38-40] further speculated that these patterns antedated the onset of the disorder and continued to support the schizophrenic condition in the affected family member. Unfortunately, the data on which these theories were based did not justify such sweeping conclusions, and the family therapy models that emerged from them did not appear effective in curing schizophrenia.[41] The implications of the aforementioned vulnerability stress model for family interaction research are profound. This model implies that researchers must investigate the interaction between intrafamilial relationships and indices of vulnerability to a particular psychiatric disorder. Ideally, researchers should have available one or more established vulnerability markers that can be investigated in the context of different family environments, some of which may be provocative of and others protective against the expression of a disorder.

Current thinking in developmental psychopathology reflects a more sophisticated view of the complex transactions[17] between parent and child as they impact upon one another sequentially from birth onward. It is now recognized that children have unique biologically based individuality that has a powerful impact on the type of parenting behavior elicited by the child, as well as determining the impact of variations in parent behavior on the child at various stages of development. The transactional model is complex and demands sophisticated research strategies to uncover factors associated with healthy or psychopathological development. It also does not lend itself to simplistic formulations in which one generation can be indicted for producing the ills of the next.

Despite the emotionality generated by attempts to isolate stressful patterns of family relationships which may interact with individual vulnerabilities to a schizophrenic disorder, the fact is that there is a very limited body of empirical evidence to support this position. The best evidence requires longitudinal prospective studies in which intrafamilial transactional processes are observed long before the onset of the disorder. Ideally, such studies should also include some indices of the vulnerability to the disorder so that interactions between vulnerability and stressors can be evaluated.

Studies of family factors also require a clear specification of the family processes believed stressful for the vulnerable offspring. Two types of variables have been suggested as particularly stressful for the vulnerable person: disordered communication among family members, termed communication deviance (CD) by Wynne et al,[42] and a negative affective climate in the family, termed high expressed emotion (high EE)[43] or, as indexed in direct interaction, negative affective style (AS).[44]

These variables, primarily measured on parents, were used in a longitudinal prospective study carried out by Goldstein and associates,[44-47] in which a sample of 64 families of mildly to moderately disturbed adolescents were studied for the 15 years after their assessment at an outpatient psychological clinic. A key part of this assessment was intensive study of parental communication style, affective attitudes, and interactive behavior as well as data on the form of adolescent behavioral disturbance.

Goldstein[46,47] reported that the incidence of schizophrenia and related disorders (schizotypal, paranoid, schizoid personality disorders) was highest in the families originally classified high in communication deviance (CD) 15 years earlier. In fact, there were no cases of schizophrenia in the low CD cases and only one case diagnosed in the extended schizophrenia spectrum (a schizoid personality). Further, the addition of measures of affective climate (high EE or negative AS) sharpened the ability to identify those cases likely to manifest schizophrenia spectrum disorders in the follow-up period.

Although these family measures did identify family units at high risk for offspring of schizophrenia or related disorders, there was also a notable number of offspring with diagnoses of borderline personality disorder in the high CD cohort, raising the question of whether the high CD, high EE, negative AS aggregation of family attributes has any specific linkage to schizophrenia spectrum disorders or if it measures high stress family units linked to severe offspring psychopathology in general. A recent study by Miklowitz et al[48] that contrasted parents of schizophrenics and parents of manic patients, in which equal levels of CD were found in both groups, argues against the specificity of high CD to schizophrenia.

One attempt to test the vulnerability stress hypothesis is the Goldstein et al study.[44-47] It involved estimates of the presence or absence of a family history of psychosis. This index of a positive or negative family history did not correlate with the CD level of the family, indicating that they were not redundant information.[47] However, it was found that the combination of a notable genetic load for psychosis and high CD greatly increased the risk that an offspring would manifest a disorder in the extended schizophrenia spectrum.

The second study that bears on this issue is that of Tienari et al[49] in Finland, which considers the vulnerability to schizophrenia by contrasting the psychiatric status of adopted-away offspring of schizophrenic mothers with adopted-away offspring of nonpsychiatric cases. The cases were drawn from a nationwide sample of schizophrenic women and matched controls all of whom gave away offspring for adoption to a nonrelative.

This study attempts to investigate both genetic and environmental factors in the development of schizophrenia as it assesses the incidence of schizophrenia in offspring as a function of the quality of the rearing envi-

TABLE 9.1. The rate of psychosis observed in adopted-away offspring of schizophrenic mothers as a function of rearing family environment (from Tienari et al[50]).

| | Adoptive family rearing environment | |
Offspring diagnosis	Healthy ($N = 49$)	Seriously disturbed ($N = 43$)
Psychotic*	0%	16.3%
Borderline Psychotic	0%	20.9%

*5 diagnosed schizophrenic, 2 paranoid psychosis.

ronment. To date, these various measures of family relationships have been reduced to categorical ratings ranging from healthy to severely disturbed. Whereas ratings of measures used in the Goldstein study cited above (CD, EE, AS) are available from the data collected in the Tienari et al study,[49] they have not been completed as yet.

The data reported so far[50] strongly support the role of genetic factors in schizophrenia, because of the 10 psychotic offspring in the sample, 8 were found in the adopted-away offspring of schizophrenic mothers (7.14%), whereas the population base rate was found in the control families (2/135 = 1.48%).

However, the Tienari et al[50] data also support a vulnerability stress model, because all of the schizophrenic cases in the 92 families rated thus far occurred in families rated as disturbed (see Table 9.1). In fact, the rates in the adopted-away offspring of schizophrenics with rearing environments rated as "healthy" have rates of schizophrenia at or below the general population rate.

These data also weaken the argument against a purely environmental etiology of schizophrenia as similar patterns of family disturbance did not relate to a notable incidence of schizophrenia in the adopted-away offspring of nonpsychiatric biological parents.

Although the study designs and data bases are quite different, both the Goldstein et al[44–47] and Tienari et al[49,50] studies are quite congruent in supporting the vulnerability stress model outlined previously in this chapter.

To summarize, only two studies relate to the question of whether one type of stress, disturbed family relationships, interacts with individual vulnerability to increase the risk for the onset of schizophrenia. Each of these studies have notable limitations, yet the congruence between them suggests that it may be premature to reject the hypothesis that family stress may be a significant component in the epigenesis of schizophrenia.

Stress Factors and the Course of Schizophrenia

A similar vulnerability stress model has been used in research on the course of schizophrenia once the disorder develops. Returning once again to Figure 9.1, we can see that personal vulnerability factors outlined related to: (1) brain biochemistry (dopaminergic dysfunction); (2) AIP dysfunction (reduced available processing capacity); (3) autonomic nervous system hyperactivity; and (4) certain personality traits, schizotypal personality, in particular.

Because evidence regarding most of these topics is covered in other chapters in this book, we will focus on what are termed environmental potentiators and stressors. Once again, most of the research in recent years has been directed to one of these stressor conditions, a critical or emotionally involved family climate, termed high expressed emotion (high EE) in the early British studies.[51] Although we focus on this one form of stress, it should be recognized that, as indicated in Figure 9.1, other nonfamilial factors (stressful life events, for example) have been hypothesized to be major risk factors for a poor course (relapse or impaired social role functioning).

It should be recognized that although most research has focused on the affective climate of the family, many schizophrenic patients are either estranged from or in minimal contact with their families and, therefore, their clinical course cannot be explained by family stress factors. It is also critical to recognize that the best predictor of risk for relapse or poor clinical course is noncompliance with antipsychotic medication, and that all studies on psychosocial stress factors must be considered within the context of medication compliance.

Research on Expressed Emotion

The concept of expressed emotion evolved from a series of studies carried out at the Medical Research Council (MRC) Social Psychiatry Unit in London over the last 30 years designed to understand why some discharged schizophrenic patients survived in the community and others did not. An excellent description of the evolution of this research is contained in Leff and Vaughn[51] and Brown.[52]

This research, which began before the widespread application of antipsychotic medication, started with the observation, not since replicated, that patients who returned to family homes relapsed more frequently than patients who went to other living arrangements.[53] This lead to an investigation of attributes of the family environment that might potentiate relapse in an already vulnerable person who had suffered a recent schizophrenic episode. Observations of families resulted in the notion that high levels of tension and emotion characterized those family units with the most relapse-prone patients, originally termed "emotional involvement"[52] (p 19). This research was facilitated by the development of an interview procedure by Rutter and Brown[54] termed the Camberwell Family Interview (CFI). This interview focuses on the 3-month period before the onset of an episode of schizophrenia and focuses upon various types of events in families (quarrels, how often household tasks were done, amount of face-to-face contact, etc), as well as the psychiatric history, irritability, and clinical symptoms of the patient. The main focus of the interviewing procedure is to get respondents to express themselves in ways that reflect their inner feelings. The whole interview is rated on a series of scales (warmth, hostility, emotional overinvolvement), and frequency counts are made on the number of critical comments and positive remarks made about the patient.

In the original study[55] it was found that 76% of patients returning to homes high on criticism and/or emotional overinvolvement relapsed, whereas only 28% of those returning to low emotional involvement homes did so. Note that by contemporary standards high and low involvement are now called high and low EE.

Since this original study a number of replications have been carried out,[43,55–60] all of which have confirmed the original trends. However, four reports exist in the literature of nonreplication.[61–64] The Hogarty publication[61] is particularly important in pointing out that most of the replications have found that high EE status is predictive predominantly for male schizophrenic patients.

The 1976 Vaughn and Leff[43] paper indicated that high EE status interacted with the patient's level of compliance with antipsychotic medication and the amount of face-to-face contract. However, recent studies have not supported these findings and have shown instead that medication and family EE status are independent and additive predictors of clinical course,[57,58,60] and that the contact effect has not been replicated.

The greatest controversy in this research has to do with the intepretation of these findings and their implications regarding the direction of effects. Both in the 1962 and 1972 Brown et al studies, relationships were found between ratings of patient "behavioral disturbance" in the 3-month prehospitalization period and relapse. However, when this patient attribute was entered into a prediction equation with EE status, it failed to add anything to prediction from EE status. The 1976 Vaughn and Leff study found that ratings of the severity of psychopathology at discharge were unrelated to EE status, a finding subsequently confirmed by Miklowitz et al[65] in the United States.

It might be expected that the patient's premorbid history would relate to the EE attitudes of relatives, as those relatives who have been faced with a socially ineffective offspring or spouse (a poor premorbid patient) might be more critical and/or emotionally overinvolved after a schizophrenic breakdown, because this is experienced as still another sign of dysfunctional adaptation in the patient. Miklowitz et al[65] failed to find such a relationship for relatives defined as high EE on the basis of the criticism criterion, but did find that relatives rated as high EE on the basis of emotional overinvolvement did have a schizophrenic offspring with a poor premorbid history.

Along a similar line of investigating a possible link between EE status of relatives and the history of the patient's illness, MacMillan et al[60] report an association between preadmission duration of illness (the time between the reported initial signs of the first episode of schizophrenia and first lifetime hospital admission for the disorder) and EE status, with longer history associated with a greater probability of high EE attitudes. These authors further conclude, from logistic regression analyses, that EE was not a significant predictor of relapse when duration of illness was also entered as a predictor.

Statistical removal of the duration of untreated illness from the predictor equation does not eliminate the significance of EE attitude for the future course of the patient's disorder. It is one thing to clarify the origins of contemporary attitudes or behaviors (high or low EE status), but quite another to assume that contemporary attitudes are irrelevant determinants of the behavior of others. It is also interesting to note that a recent report by Nuechterlein et al[59] of preliminary data from a comparable sample of recent onset, predominantly first admission schizophrenic patients, failed to replicate the association between EE status of relatives and duration of illness. Also, a reanalysis of the data for first lifetime admission cases in the Nuechterlein study[66] revealed that the relationship of EE to duration in the MacMillan et al[60] study was an artifact of differential exposure by relatives to the early stages of their relative's disorder.

The relationship between relatives' EE status and relapse in schizophrenic patients does not clarify the nature of mediating mechanism between family attitude and patient response. A number of studies have attempted to address this problem by observing actual interactional patterns among patients and relatives. Three studies[67-69] have indicated that high EE relatives do, in fact, express more negative affect (coded by the affective style coding system[44]) in experimentally induced interactional sessions. Further, the type of negative affective messages parallel the subtypes of high EE attitudes as relatives classified as high EE on criticism express more criticism, but those high EE on emotional overinvolvement do not and instead are more intrusive.

A critical issue in EE research is whether these family attitudes are state dependent or are consistent across time, independent of the patient's clinical state. In a recent study, Miklowitz et al[70] estimated EE in the conventional way by administering the CFI during the patient's hospitalization. A brief measure of EE, the Five Minute Speech Sample (FMSS)[71] was used as a probe for the stability of EE 5 to 6 weeks after the patient had been discharged and returned home. These investigators found that more than half of the original high EE relatives were low EE after remission, whereas few if any low EE relatives had changed. They further found that the most negative interaction patterns were found in the families rated as consistently high EE, whereas those where relatives shifted from high to low EE were not discriminable from those with consistently low EE relatives. These data suggest that it is valuable to obtain estimates of EE over time to separate those relatives whose high EE attitudes are largely state dependent from those who maintain this attitude consistently from acute episode to remission phases of the disorder.

A number of studies have found that these verbal interchanges are paralleled by increasing psychophysiological arousal and reactivity[72,73] in the patient and, in one study with disturbed teenagers hypothesized to be at risk for schizophrenia, in both parents and offspring.[67] These data suggest that a negative affective climate in the family may enhance the likelihood of relapse by raising the level of arousal in the patient beyond the limits of his vulnerable postpsychotic coping mechanisms.

That the affective climate of the family may be causally related to relapse has been investigated within the framework of the Falloon et al[74] aftercare intervention study. This study contrasted a behavioral family management program with a comparable patient-focused one where all patients received regular maintenance antipsychotic medication. The direct interaction task used in the Miklowitz et al[65] study was repeated two times in the Falloon et al study, before entry into the study and after 3 months of intensive treatment. The parental data were coded by the affective style system at both times. Pre- and posttreatment comparisons[75,76] indicated that not only did the family management program on the average produce a greater reduction of negative affect in the family than did the patient-focused intervention, and that those families where this reduction occurred were least likely to experience a relapse by their young adult schizophrenic offspring by the 9-month follow-up point.

Similar findings were recently reported by Hogarty et al[77] using the original Camberwell Family Interview method of EE assessment before and after 1 year of either family management, social skills training for the patient, a combination of the two, or regular maintenance drug therapy. All families in these studies were originally selected as being high EE. The rate of change from high to low EE status was greatest in the family treatment groups (family alone or family and social skills) and lowest in the drug-only condition. However, regardless of the assigned treatment condition, when relatives did shift to a low EE status, patient relapse rate was 0%, whereas when this did not occur, the rate averaged 40%.

While studies carried out to date suggest that relatives' affective attitudes toward a recently discharged schizophrenic patient may play some role in the subsequent course of the patient's disorder, there are still a number of unanswered questions in this area. First, whereas there is little evidence that high EE attitudes are simply reactions to variations in the clinical state of the patient, many of the direct interaction studies have not carefully examined the more subtle aspects of how patients relate to their family members. Given that EE is measured when family members are going through a major crisis involving either the hospitalization or rehospitalization of a spouse or offspring, there may be attributes of the crisis or its history, as suggested by MacMillan et al,[60] that can help us understand variations in these responses to the patient's disorder. It is very likely that high EE attitudes and negative affective behaviors toward patient relatives have complex origins, as suggested by Leff and Vaughn.[51] Investigators should go beyond the convenient high-low EE typology to understand not only the natural history of a schizophrenic disorder, but the natural history of relatives' varying efforts to cope with the many difficult demands of a close relative with schizophrenia residing in or near their home. Two recent studies[78,79] have attempted a more sophisticated look at this issue by examining the behavior of patients toward relatives defined as either high or low EE. These studies have found that the pattern of negative escalation, observed in high EE families, reflects complex reciprocal transactions between patients and relatives and cannot be accounted for by a simple linear model in which the affective tone of interactions is determined solely by the relatives' behavior. This literature will ultimately profit from a reinterpretation of the data within the framework of a vulnerability stress model applied to the relatives of schizophrenics as well.

Family Intervention Studies

The burden experienced by relatives of schizophrenics who are frequently required to care for their patient relative after discharge following a relatively brief hospitalization, has generated considerable interest in the development of family intervention programs designed to reduce stress on all family members and thereby reduce the risk of patient relapse. Unquestionably, the development of these programs and the controlled clinical trials that were carried out, received considerable impetus from the EE research as these studies specified family attributes that were likely targets for effective modification. However, the programs that have been tested so far cannot be seen as strictly derived from the EE model, as they frequently involve a complex set of interventions that involve information, support, communication training, and instruction in the development of new coping skills for all family members.[80] However, as noted, one consequence of these programs has been the reduction of the negative affective messages in the family.

Despite wide variations in format and theoretical model (in one study by Leff et al[82] only relatives were involved in groups), the four controlled clinical trials carried out to date[74,77,81,82] found outcomes remarkably consistent with one another in revealing a substantial reduction in relapse rates for the family-based intervention when contrasted to either regular drug treatment or, in the Falloon et al[74] study, with drug plus individual therapy. A noteworthy finding in the Hogarty et al study was that the combination of family management, social skills training for the patient, and regular drug treatment produced the lowest rate of relapse (0%) at 1 year postdischarge. This finding is particularly important, as previous research on individually based treatments for schizophrenia have not produced encouraging results, and this is the first positive evidence on this score. All of these family intervention programs are superimposed on regular maintenance antipsychotic drug treatment, and appear to add something of significance to the protection provided by drug treatment.

There are a number of unresolved issues regarding these family programs, namely: (1) how much of the efficacy is due to the provision of information and support, and how much to the specific behavioral alterations targeted by the model of treatment, (2) do these programs actually prevent relapse or merely delay its occurrence, and (3) how, and in what ways, do these family programs designed to reduce family stress, interact with different pharamacological strategies for maintenance treatment? If the vulnerability stress model is an accurate one for accounting for risk of relapse, then factors that reduce stress should permit variation in the protection required against vulnerability in the patient. This suggests that variations in dose (so-called low-dose strategies) or pattern of medication (targeted or intermittent medication) would be more likely to be effective when the stress level is lowered. This is the basic design of the NIMH Treatment Strategies in Schizophrenia Cooperative Agreement Program,[83] and the results of that study will shed considerable light on this question.

In summary various studies have supported the view that a negative affective climate in the family is predictive of relapse in a patient relative in the short term. The origins of these attitudes are quite complex and warrant careful investigation to determine whether they antedate the onset of the disorder, are reactive to or provoked by attitudes of the patient's premorbid and postmorbid social and clinical behavior, and how they relate to coping mechanisms used by relatives to handle the very real difficulties of having a remitted schizophrenic person at home.

The controlled clinical trials contrasting family intervention and drug therapy programs with regular maintenance drug treatment only, have produced clear and consistent evidence of effectiveness for the additive effects of a family management program. However, the evidence regarding duration of these effects beyond 9 months to 1 year postdischarge have not been consistent. Further research in this area should involve studies of other modalities of psychosocial treatment (as in the social skills training module of Hogarty et al[77] that could be added to or extended beyond the typical period of family management studies to date, to develop a comprehensive rehabilitation program for schizophrenic patients. A successful family management program may merely stabilize the patient at a level of clinical and social functioning that permits the introduction of patient-focused, psychosocial rehabilitation programs designed to go beyond relapse prevention. New and innovative models of patient-focused psychosocial rehabilitation programs are urgently needed to extend and amplify the family-based programs tested to date.

Summary

This chapter uses a version of the vulnerability stress model to examine psychosocial factors related to the onset, course, and treatment of schizophrenia. High-risk studies, most of which study offspring of a schizophrenic parent, suggest that signs of vulnerability to the disorder may emerge in early to middle childhood in neuromotor integration, attentional and information-processing abilities, and deviant social behavior. It is still not clear that these markers are specific to the subsequent development of schizophrenia. The evidence suggests that further investigation is warranted.

Stressors, particularly those arising from within the family, are also examined as they relate to the course of schizophrenia. The data on expressed emotion (EE) have been replicated more often than not, although the origins of high EE attitudes are not precisely understood. These attitudes do not arise as reactions to the form or severity of a relative's disorder, but they may relate to the length of time between initial onset of the disorder and first hospitalization.

Family-based intervention programs, overlaid on regular antipsychotic drug treatment, appear to reduce the risk for relapse in the short term. At least one of the mechanisms of action of these programs is to reduce the negative affective climate in the family.

Acknowledgments.   Preparation of this chapter was greatly facilitated by grants from NIMH (MH08744) and the John D. and Catherine T. MacArthur Foundation for the Network on Risk and Protective Factors in the Major Mental Disorders. The author is also greatly indebted to Joan Asarnow, PhD, for her analyses of high-risk research literature.

References

1. Goldstein MJ, Asarnow JR: Prevention of schizophrenia: what do we know?, in Barter JT, Talbot SW (eds): *Primary Prevention in Psychiatry: State of the Art.* Washington, DC, American Psychiatric Press, 1986; pp 87–115.
2. Goldstein MJ, Tuma AH: High-risk research: editor's introduction. *Schizophr Bull* 1987;13:369–371.
3. Zubin J, Spring BJ: Vulnerability: a new view of schizophrenia. *J Abnorm Psychol* 1977;86:103–126.
4. Nuechterlein K: Vulnerability models for schizophrenia: state of the art, in Hafner H, Gattaz WF, Janzarik (eds): *Search for the Causes of Schizophrenia.* Heidelberg, Springer–Verlag, 1987, pp 296–316.
5. Asarnow JR, Goldstein MJ: Schizophrenia during adolescence: a developmental perspective on risk research. *Clin Psychol Rev* 1986;6:211–235.
6. Walker E, Emory E: Infants at risk for psychopathology: offspring of schizophrenic parents. *Child Devel* 1983;54:1269–1285.
7. McNeil TF, Kaij L, Malmquist-Larsson A, et al: Development of a longitudinal study of children at high risk. *Acta Psychiatr Scand* 1983;68:234–250.
8. Fish B: Characteristics and sequelae of the neurointegrative disorder in infants at risk for schizophrenia: 1952–1982, in Watt N, Anthony EJ, Wynne L, Rolf J (eds): Children at risk for schizophrenia: a longitudinal perspective. New York, Cambridge University Press, 1984, pp 423–439.
9. Ragins N, Schacter J, Elmer E, et al: Infants and children at risk for schizophrenia. *J Am Acad Child Psychiatr* 1975;14:150–177.
10. Fish B: Infant predictors of the longitudinal course of schizophrenic development. *Schizophr Bull* 1987;13:395–409.

11. Marcus J, Hans S, Lewow E, et al: Neurological findings in the offspring of schizophrenics: childhood assessment and 5-year follow-up. *Schizophr Bull* 1985;11:85–100.

12. Marcus J, Hans SL, Nagler S, et al: Review of the NIMH Israeli Kibbutz-City study and the Jerusalem infant development study. *Schizophr Bull* 1987;13:425–438.

13. Parnas J, Schulsinger F, Schulsinger H, et al: Behavioral precursors of schizophrenia spectrum. *Arch Gen Psychiatry* 1982;39:658–644.

14. Parnas J, Schulsinger F, Teasdale TW, et al: Perinatal complications and clinical outcome within the schizophrenia spectrum. *Br J Psychiatry* 1982;140: 416–420.

15. Nasland R, Persson-Belnnow I, McNeil T, et al: Offspring of women with nonorganic psychosis: fear of stranger during the first year of life. *Acta Psychiatrica Scand* 1984;69:435–444.

16. Ainsworth MD, Wittig, BA: Attachment and exploratory behavior of 1-year-olds in a strange situation, in Foss BM (ed): *Determinants of Infant Behavior IV*. London, Methuen, 1969, pp 111–136.

17. Sameroff AJ, Barocas R, Seifer R: The early development of children born to mentally ill women, in Watt NF, Anthony EJ, Wynne LC, Rolf JE (eds): *Children at Risk for Schizophrenia: A Longitudinal Perspective*. New York, Cambridge University Press, 1984, pp 482–514.

18. Hanson D, Gottesman I, Heston L: Some possible childhood indicators of adult schizophrenia inferred from children of schizophrenics. *Br J Psychiatry* 1976;129:142–154.

19. Goodman SH: Emory University Project on children with disturbed parents. *Schizophr Bull* 1987;13:411–423.

20. Erlenmeyer-Kimling L, Cornblatt BA, Golden R: Early indicators of vulnerability to schizophrenia in children at high genetic risk, in Guze SB, Earls FJ, Barrett JE (eds): *Childhood Psychopathology and Development*. New York, Raven Press, 1983, pp 247–261.

21. Reider RO, Nichols PL: The offspring of schizophrenics. Part III. *Arch Gen Psychiatry* 1979;36:665–674.

22. Orvaschel H, Mednick S, Schulsinger F, et al: The children of psychiatrically disturbed parents. *Arch Gen Psychiatry* 1979;36:691–695.

23. Asarnow JR: Schizophrenia, in Tarter R (ed) *The Child at Psychiatric Risk*. New York, Oxford University Press, 1983, pp 150–194.

24. Harvey P, Weintraub S, Neale J: Span of apprehension deficits in children vulnerable to psychopathology: a failure to replicate. *J Abnorm Psychol* 1985;94:410–413.

25. Cornblatt BA, Erlenmeyer-Kimling L: Global attentional deviances as a marker of risk for schizophrenia: specificity and predictive validity. *J Abnorm Psychol* 1985;94:470–486.

26. Nuechterlein K: Signal detection in vigilance tasks and behavioral attributes among offspring of schizophrenic mothers and among hyperactive children. *J Abnorm Psychol* 1983;92:4–28.

27. Rutschmann J, Cornblatt B, Erlenmeyer-Kimling L: Sustained attention in children at risk for schizophrenia: report on a continuous performance test. *Arch Gen Psychiatry* 1977;34:571–575.

28. Wynne LC: The University of Rochester Child and Family Study: overview of research plan, in Watt NF, Anthony EJ, Wynne LC, Rolf JE (eds): *Children*

at Risk for Schizophrenia: A Longitudinal Perspective. New York, Cambridge University Press, 1984, pp 335–347.

29. Wynne LC, Cole RE, Perkins P: University of Rochester Child and Family Study: risk research in progress. *Schizophr Bull* 1987;13:463–476.

30. Rolf JE: The social and academic competence of children vulnerable to schizophrenia and other behavior pathologies. *J Abnorm Psychol* 1972;80: 225–243.

31. Fisher L, Harder D, Kokes R, et al: School functioning of children at risk for behavioral pathology, in Baldwin A, Cole R, Baldwin C (eds): *Parental Pathology, Family Interaction, and the Competence of the Child in School.* Monographs of the society for research in child development, 1982; 47:12–16.

32. Watt NF: Patterns of childhood social development in adult schizophrenics. *Arch Gen Psychiatry* 1978;35:160–165.

33. Weintraub S, Neale J: The Stony Brook high-risk project, in Watt NF, Anthony EJ, Wynne LC, Rolf JE (eds): *Children at Risk for Schizophrenia: A Longitudinal Perspective.* New York, Cambridge University Press, 1984, pp 243–263.

34. Marcuse Y, Cornblatt B: Children at high risk for schizophrenia: predictions from infancy to childhood functioning, in Erlenmeyer-Kimling L, Miller N (eds): *Life Span Research on the Prediction of Psychopathology.* New Jersey, Lawrence Earlbaum and Associates, 1986, pp 84–100.

35. Erlenmeyer-Kimling L, Cornblatt B: The New York high-risk project: a follow-up report. *Schizophr Bull* 1987;13:451–461.

36. Mednick SA, Schulsinger F: Some premorbid characteristics related to breakdown in children with schizophrenic mothers, in Rosenthal D, Kety SS (eds): *The Transmission of Schizophrenia.* New York, Pergamon Press, 1968, pp 267–291.

37. Dawson ME, Nuechterlein KH: Psychophysiological dysfunctions in the developmental course of schizophrenic disorders. *Schizophr Bull* 1984;10:204–232.

38. Lidz T, Cornelison AR, Fleck S, et al: The intrafamilial environment of schizophrenic patients: II. Marital schism and marital skew. *Am J Psychiatry* 1957;114:241–248.

39. Bowen M: A family concept of schizophrenia, in Jackson DD (ed): *The Etiology of Schizophrenia.* New York, Basic Books, 1960, pp 346–372.

40. Bateson B, Jackson D, Haley J, et al: Toward a theory of schizophrenia. *Behav Sci* 1956;1:252–264.

41. Massie HN, Beels CC: The outcome and family treatment of schizophrenia. *Schizophr Bull* 1972;(Fall):24–36.

42. Wynne LC, Singer, MT, Bartko JJ, et al: Schizophrenics and their families: research on parental communication, in Tanner JM (ed): *Developments in Psychiatric Research.* London, Hodder & Stroughton, 1977, pp 254–286.

43. Vaughn CE, Leff JP: The influence of family and social factors on the course of psychiatric illness: a comparison of schizophrenic and depressed neurotic patients. *Br J Psychiatry* 1976;129:125–137.

44. Doane JA, West KL, Goldstein MJ, et al: Parental communication deviance and affective style: predictors of subsequent schizophrenia spectrum disorders in vulnerable adolescents. *Arch Gen Psychiatry* 1981;38:679–685.

45. Goldstein MJ, Judd LL, Rodnick EH, et al: A method for the study of social

influence and coping patterns in the families of disturbed adolescents. *J Nerv Ment Dis* 1968;147:233–251.

46. Goldstein MJ: Family factors that antedate the onset of schizophrenia and related disorders: the results of a fifteen year prospective longitudinal study. *Acta Psychiatr Scand* 1985;71:7–18.
47. Goldstein MJ: The UCLA high risk project. *Schizophr Bull* 1987;13:505–514.
48. Miklowitz DJ, Goldstein MJ, Nuechterlein KH, et al: Family factors and the course of bipolar affective disorder. *Arch Gen Psychiatry* 1988;45:225–231.
49. Tienari P, Sorri A, Naarala M, et al: The Finnish adoptive and family study: adopted-away offspring of schizophrenic mothers, in Stierlin H, Wynne LC, Wirsching M (eds): *Psychosocial Intervention in Schizophrenia.* Berlin, Springer–Verlag, 1983, pp 21–34.
50. Tienari P, Sorri A, Lahti I, et al: Genetic and psychosocial factors in schizophrenia: the Finnish adoptive family study. *Schizophr Bull* 1987;13:477–484.
51. Leff J, Vaughn C: *Expressed Emotion in Families.* new York, Guilford Press, 1985.
52. Brown GW: The discovery of expressed emotion: induction or deduction? in Leff J, Vaughn C (eds): *Expressed Emotion in Families.* New York, Guilford Press, 1985, pp 7–25.
53. Brown GW: Experiences of discharged chronic schizophrenic mental hospital patients in various types of living groups. *Millbank Memorial Fund Quarterly* 1959;37:105–131.
54. Rutter M, Brown GW: The reliability and validity of measures of family life and relationships in families containing a psychiatric patient. *Soc Psychiatry* 1966;1:38–53.
55. Brown GW, Monck EM, Carstairs GM, et al: Influence of family life on the course of schizophrenic illness. *Br J Prevent Social Medicine* 1962;16:55–68.
56. Brown GW, Birley JLT, Wing JK: Influence on the course of schizophrenic disorders: a replication. *Br Psychiatry* 1972;121:241–258.
57. Vaughn CE, Snyder KS, Jones S, et al: Family factors in schizophrenic relapse: replication in California of the British research on expressed emotion. *Arch Gen Psychiatry* 1984;41:1169–1177.
58. Jenkins JH, Karno M, de la Selva A, et al: Expressed emotion, maintenance pharmacotherapy, and schizophrenic relapse among Mexican-Americans. *Psychopharmacol Bull* 1986;22:621–627.
59. Nuechterlein KH, Snyder KS, Dawson ME, et al: Expressed emotion, and fixed-dose fluphenazine decanoate maintenance, and relapse in recent-onset schizophrenia. *Psychopharmacol Bull* 1986;22:633–639.
60. MacMillan JF, Gold A, Crow TJ, et al: Expressed emotion and relapse. *Br J Psychiatry* 1986;148:133–143.
61. Hogarty GE: Expressed emotion and schizophrenic relapse: implications from the Pittsburgh study, in Alpert M (ed): *Controversies in Schizophrenia.* New York, Guilford Press, 1985, pp 354–365.
62. Dulz B, Hand I: Short-term relapse in young schizophrenics: can it be predicted and affected by family (CFI), patient and treatment variables? An experimental study, in Goldstein MJ, Hand I, Hahlweg K (eds): *Treatment of Schizophrenia: Family Assessment and Intervention.* Berlin, Springer–Verlag, 1986, pp 59–75.

63. McCreadie RG, Phillips K: 1988: The Nithsdale schizophrenia survey. VII. Does relatives' high expressed emotion predict relapse? *Br J Psychiatry* 1988;152:477–481.
64. Parker, G, Johnston P, Hayward: Parental expressed emotion as a predictor of schizophrenic relapse. *Arch Gen Psychiatry* 1988;45:806–813.
65. Miklowitz DJ, Goldstein MJ, Falloon IRH: Premorbid and symptomatic characteristics of schizophrenia from families with high and low levels of expressed emotion. *J Abnorm Psychol* 1983 92:359–367.
66. Mintz LI, Nuechterlein KH, Goldstein MJ, et al: The initial onset of schizophrenia and family expressed emotion: some methodological considerations. *Br J Psychiatry* 1989; 154;212–217.
67. Valone K, Norton JP, Goldstein MJ, et al: Parental expressed emotion and affective style in an adolescent sample at risk for schizophrenia spectrum disorders. *J Abnorm Psychol* 1983;92:399–407.
68. Miklowitz DJ, Goldstein MJ, Falloon IRH, et al: Interactional correlates of expressed emotion in the families of schizophrenics. *Br J Psychiatry* 1984;144:482–487.
69. Strachan AM, Leff JP, Goldstein MJ, et al: 1986: emotional attitudes and direct communication in the families of schizophrenics. *Br J Psychiatry* 1986;149: 279–287.
70. Miklowitz DJ, Goldstein MJ, Doane JA, et al: Does expressed emotion index a transactional process? I: Relative's affective style. *Fam Process* 1989; 28:153–167.
71. Magana AB, Goldstein MJ, Karno M, et al: A brief method for assessing expressed emotion in relatives of psychiatric patients. *Psychiatr Res* 1986;17:203–212.
72. Tarrier N, Vaughn, C, Lader MH, et al: Bodily reactions to people and events in schizophrenia. *Arch Gen Psychiatry* 1979;36:311–315.
73. Sturgeon D, Kuipers L, Berkowitz R, et al: Psychophysiological responses of schizophrenic patients to high and low expressed emotion relatives. *Br J Psychiatry* 1981;138:40–45.
74. Falloon IRH, Boyd JL, McGill CW, et al: Family management in the prevention of exacerbations of schizophrenia: a controlled study. *N Engl J Med* 1982;306:1437–1440.
75. Doane JA, Falloon IRH, Goldstein MJ, et al: Parental affective style and the treatment of schizophrenia: predicting the course of illness and social functioning. *Arch Gen Psychiatry* 1985;42:34–42.
76. Doane JA, Goldstein MJ, Miklowitz DJ, et al: The impact of individual and family treatment on the affective climate of families of schizophrenics. *Br J Psychiatry* 1986;148:279–287.
77. Hogarty GE, Anderson CM, Reiss DJ, et al: Family psychoeducation, social skills training, and maintenance chemotherapy in the aftercare treatment of schizophrenia. *Arch Gen Psychiatry* 1986;43:633–644.
78. Hahlweg K, Goldstein MJ, Nuechterlein KH, et al: Expressed emotion and patient-relative interaction in families of recent-onset schizophrenics. *J Consult Clin Psychol* 1989;57:11–18.
79. Strachan AM, Feingold D, Goldstein MJ, et al: Does expressed emotion index a transactional process? II. Patient's coping style. *Fam Process* 1989;28:169–181.

80. Goldstein MJ (ed): *New Developments in Interventions with Families of Schizophrenics.* San Francisco, Jossey–Bass, 1981.
81. Goldstein MJ, Rodnick EH, Evans JR, et al: Drug and family therapy in the aftercare of acute schizophrenics. *Arch Gen Psychiatry* 1978;35:1169–1177.
82. Leff JP, Kuipers L, Berkowitz R, et al: A controlled clinical trial of social intervention in the families of schizophrenic patients. *Br J Psychiatry* 1982;141:121–134.
83. Schooler NR, Keith SJ: *Treatment Strategies in Schizophrenia Study Protocol.* Rockville, MD, National Institute of Mental Health, 1983.

10
Psychosocial Interventions in Schizophrenia

KIM T. MUESER, ROBERT P. LIBERMAN, AND
SHIRLEY M. GLYNN

Schizophrenia is a complex and multifaceted illness that has a pervasive impact on a wide range of human experience, including social and vocational functioning, the ability to maintain basic living skills such as grooming and personal hygiene, the affects and emotions, and the perception of reality. Problems in social functioning are axiomatic to the diagnosis of schizophrenia, because such difficulties are necessary to establish the illness according to recent diagnostic criteria.[1] (The impairments in schizophrenic patients' functioning and interactions may reflect a variety of influences, including: the primary impact of the illness on the drive and ability to experience and enjoy interpersonal relationships (ie. negative symptoms); effects of an altered perception of reality and affect (ie, positive symptoms); inadequate learning experiences (ie, poor premorbid adjustment); and mild adaptive responses to adverse environmental events or contingencies (eg, life events, excessive criticism). Thus, deficiencies in social functioning can be the result of paranoid or other delusions, anhedonia or asociality, and avoidance of interpersonal stress or difficulty initiating and maintaining social interactions.

Stress Vulnerability Coping Model

To guide the clinician through the maze of primary and secondary effects of schizophrenia on social functioning to the point of identifying effective strategies for intervention, a brief review of the stress vulnerability coping skills model[2-4] is useful. Positive and negative symptoms and their associated social and personal disabilities are the consequences of stress impinging upon an individual's enduring psychobiological vulnerability to a schizophrenic disorder. This vulnerability is thought to be determined by genetic loading,[5] putative neurotransmitter dysfunctions,[6] and structural[6,7] or lesional[8] brain abnormalities, and may result in cognitive, autonomic, or attentional impairments.[9,10] Coping skills are the ability to reduce or adapt successfully to environmental stress, and hence modulate the noxious effects of stress on an individual's vulnerability.[11] Evidence abounds documenting that premorbid and morbid social competence and coping skill contribute to adequate social adjustment[12,13] and are predictive of a favorable outcome of the illness.[14,15] According to this model, the functioning of a schizophrenic patient is reflected by the dynamic balance of protective factors (coping skill, antipsychotic medication, social support) on the one hand, and stress and vulnerability on the other.

The role of protective factors in mitigating the impact of stressors on vulnerability has broad implications for psychosocial interventions. The interactional nature of coping skill, social support, stress, and vulnerability clearly identifies the therapeutic objectives and modalities for interventions. Neuroleptic drugs may be prescribed to lessen vulnerability and to buffer against the effects of stress. Environmental modification can ameliorate the noxious effects of stress on the individual by reducing the stressor itself. This may account for some of the benefit of hospitalization, in which the patient is temporarily removed from stressors in the family and community. Structured community-based aftercare environments, such as day treatment programs, social clubs, and sheltered workshops, can be effective in providing patients with support to compensate for deficits in community living skills and opportunities for improving their interactions with others. In addition, interventions such as case management, social skills training, and family therapy may further strengthen social support networks and improve patients' skills at coping with a range of stressors.

Effective psychosocial rehabilitation of schizophrenia must attempt to remediate impairments, disabilities, and handicaps arising from the illness.[16,17] Impairments refer to abnormalities of physiological or psychological function, such as reflected by distractibility and positive or negative symptoms. Disabilities are the restrictions of ability to perform activities in a manner consistent with adaptive human functioning, such as deficits in social skills. Handicaps are related to a person's overall social competence, and are defined as the disadvantages individuals experience in fulfilling social and instrumental roles, and that are the consequences of impairments and disabilities caused by the disease. Within this framework interventions aimed at remediating impairments are the most basic and least social in nature (eg. pharmacotherapy and hospitalization), although social skills training may produce partial remediation of negative symptoms.[18] Interventions that focus on disabilities aim at improving patient competencies mainly by the application of principles of social learning and reinforcement, but also by providing social support and a therapeutic milieu. Efforts to modify handicaps focus more exclusively on the environment and providing community supports that enable a partial and gradual assumption of more demanding roles.

Psychosocial interventions can be catalogued according to whom the focus of the treatment is upon, its locus (location), modus (method), and the goals and objectives of the therapy. The *focus* can be on the individual as in one-on-one psychotherapy, in groups, in families, or in a total milieu. The locus of therapeutic and rehabilitative efforts can be the hospital, private office, clinic, mental health center, natural home, board and care home, or social club. The modus of intervention can derive from one or more explicit or implicit theoretical orientations, such as cognitive-behavioral, psychodynamic, systems-strategic, client-centered, or supportive therapy. There may be considerable overlap among modalities of treatment. It must also be recognized that much therapeutic impact of any psychiatric or medical treatment derives from so-called nonspecific and placebo effects that are inherent in any therapy that is offered in a credible, hopeful, and positive manner. Focus, locus and modus of treatment may change over time as the specific problems and needs of the patient and available resources change. At any point in time, multiple foci, loci, and modalities may be harnessed to implement a comprehensive rehabilitation plan.

A wide spectrum of goals and objectives are reflected in the variety of psychosocial interventions brought to bear on persons suffering from schizophrenia, including those that aim primarily to maintain a person at a marginal level of functioning with minimal stress and relapses, those that provide crisis intervention when needed, and those that attempt to build social and independent living skills. Thus, the process of designing, employing, and evaluating psychosocial interventions requires reference to at least four mutually exclusive domains of attributes; for example, family therapy (focus) may be provided in the home (locus), with a behavioral orientation (modus) that aims to improve the problem-solving and communication skills (goals) of the patient and relatives. We first provide an overview of traditional psychosocial treatments for schizophrenia before focusing more extensively on behavioral rehabilitation.

Traditional Psychosocial Therapies

Individual Psychotherapy

A wide variety of different psychotherapies have been tried for schizophrenic patients. However, most attempts to improve the outcome of schizophrenia by traditional individual therapy approaches have met with limited success. Client-centered therapy has not been found to be helpful in controlled clinical trials.[19] With few exceptions,[20] psychoanalytic, psychodynamic, or exploratory and insight-oriented therapies also have demonstrated little therapeutic impact on schizophrenic patients in controlled clinical outcome studies[21-23] or longer-term naturalistic treatment studies.[24,25] Early applications of cognitive therapy for schizophrenia have shown promising results,[26] but this treatment remains experimental at this time.

Family Therapy

Most early approaches to family therapy were based on the theory that schizophrenia was the result of disordered communication within the family,[27,28] such as the "double-bind" hypothesis.[29] Few successes were achieved with these methods,[30] and some have argued that families and patients experienced deleterious effects from interventions based on family etiologic theories.[31,32] The increased evidence for a genetic role in the development of schizophrenia[5] and the failure of family therapy approaches designed to correct pathological communication shifted research priorities from examining the role of the family as a determinant of the illness to examining its influence on the course of the illness.

"Expressed emotion",[33] the communication of critical, hostile, and/or emotionally overinvolved feelings by relatives to patients, has been found to be an important predictor of relapse in schizophrenia in numerous studies conducted over the past 25 years in the United States and abroad.[34] As the impact of negative affect in the family on the course of schizophrenia was discovered, several new modes of family therapy were developed and empirically validated for their ability to change the emotional climate of the family and reduce the incidence of such relapses. The newer family therapy approaches embrace the family as an important resource in the rehabilitation of schizophrenics, making them and patients together extended members of the patient's own treatment team. Two different family therapy approaches whose major aims are educational have been found to significantly reduce risk of relapse in controlled studies.[35-37] Furthermore, a behavioral approach that focuses on communication and problem-solving skill in addition to education has been found to reduce risk of relapse.[38] This approach is described in the Behavioral Methods section.

Group Therapy

Group psychotherapy evolved from individual psychotherapy, so there are as many schools of group psychotherapy as there are of individual therapy. Although many different types of group therapy exist for schizophrenia, groups are most likely to be beneficial when they focus on providing support and attention to the practical problems of daily living experienced by patients trying to adjust to the community, rather than on insight and interpretation.[39] Group therapy has been subjected to relatively few controlled clinical trials,[40] although it continues to be an important treatment modality for most patients.

Therapeutic Milieus

Milieu therapy can be based on any of a number of modalities, ranging from structured behavior therapy to spontaneous humanistically-oriented approaches. In a controlled clinical study, intensive milieu therapy for chronically ill schizophrenic inpatients was found to improve social functioning and discharge rates compared with traditional custodial care.[41] As an alternative to and transition from more costly inpatient care, the day treatment center has become a focal point for treatment of schizophrenia in the community. Treatment programs that include a high level of staff-patient interaction, and that are structured and focus on adaptive, practical aspects of everyday behavior and functioning, are associated with better outcomes than less structured programs with emphasis on symptoms and the development of "insight."[42–44]

The self-help movement created another modality of milieu therapy in the late 1940s, when former patients began to meet together in a social club in New York City to satisfy their needs for acceptance and emotional support. The original program, Fountain House,[45] has spawned hundreds of similar programs that emphasize self-help, mutual interdependence, and reliance on personal assets. The main assumption of the approach is that patients (or members as they call one another) have a right to work, and that employment suppresses symptoms of the illness and promotes community adaptation. Employment opportunities are provided both in the clubhouse (eg, food preparation, switchboard) and transitional jobs are available in the community, with no limitation on the length of participation in the program. Outcome results suggest that club members are much less likely to be rehospitalized after participation in the program than controls.[46] Despite these positive results, methodological difficulties with self-selection, nonrandomly assigned control groups, and lack of diagnostic clarity limit the conclusions that can be drawn from these studies.

Psychosocial Outreach Programs

Effective strategies for reducing rehospitalization rates and improving rehabilitation outcomes have been developed that use assertive outreach services to aid schizophrenics functioning in the community. The hallmark of these approaches is the locus of treatment, which is almost invariably in the community, at locales such as homes, streets, day programs, and bars where the basic focus is on helping patients meet their basic living needs. In addition, intervention is provided on an as-needed basis by an interdisciplinary team, 7 days a week, with intensive case management, crisis intervention, and patient advocacy being the main modalities of treatment. The most widely disseminated and emulated program has been the Training in Community Living program,[47,48] which, in controlled studies, has reduced symptoms and rates of rehospitalization, increased independent living skills and the capacity to work, and has been cost effective.[49–51] With promising results, these programs have been successfully "exported" to many urban and rural settings in the United States, United Kingdom, Canada, and Australia.

Case Management and Community Support

The comprehensive management of schizophrenia must include: treatments for the primary impairments (symptoms); rehabilitation of social and self-care skills; access to necessary medical, housing, and social services; and continuity of care.[52] Over the lifelong course of schizophrenia, patients' needs often change.[53] Linking these needs for treatment and community support with available resources is the process of case management. Assisting chronic mental patients to maximize their use of existing resources can enable them to increase their independence and the quality of their lives. Case management helps to ensure accountability, accessibility, efficiency, and continuity of care.[54] Effective case management must include the following functions: (1) client identification and outreach; (2) individual assessment; (3) service planning; (4) linkage with required services; (5) monitoring service delivery; and (6) patient advocacy.

An important facet of case management and the coordination of treatment for schizophrenia is the development of social supports that will act as a buffer against the aversive effects of environmental stress,[55] including symptom exacerbations and rehospitalizations. Schizophrenics are particularly prone to disruptions in their social networks. Patients recovering from the acute phase of the illness often fail to reestablish their former network because of the social stigma of the illness and their deficits in social skills.[56]

A multilevel approach must integrate diverse elements of treatment tailored to different stages of the illness to strengthen social supports and improve the outcome of schizophrenia. The many different facets of psychosocial treatment can be conceptualized as fitting into three dimensions of comprehensive rehabilitation: the stage or type of disorder; interventions aimed at reducing impairments and disabilities; and community support programs aimed at minimizing handicap.[57] These facets of treatment are illustrated in Figure 10.1, which depicts the "complex cube" of psychiatric rehabilitation. Research is only beginning to identify the elements in case management, community support, and other comprehensive rehabilitation programs that are responsible for sustaining community tenure, lower relapse rates, and a better quality of life.[58]

Behavioral Therapies

Behavioral or cognitive-behavioral interventions play an increasingly important role in modifying symptomatic characteristics of schizophrenia and for retraining adaptive interpersonal and living skills through structured learning experiences.[59,60] The principal distinction between behavioral and other treatment approaches to schizophrenia is the firm adher-

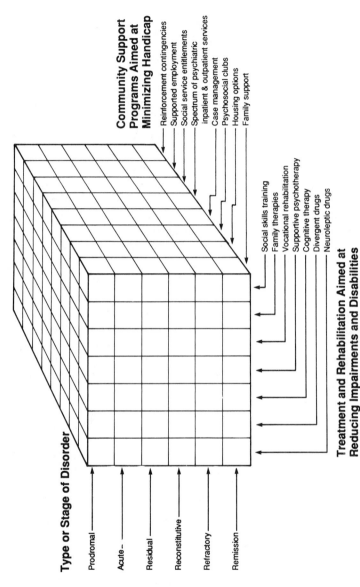

FIGURE 10.1. The complex cube of psychiatric rehabilitation. To assure optimal benefit from treatment and rehabilitation, persons with schizophrenia need to have their services keyed to their stage of disorder. Treatments appropriate for acute episodes of illness are not necessarily the forms or doses of therapy best for those in remission or residual stages of their disorder. In prior eras, social support was provided by the total institution of public psychiatric hospitals; now, such supportive services must be patched together through case management in the community. Without a matrix of social, medical, housing, and family support, specific modalities of drug or psychosocial treatment will be less effective.

ence to specification and measurement by practitioners of behavioral analysis and therapy. In this theoretical framework, psychotic dysfunctions are analyzed in terms of behavioral excesses (eg, delusional verbalizations), behavioral deficits (eg, inadequate social skills), and poor behavior-environment fit (eg, inappropriate affect). Psychosocial treatment involves a combination of altering antecedent and consequent stimuli that surround the problem areas, to supplant and suppress psychotic behaviors, and teaching and strengthening adaptive living skills.

Persons with schizophrenia spectrum illnesses may require repeated prompts, gradual and prolonged shaping of new responses, tangible reinforcement, and other socioenvironmental aids for rehabilitative training. However, their behavior is influenced and determined by the same learning and motivational processes as those that govern the actions of other human beings.[61] The modifiability of psychotic behaviors is constrained by the degree of biological vulnerability and the limitations of environmental resources and consistency.[62] Although most psychosocial rehabilitation programs currently define their efforts as educational and skill building, they differ widely in the degree to which they systematically apply behavioral learning principles, and thus in their effectiveness. Positive reinforcement may naturally occur for appropriate social behavior in a self-help social club or foster home, but unless it is provided consistently and frequently following that behavior, only schizophrenics who are higher functioning and more motivated are likely to benefit.

Behavioral rehabilitation techniques are drawn from learning theory,[63] and are optimally applied in schizophrenia when provided in conjunction with psychotropic medication, and in an environment likely to reinforce positively therapeutic changes. Attributes of behavioral rehabilitation that distinguish it from other interventions, including methods of assessment, therapeutic strategies, environmental supports, and planned generalization, are summarized in Table 10.1.

The stress vulnerability coping skills model of schizophrenia points to several different avenues for intervention based upon behavioral methods. As coping skills are defined in terms of their ability to successfully ward off noxious stressors and maximize patient-environment fit, one fruitful strategy has been to endeavor to improve these skills in patients by engaging them directly in skills training, either individually, in groups, or in the context of family therapy. Another approach, not mutually exclusive of skills training, has been to modify the ability of the family to manage the illness by providing information, and focusing on communication and problem-solving skills of all family members, including the patient. A final behavioral approach that derives from the stress vulnerability model is the actual manipulation of environmental antecedents and consequences via reinforcement contingencies that maintain maladaptive behaviors, to reinforce progressively behavior changes to more socially appropriate and self-regulatory behaviors (eg, token economy and contingency contracting).

TABLE 10.1. Attributes of behavioral psychosocial intervention.

Assessment
  Individualized specification and targeting of problems and goals in behavioral and
    operational terms
  Measurement and monitoring of behavioral progress
  Functional analysis of environmental antecedents and consequences that may be
    maintaining behavioral problems and deficits
  Identification of positive and negative reinforcers that influence target behaviors
  Naturalistic and simulated assessment of targeted behavioral skills
Strategies for behavior change
  Environmental modification (eg, material rewards, changing communication patterns of
    significant others)
  Therapeutic instructions and positive expectation for change
  Social modeling—"life" and video
  Repeated practice and overlearning
  Positive reinforcement of small increments of adaptive behavior (shaping)
  Active prompting and coaching
  Adaptable curriculum to address range of behavior deficits and excesses
  Teaching problem-solving skills for novel situations
Environmental supports
  Therapeutic alliance with patient and significant others
  Optimal psychotropic drugs
  Adequate social and material supports
  Coordination with a comprehensive treatment program
Planned generalization
  Homework assignments
  Multiple models, trainers, and learning settings
  Problem-solving strategy
  Fading of training structure, frequency, and supervision
  Recruitment of environmental supports to maintain gains

Social Skills Training

Social skills training (SST) is a treatment approach whose origins date back to conditioned reflex therapy[64] and assertion training.[65] The goal of SST is to teach patients specific interpersonal and self-care skills that enable them to cope with stressors impinging on them and to attain instrumental and socioemotional goals relevant to more independent living and an improved quality of life.[66,67] Social skill deficits are assumed to reflect the combined influences of the illness itself, learning history before the onset of the illness, lack of environmental stimulation, and the loss of skill due to prolonged disuse.[11] Deficits in social skill can be remediated through the application of highly structured experiential learning procedures with a strong emphasis on social learning.[63]

Social skills training is usually conducted with groups of patients, ranging from 4 to 10 patients, either in inpatient or outpatient settings, preferably with two trainers or therapists. The treatment is highly structured, employing preplanned agendas, audiovisual aids, written handouts, and homework assignments. Problem areas are broken down into small behavioral components to facilitate learning. For example, expressing a positive feeling can be broken down into: look at the person, show a pleasant facial expression, tell them what pleased you, tell how you felt. Social skills training is characterized by a high degree of active involvement by both patients and trainers, with an explicit focus on developing new skill competencies for obtaining practical goals (set by patients), rather than the development of insight or catharsis.

Problems and goals are selected in recurring fashion from session to session, with less complex and challenging skills usually preceding more difficult ones. Groups (or individual sessions) typically last between 45 and 90 minutes, and can be conducted either weekly or more often, although more frequent sessions result in superior learning and generalization of skills. Groups consisting of patients with heterogeneous levels of functioning and homogeneous skill competencies are desirable because patients are able to model the targeted skill for each other, increasing the availability of role models.

Several different models of SST have been developed,[68] but they all share the following basic elements instrumental to changes in interpersonal behavior: (1) assessment of patient's deficits and excesses in interpersonal situations; (2) providing a rationale for learning a particular skill; (3) modeling of the skill by therapist(s) in simulated social interactions; (4) provision of focused instruction to patients practicing a skill; (5) patient behavioral rehearsal of skill (ie, role playing); (6) positive and corrective feedback to patient from therapists and group members; (7) repeated rehearsal and feedback; and (8) homework to promote generalization.

The process of interpersonal communication can be conceptualized as involving three types of skills, each corresponding to a stage of the interaction: receiving, processing, and sending skills.[66] Receiving skills are those skills involved in accurate social perception[69]—the ability to accurately recognize relevant social parameters that constrain the range of socially appropriate behavior, such as the other person's emotional expression or the situational context. Processing skills, also referred to as problem-solving skills, entail the cognitive ability to identify a problem or goal area, generate and evaluate potential solutions, anticipate the probable outcomes of different response options, and select a "best" solution or combination thereof. Sending skills are the actual overt behaviors that a person uses to communicate with others, and include nonverbal behaviors (eg, facial expression, posture, gestures), paralinguistic features (eg, voice volume, tone, affect, fluency, latency, length of utterance), and verbal content. Because individuals with schizophrenia frequently have core psychobiological dysfunctions that appear to be trait markers of the illness,[10] any attempt to modify their interpersonal behavior must attend to and remediate receiving and processing skills in addition to sending skills.

Social skills training procedures incorporate rehabilitation of all three types of skills into a single method that is applied sequentially to develop new skill repertoires. Interpersonal scenes relevant to patients' skill deficits are identified and role played by the therapist(s), who then engage the patient in a behavioral rehearsal. After the role play, the patient is given feedback regarding his or her performance, and asked specific questions to assess, reinforce, and correct his or her receiving and processing skills. For example, in a friendship situation where a patient was inviting his friend John to the movies, a receiving question might be: "What emotion was John feeling when he said he didn't want to go to the movies?" An example of a processing question in the same situation might be: "How do you think John would respond if you asked him to go out and eat with you?" Then, the patient role plays the situation again and is given more feedback. The steps of SST are outlined in a flow chart in Figure 10.2.

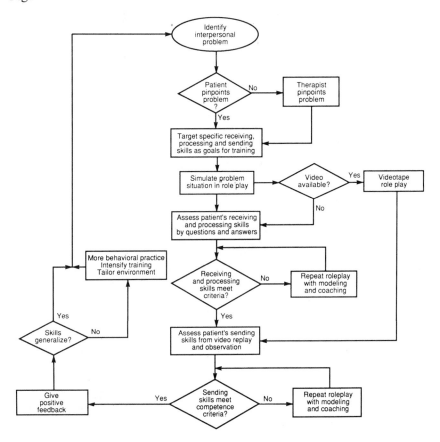

FIGURE 10.2. Steps in conducting social skills training. The training of social skills is carried out with ongoing assessment of progress and repetition of training steps until the patient demonstrates criterion levels of skill acquisition and generalization. One should not assume that transfer of skills to the natural environment will occur "spontaneously"; rather, the therapist must design specific programs and principles to promote transfer and generalization. (Reprinted with permission from Liberman and Mueser.[3] Copyrighted © 1989 Williams and Wilkins Co.)

A recent innovation in SST has been the packaging of a group of functionally related skills into training "modules." Modules have been developed for areas such as medication management, symptom self-management, personal hygiene and grooming, conversational skills, friendship and dating, social problem solving, and leisure and recreational skills. Modules consist of a patient's workbook, a trainer's manual, and a demonstration videocassette that provides adaptive models for the patients to learn from. Each module contains a set of sequential exercises designed to teach patients the skills that constitute the module, train them to solve problems they might encounter when using the skills, and have them practice the skill in both training sessions and the real world.[66,68,69]

More than 40 studies have been conducted on SST with schizophrenic or other chronically mentally ill persons,[70,71] although many of these studies were limited by the absence of controls, lack of diagnostic clarity, or failure to use broadly accepted criteria to assess outcome. However, there is convergence across studies with respect to several findings. First, schizophrenic patients can be trained to improve a wide range of social skills in specific situations, including assertive responses,[72,73] nonverbal behaviors such as eye contact and smiles,[74,75] paralinguistic behaviors[76,77] conversational skills,[78,79] and job interview skills.[80,81] Second, moderate generalization of acquired skills to similar situations can be expected from training, with more complex skills showing less generalization,[82,83] and highly symptomatic and distractible patients acquiring fewer skills. Last, participants in SST consistently report decreases in social anxiety after training. These positive results are bolstered by recent controlled outcome studies that have reported a decreased risk of relapse, and improved social and community functioning for schizophrenic patients who have received SST, either individually[37] or in groups.[84,85]

Behavioral Family Therapy

Behavioral family therapy (BFT)[86–89] has emerged as an important treatment modality that represents a combination of family support and education[35–38] with social skills training involving the entire family. The goals of BFT are to improve the collective ability of the family to manage the schizophrenic patient's illness, while minimizing stress on the patient and maximizing the progress of each family member toward personally identified goals. Improving the problem-solving and coping capacities of the family and reducing the burden of the illness of schizophrenia on the family[90] are as important to the success of BFT as is lowering a negative affective climate in the family. Ultimately, the purpose of BFT is to enable the family to manage independently most of the daily stresses involved in living with a person with a chronic illness without ongoing family therapy, although in some cases maintenance therapy may be necessary. Thus, this intervention is time limited, and focuses on teaching practical information and skills to enhance family coping and goal attainment.

Like social skills training, BFT is a specified and structured intervention, in some ways resembling more of a classroom than a traditional therapy setting. Sessions are based on preplanned agendas and involve the active participation of all family members and the therapist. Homework is routinely given to foster generalization of skills to the natural environment. Sessions can be conducted either with individual families, or in multiple family groups, and are usually offered on a declining contact basis to gradually fade the structure of the family session. Behavioral family therapy can be provided in a variety of different settings, including the hospital, day treatment program, or in the home.

Behavioral family therapy can be divided into five components: (1) assessment of each family member, (2) education about schizophrenia, (3) communication skills training, (4) problem-solving training, and (5) special techniques. Although the components of the model are followed sequentially, considerable recycling of each stage occurs throughout therapy. The behavioral analysis of the family system is an ongoing process that is interwoven throughout treatment. Behavioral analysis requires the therapist to identify assets and deficits of family members and of the family as a unit, as well as the role that specific problem behaviors play in the functioning of the family. Assessment information is gathered through individual interviews, observing family members interact with each other during sessions, and family performance on specific problem-solving tasks.

During the educational sessions, common misconceptions about the cause of schizophrenia are refuted, such as the schizophrenic having a "split personality" or the family being the cause of the illness. Families are informed about the symptoms and diagnosis of schizophrenia, its prevalence, course, biological theories, the influence of drug abuse, and the relationship between stress and vulnerability in causing symptom exacerbations. The role of neuroleptic medications in reducing biological vulnerability and preventing rehospitalization is emphasized, and families are taught to recognize the prodromal signs of a relapse. Information is conveyed to family members with handouts and visual aids such as posters, blackboards, videos, and films.

Communication skills training attempts to alleviate family tensions by teaching empathic listening, effective ways of expressing positive feelings, making requests of others, and expressing negative feelings. Training in these skills is conducted following the procedures of social skills training, employing modeling, behavioral rehearsal, feedback, social reinforcement, and specific homework instructions. Additional communication skills are taught when needed, such as "compromise and negotiation," and "requesting a time out" (ie, time to be alone). Communication deficits are assessed in an ongoing fashion within each family, and targeted interventions are systematically implemented throughout the therapy.

Problem-solving training builds on the ability to use communication skills and consists of teaching a set of steps for resolving a problem or conflict that minimizes the negative emotional undercurrents while maximizing the identification and implementation of an effective solution. These steps are: (1) define the problem to everyone's satisfaction, (2) brainstorm possible solutions, (3) evaluate the advantages and disadvantages of each solution, (4) choose the best solution or combination of solutions, (5) formulate a plan on how to implement the best solution, and (6) review progress on implementation and reinforce approximations toward goal achievement. For problem-solving training each family member takes turns "chairing" the family discussion, recording the various solutions, and writing and monitoring the steps necessary to implement the best solution. Families are taught to have weekly family meetings during which time they problem solve on family and individual goals, resolve conflict between members, and pinpoint stressors.

The last stage of therapy is oriented toward teaching the skills necessary for resolving the problems that remain. This may involve teaching a range of behavioral techniques, depending on the needs of the family, such as contingency contracting for marital discord, social skills training for social inadequacy, token economy for severe social withdrawal, or relaxation and exposure for anxiety. In most instances, the entire family is involved in planning and implementing these special interventions.

The clinical efficacy of BFT for schizophrenia has been supported in one carefully controlled outcome study that compared it with individual treatment and case management.[38,91] A 2-year follow-up revealed that 83% of the individually treated patients but only 17% of the BFT patients had experienced exacerbations of psychotic symptoms. In addition, family participants in BFT reported significantly greater reductions in mental and physical problems and burden of the illness than those in the individual treatment. Behavioral family therapy is currently under replication investigation in several outcome studies, preliminary results of which show good promise for this method.

Token Economy

For chronic, treatment-refractory, long-stay schizophrenic patients who have resisted all efforts at deinstitutionalization, the psychosocial strategy of choice is the token economy. Utilizing behavioral assessment and therapy, highly trained paraprofessionals and nursing staff have been successful in remediating the bizarre symptoms and social and self-care deficits of the most chronic schizophrenic patients. In the most rigorous study conducted on the token economy, Paul and Lentz[41] compared a token economy-social learning program with an equally intensive therapeutic milieu, and a custodial hospital care group. The token economy program was highly structured with many hours of educational activities throughout the day. Patients were positively reinforced with praise and tokens for productive, appropriate behavior (eg, grooming) and fined tokens and/or ignored for inappropriate behaviors (eg, assaults). They could exchange tokens for primary reinforcers, such as food and cigarettes or privileges (eg, grounds pass). Patients were held accountable for their behavior and were provided with training in social skills to help them prepare for community living. Activities in the therapeutic milieu were equally structured, with peer pressure and democratic decision making as the main vehicles for promoting behavior change.

Differences in clinical outcome strongly favored the token economy program over both the therapeutic milieu and custodial hospital treatments. More patients in the token economy program were successfully discharged into the community, experienced greater reductions in symptoms, and were able to be withdrawn from psychotropic medications than in either of the other two groups. In addition to better overall patient functioning and less behavioral disturbance, the token economy program also was more cost effective than either of the other programs, as the increased community tenure resulted in much lower hospital costs.

There are relatively few token economy-social learning inpatient units for adult psychiatric patients nationwide, in contrast to many existing for the developmentally disabled and for children and adolescents.[92] One such program is located at the Clinical Research Unit (CRU) at Camarillo State Hospital. The unit's day-to-day programming and token economy are very similar to those used in the Paul study.[41] Patients are referred to the CRU when standard hospital programming proves ineffective to participate in studies of treatment refractory schizophrenia. On the unit they are provided with training in personal grooming, social skills, room clean-up, and appropriate meal behavior. Special programs are developed for each patient's unique behavioral problems (eg, verbal aggression, polydipsia) as well, thus increasing the likelihood of discharge.[93]

Most of the patients' awake hours are filled with learning and recreational activities, and frequent training sessions, as a number of studies have indicated that patients engage in less deviant or bizarre behavior when they are engaged in structured activities.[94–96] During its 17 years of operation, 42% of the patients referred to the CRU as refractory have been discharged into the community, with half of them being successfully maintained in the community postdischarge.[97] The therapeutic impact of the CRU on even the most intractable state hospital patients is reviewed in Table 10.2, which describes the level of improvement for different behavior problems among 211 consecutive patients treated at the unit.

Bridging the Gap from Innovation to Practice

The past 15 years have witnessed an explosion in the development of new and effective psychosocial interventions for schizophrenia, with behavioral interventions including social skills training, behavioral family therapy, and the token economy. As with all innovations, there is a time lag

TABLE 10.2. Clinical Research Unit (CRU) treatment evaluation.*

Behavioral problems	No. of patients with problem behaviors	Average improvement level
Self-care, grooming	145	1.90
Assaults and property destruction	91	2.17
Social skills deficit	70	1.96
Work and leisure skills	48	1.84
Verbal aggression	38	1.69
Stereotypic movements and posturing	32	1.97
Delusional speech	21	2.19
Self-injury	20	1.65
Peskiness, demandingness	18	1.67
Social isolation	16	2.13
Depression	13	1.92
Prader–Willi syndrome (obesity)	9	1.00
Sexual deviance	9	2.11
Hallucinations, self-talk	5	2.60
Incontinence	4	2.72
Spitting and mucous smearing	4	1.00
Inactivity, amotivation	3	2.67
Screaming, tantrums	2	2.00
Obsessive-compulsive behavior	2	3.00
Mutism	2	2.50
Incoherent speech	2	2.50
Antisocial behavior (stealing, breaking and entering, disruption)	2	2.00
Entering restricted areas	1	1.00
Psychogenic polydipsia	1	1.00
Vomiting	1	1.00
Anxiety	1	1.00
Total number of patient behaviors treated	546	
Overall average improvement level		1.92

*Levels of improvement for different categories of behavioral problems targeted for treatment in the 211 patients treated on the CRU between 1970–1987. The improvement ratings are based on the following criteria: marked improvement (1) = 75–100% change from baseline; moderate improvement (2) = 50–75% change from baseline; slight improvement (3) = 25–50% change from baseline; and no improvement (4) = less than 25% improvement.

between the empirical validation of a treatment method and its adoption and implementation by on-line practitioners. Recent advances in social skills training and behavioral family therapy have emphasized establishing refined, specific, core curriculum areas for skills training—modules—to which patients can be referred depending on their behavioral deficits and presenting problems.[98,99] This modular approach to psychosocial treatment may both target the full spectrum of social and independent living skills needs of chronic schizophrenics, as well as facilitate dissemination by the specificity of the training procedures and the establishment of readily usable curricula. By providing practitioners with empirically validated methods and curricula for engaging schizophrenics and their families in skill enhancement programs, they are freed of having to "re-invent the wheel" when they attempt to provide state-of-the-art treatment without adequate resource materials. The packaging of psychosocial interventions into readily trainable and testable modules holds much promise for the rapid dissemination and adoption of novel and efficacious treatments.[100]

Summary

Psychological interventions for schizophrenic patients have made dramatic advances in recent years, with the emergence of several empirically validated methods. Treatments are based upon the stress-vulnerability-coping skills model of schizophrenia. This model proposes that schizophrenic symptoms are the consequence of stress impinging on psychobiological vulnerability, and that coping and social skills can protect the patient from the noxious effects of stressors on vulnerability. Social support is also hypothesized to reduce the adverse effects of stress on schizophrenic patients.

Based on this model, the primary aim of psychosocial interventions is to either build up patients' individual skill competencies as through social skills training, or to decrease ambient stress in their environment as in behavioral family therapy. Treatments focusing on developing new skills and designed to improve patients' and relatives' understanding of the illness and ability to manage it effectively have received strong empirical support.

An assertive outreach program providing supportive therapy and patient advocacy has been replicated in several locales as an effective alternative to hospital treatment. The characteristic features accounting for the success of these programs are: the flexible community locus of treatment; seven days a week availability of staff intervention; and an emphasis on practical issues related to basic living needs and everyday functioning.

Token economy programs that emphasize social learning have also been found to be effective with treatment-refractory, institutionalized schizophrenics who are unresponsive to more socially-oriented interventions. Utilizing behavioral assessment and therapy techniques, highly trained paraprofessionals and nursing staff have been successful in remediating the bizarre symptoms and social and self-care deficits of even the most chronic schizophrenic patients.

The empirical support for the effectiveness of traditional psychosocial interventions is skimpy, including individual psychotherapy, insight-oriented or systems-strategic family therapy, group therapy, milieu therapy, and case management.

Studies of the effects of social skills training on schizophrenic patients have demonstrated a number of positive findings: improvement in a wide range of social skills in specific situations; a moderate generalization of acquired skills; decreases in social anxiety; a decreased risk of relapse; and improved social and community functioning. Deficits in social skills appear to reflect the combined influence of: the illness itself; learning history prior to the onset of the illness; lack of environmental stimulation; and the loss of skills secondary to prolonged disease. A recent innovation in social skills training has been the packaging of a group of functionally related skills into training "modules": medication management; symptom self-management; personal hygiene and grooming; conversational skills; friendship and dating; social problem solving; and leisure and recreational skills.

References

1. American Psychiatric Association: *Diagnostic and Statistical Manual—III-R.* Washington, DC, American Psychiatric Association Press, 1987.
2. Zubin J, Spring B: Vulnerability: a new view of schizophrenia. *J Abnormal Psychol* 1977;96:103–126.
3. Liberman RP, Mueser KT: Schizophrenia: psychosocial treatment, in Kaplan HI, Saddock BJ (eds): *Comprehensive Textbook of Psychiatry/V.* Baltimore, Williams & Wilkins, 1989, pp 792–806.
4. Ciompi L: Toward a coherent multidimensional understanding and therapy of schizophrenia: converging new concepts, in Strauss JS, Boker W, Brenner HD (eds): *Psychosocial Treatment of Schizophrenia.* Toronto, Hans Huber Pub, 1987, pp 48–62.
5. Farmer AE, McGuffin P, Gottesman II: Twin concordance for DSM-III schizophrenia. *Arch Gen Psychiatr* 1987;44:634–641.
6. Crow TJ: Molecular pathology of schizophrenia: more than one disease pathology? *Br Med J* 1980;280:66–68.
7. Andreason NC, Olsen S: Negative *vs* positive schizophrenia: definition and validation. *Arch Gen Psychiatr* 1982;39:789–794.
8. Weinberger DR: Implications of normal brain development for the pathogenesis of schizophrenia. *Arch Gen Psychiatr* 1987;44:660–669.
9. Dawson ME, Nuechterlein KH: Psychophysiological dysfunctions in the developmental course of schizophrenic disorders. *Schiz Bul* 1984;10:204–232.
10. Nuechterlein KH, Dawson ME: Information processing and attentional functioning in the developmenal cause of schizophrenic disorders. *Schiz Bul* 1984;10:160–202.
11. Liberman RP, DeRisi WR, Mueser KT: Social skills training for psychiatric patients. New York, Pergamon, 1989.
12. Zigler E, Glick M: A developmental approach to adult psychopathology. New York, Wiley, 1986.
13. Serban G: Functioning in schizophrenia and "normal" subjects. *Compr Psychiatr* 1975;16:447–456.
14. Strauss JS, Carpenter WT: Prediction of outcome in schizophrenia. *Arch Gen Psychiatr* 1977;34:159–163.

15. DeJong A, Giel R, Slooff CJ, et al: Social disability and outcome in schizophrenic patients. *Br J Psychiatr* 1985;147:631–636.
16. Anthony WA: A rehabilitation model for rehabilitating the psychiatrically disabled. *Rehabilitation Counseling Bulletin* 1980;24:6–21.
17. Anthony WA, Liberman RP: The practice of psychiatric rehabilitation: historical, conceptual, and research base. *Schiz Bul* 1986;12:542–559.
18. Wixted JT, Morrison RL, Bellack AS: Social skills training in the treatment of negative symptoms. *Int J Mental Health* 1988;17:3–21.
19. Rogers CR, Gendlin EG, Keisler DJ, et al, (eds): *The Therapeutic Relationship and Its Impact: Study of Psychotherapy with Schizophrenics*. Madison, University of Wisconsin Press, 1967.
20. Karon BP, VandenBos GR: The consequences of psychotherapy for schizophrenic patients. *Psychother Theory, Research and Practice* 1972;9:111–119.
21. May PRA: *Treatment of Schizophrenia: A Comparative Study of Five Treatment Methods*. New York, Science House, 1968.
22. Grinspoon L, Ewalt JR, Shader RI: *Schizophrenia: Pharmacotherapy and Psychotherapy*. Baltimore, Williams & Wilkins, 1972.
23. Gunderson JG, Frank A, Katz HM, et al: Effects of psychotherapy in schizophrenia: II. Comparative outcome of two forms of treatment. *Schiz Bul* 1984;10:564–598.
24. McGlashan TH: The Chestnut Lodge follow-up study II. Long-term outcome of schizophrenia and the affective disorders. *Arch Gen Psychiatr* 1984; 41:586–601.
25. Stone MH: Exploratory psychotherapy in schizophrenia-spectrum patients. *Bul Menninger Clinic* 1986;50:287–306.
26. Perris C: *Cognitive Therapy of Schizophrenia*. New York, Guilford Press, 1989.
27. Lidz T, Fleck S, Cornelison A (eds): *Schizophrenia and the Family*. New York, International Universities Press, 1965.
28. Bowen M: The family as a unit of study and treatment. *Am J Orthopsychiat* 1961;31:40–60.
29. Bateson G, Jackson DD, Haley J, et al: Toward a theory of schizophrenia. *Behav Sci* 1956;1:251–264.
30. Massie HN, Beels CC: The outcome of the family treatment of schizophrenia. *Schiz Bul* 1972;6:26–36.
31. Terkelsen KG: Schizophrenia and the family: II. Adverse effects of family therapy. *Family Process* 1983;22:191–200.
32. Appleton WS: Mistreatment of patients' families by psychiatrists. *Am J Psychiatr* 1974;131:655–657.
33. Leff J, Vaughn C: *Expressed Emotion in Families*. New York, Guilford Press, 1985.
34. Koenigsberg HW, Handley R: Expressed emotion: from predictive index to clinical construct. *Am J Psychiatr* 1986;143:1361–1373.
35. Leff J, Kuipers L, Berkowitz R, et al: A controlled trial of social intervention in the families of schizophrenic patients: two-year follow-up. *Br J Psychiatr* 1985;46:594–600.
36. Anderson CM, Reiss DJ, Hogarty GE: *Schizophrenia and the Family*. New York, Guilford Press, 1986.

37. Hogarty GE, Anderson CM, Reiss DJ, et al: Family psychoeducation, social skills training and maintenance chemotherapy. I. One-year effects of a controlled study on relapse and expressed emotion. *Arch Gen Psychiatr* 1986;3:633–642.

38. Falloon IRH, Boyd JL, McGill CW, et al: Family versus individual management in the prevention of morbidity of schizophrenia. *Arch Gen Psychiatr* 1985;2:887–896.

39. Linn MW, Klett J, Caffey FM: Foster home characteristics and psychiatric patient outcomes. *Arch Gen Psychiatr* 1980;37:129–132.

40. Keith SJ, Matthews SM: Group, family, and milieu therapies and psychosocial rehabilitation in the treatment of the schizophrenic disorders, in Grinspoon L (ed): *Psychiatry 1982 Annual Review*. Washington, DC, American Psychiatric Press, 1982.

41. Paul G, Lentz R: *Psychosocial Treatment of Chronic Mental Patients: Milieu vs Social-Learning Programs*. Cambridge, MA, Harvard University Press, 1977.

42. Austin NK, Liberman RP, King LW, et al: A comparative evaluation of two-day hospitals. *J Nerv Ment Dis* 1976;163:253–262.

43. Spiegler MD, Agigian H: *The Community Training Center: An Educational-Behavioral Social Systems Model for Rehabilitating Psychiatric Patients*. New York, Brunner/Mazel, 1977.

44. Milne D: A comparative evaluation of two psychiatric day hospitals. *Br J Psychiatr* 1984;145:533–537.

45. Beard JH, Propst RN, Malamud TJ: The Foundation House model of psychiatric rehabilitation. *Psychosoc Rehab J* 1982;5:47–53.

46. Beard JH, Malamud TJ, Rossman E: Psychiatric rehabilitation and long-term rehospitalization rates: the findings of two research studies. *Schiz Bul* 1978;4:622–635.

47. Test MA, Stein LI: Alternative to mental hospital treatment III. Social Cost. *Arch Gen Psychiatr* 1980;37:409–412.

48. Stein LI, Test MA (eds): *The Training in Community Living Model: A Decade of Experience*. San Francisco, Jossey-Bass, 1985.

49. Hoult J, Reynolds I: Schizophrenia: a comparative trial of community-oriented and hospital-oriented psychiatric care. *Acta Psychiatr Scand* 1984;69:359.

50. Dincin J, Witheridge TF: Psychiatric rehabilitation as a deterrent to recidivism. *Hosp Comm Psychiatr* 1982;33:645–650.

51. Bond GR, Witheridge TF, Setze PJ, et al: Preventing rehospitalization of clients in a psychosocial rehabilitation program. *Hosp Comm Psychiatr* 1985;36:993–995.

52. Bellack AS, Mueser KT: A comprehensive treatment program for schizophrenia and chronic mental illness. *Comm Ment Health J* 1986;22:175–189.

53. Liberman RP, Falloon IRH, Wallace CJ: Drug-psychosocial interactions in the treatment of schizophrenia, in Mirabi M, (ed): *The Chronically Mentally Ill: Research and Services*. New York, SP Medical Scientific Books, 1984.

54. Intagliata J: Improving the quality of community care for the chronically mentally disabled: the role of case management. *Schiz Bull* 1982;8:655–674.

55. Cohen S, Wills TA: Stress, social support, and the buffering hypothesis. *Psychol Bull* 1985;98:310–357.

56. Beels CC: Social support and schizophrenia. *Schiz Bul* 1981;7:58–72.
57. Liberman RP, Glynn S, Phipps CC: Rehabilitation of schizophrenic disorders, in *Treatment of Psychiatric Disorders: A Report of the American Psychiatric Association Task Force on Treatment of Psychiatric Disorders*. Washington, DC, American Psychiatric Press, 1988.
58. Franklin JL, Solovitz B, Mason M, et al: An evaluation of case management. *Am J Public Health* 1987;77:674–678.
59. Liberman RP: Behavior therapy for schizophrenia, in West LJ, Flinn D (eds): *Treatment of Schizophrenia*. New York, Grune & Stratton, 1976.
60. Wong SE, Massel HK, Mosk MD, et al: Behavioral approaches to the treatment of schizophrenia, in Burrows GD, Norman TR, Rubinstein G (eds): *Handbook of Studies on Schizophrenia*. Amsterdam, Elsevier, 1986.
61. Ullman LP, Krasner L: *A Psychological Approach to Abnormal Behavior*. Englewood Cliffs, NJ, Prentice–Hall, 1969.
62. Liberman RP: Sociopolitics of behavioral programs in institutions and community agencies. *Analysis and Intervention in Development Disabilities* 1983;3:131–159.
63. Bandura A: *Principles of Behavior Modification*. New York, Holt, Rinehart, & Winston, Inc., 1979.
64. Salter A: *Conditioned Reflex Therapy*. New York, Farrar, Straus, 1949.
65. Wolpe J: Psychotherapy by reciprocal inhibition. Stanford, Stanford University Press, 1958.
66. Liberman RP, Mueser KT, Wallace CJ, et al: Training skills in the psychiatrically disabled: learning coping and competence. *Schiz Bul* 1986;12:631–647.
67. Liberman RP, Foy DW: Psychiatric rehabilitation for chronic mental patients. *Psychiat Annals* 1983;13:539–545.
68. Liberman RP, Massel HK, Mosk MD, et al: Social skills training for chronic mental patients. *Hosp Common Psychiatr* 1985;36:396–403.
69. Morrison RL, Bellack AS: The role of social perception in social skill. *Behav Ther* 1981;12:69–79.
70. Brady JP: Social skills training for psychiatric patients, I: Concepts, methods, and clinical results. *Am J Psychiatr* 1984;141:333–340.
71. Brady JP: Social skills training for psychiatric patients, II: Clinical outcome studies. *Am J Psychiatr* 1984;141:491–498.
72. Hersen M, Bellack AS, Turner SM: Assessment of assertiveness in female psychiatric patients: motor and autonomic measures. *J Behav Ther Exp Psychiat* 1978;9:11–16.
73. Eisler RM, Blanchard EB, Fitts H, et al: Social skill training with and without modeling for schizophrenic and nonpsychotic hospitalized psychiatric patients. *Behav Mod* 1978;2:147–172.
74. Edelstein BA, Eisler RM: Effects of modeling and modeling with instructions and feedback on the behavioral components of social skills. *Behav Ther* 1976;7:382–389.
75. Kolko DJ, Dorsett PG, Milan MA: A total assessment approach to the evaluation of social skills training: the effectiveness of an anger control program for adolescent psychiatric patients. *Behav Assess* 1981;3:383–402.
76. Eisler RM, Hersen M, Miller PM: Effects of modeling on components of assertive behavior. *J Behav Ther Exp Psychiatr* 1973;4:1–6.

77. Finch BE, Wallace CJ: Successful interpersonal skills training with schizophrenic inpatients. *J Consult Clin Psychol* 1977;45:885–890.
78. Urey JR, Luaghlin C, Kelly JA: Teaching heterosocial conversational skills to male psychiatric inpatients. *J Behav Ther Exp Psychiatr* 1979;10:323–328.
79. Holmes MR, Hansen DJ, St. Lawrence JS: Conversational skills training with aftercare patients in the community: social validation and generalization. *Behav Ther* 1984;15:84–100.
80. Kelly JA, Laughlin C, Claiborne M, et al: A group procedure for teaching job interviewing skills to formerly hospitalized psychiatric patients. *Behav Ther* 1979;10:79–83.
81. Furman W, Geller M, Simon SJ, et al: The use of a behavioral rehearsal procedure for teaching job interview skills to psychiatric patients. *Behav Ther* 1979;10:157–167.
82. Bellack AS, Hersen M, Turner SM: Generalization effects of social skills training with chronic schizophrenics: an experimental analysis. *Behav Res Ther* 1976;14:391–398.
83. Frederickson LW, Jenkins JO, Foy DW, et al: Social skills training to modify abusive verbal outbursts in adults. *J Applied Behav Analysis* 1976;9:117–127.
84. Liberman RP, Mueser, KT, Wallace CJ: Social skills training for schizophrenics at risk for relapse. *Am J Psychiatr* 1986;143:523–526.
85. Bellack AS, Turner SM, Hersen M, et al: An examination of the efficacy of social skills training for chronic schizophrenic patients. *Hosp Comm Psychiatr* 1984;35:1023–1028.
86. Falloon IRH, Boyd JL, McGill CW: *Family Care of Schizophrenia.* New York, Guilford Press, 1984.
87. Mueser KT: Behavioral family therapy, in Bellack AS (ed): *A Treatment Guide for Schizophrenia.* New York, Grune & Stratton, in press.
88. Liberman RP, Falloon IRH, Aitchison RA: Multiple family therapy for schizophrenia: a behavioral, problem-solving approach. *Psychosoc Rehab J* 1984;4:60–77.
89. Liberman RP, Mueser KT, Glynn S: Modular behavioral strategies, in Falloon IRH (ed): *Handbook of Behavioral Family Therapy.* New York, Guilford Press, 1988.
90. Hatfield AB, Lefley HP (eds): *Families of the Mentally Ill: Coping and Adaption.* New York, Guilford Press, 1987.
91. Falloon IRH: *Family Management of Schizophrenia: A Study of Clinical, Social, Family, and Economic Benefits.* Baltimore, Johns Hopkins University Press, 1985.
92. Boudewyns PA, Fry TJ, Nightingale T: Token economy programs in VA medical centers: where are they today? *The Behavior Therapist* 1986;9:126–127.
93. Liberman RP, DeRisi WJ, King LW, et al: Behavioral measurement in a community mental health center, in Davidson P, Clark F, Hamerlynck L (eds): *Evaluating Behavioral Programs in Community, Residential and Educational Settings.* Champaign, IL, Research Press, 1974.
94. Rosen AJ, Sussman S, Mueser KT, et al: Behavioral assessment of psychiatric patients and normal controls across different environmental contexts. *J Behav Assess* 1981;3:25–36.

95. Liberman RP, Wallace CJ, Teigen J, et al: Interventions with psychotics, in Calhoun KS, Adams HE, Mitchell EM (eds), *Innovative Treatment Methods in Psychopathology*. New York, Wiley, 1974.
96. Wong SE, Terranova MD, Bowen L, et al: Providing independent recreational activities to reduce steroetypic vocalizations in chronic schizophrenics. *J Applied Behav Analysis* 1987;20:77–81.
97. Banzett LK, Liberman RP, Moore JW, et al: Long-term follow-up of the effects of behavior therapy. *Hosp Comm Psychiatr* 1984;35:277–279.
98. Liberman RP: *Psychiatric Rehabilitation of Chronic Mental Patients*. Washington, DC, American Psychiatric Press, 1987.
99. Liberman RP, Evans C: Behavioral rehabilitation of chronic mental patietns. *J Clin Psychopharm* 1985;5:8S–14S.
100. Backer TE, Liberman RP, Kuehnel TG: Dissemination and adoption of innovative psychosocial interventions. *J Consult Clin Psychol* 1986;54:111–118.

11
Clozapine: Mechanism of Action in Relation to its Clinical Advantages

HERBERT Y. MELTZER

Clozapine, a dibenzodiazepine, is the prototype of an atypical antipsychotic drug. A generally accepted definition of an atypical antipsychotic drug is one that produces weak catalepsy in rodents, minimal extrapyramidal side effects (EPS) at clinically effective doses, and minimal plasma prolactin (PRL) elevations in humans.[1] Almost all such agents are dopamine (DA) receptor antagonists, and block stereotypy or locomotor activity in rodents due to stimulation of DA receptors by direct-acting DA agonists, (eg, apomorphine) or indirect DA agonists (eg, d-amphetamine). Atypical antipsychotic drugs block the conditioned avoidance response, another test which indicates their antipsychotic potential. Clozapine clearly fits this definition.[1-3]

Extrapyramidal side effects of neuroleptic drugs include: acute reactions, such as torticollis and opisthotonous; subacute effects, such as rigidity, akinesia, drooling, and akathisia; and chronic, sometimes irreversible effects, (eg, tardive dyskinesia and tardive dystonia). Extrapyramidal side effects of any kind may be very disturbing to patients and are a major factor in noncompliance. For these reasons, there has been intense interest in developing neuroleptic drugs without EPS. There is abundant evidence that clozapine produces less EPS than typical antipsychotic drugs.[4,5] The same is true of other atypical drugs such as melperone,[6] fluperlapine,[7] and RMI-81582.[8] Furthermore, there are no published reports that either clozapine or melperone, the two atypical antipsychotics which have been extensively used in western countries for more than a decade, produces tardive dyskinesia or tardive dystonia. However, because clozapine can block the symptoms of tardive dyskinesia,[9] it is not possible to rule out that it might produce tardive dyskinesia, especially in some vulnerable individuals.

Clozapine has other advantages as well. Recent multicenter trials have shown that clozapine may be a more effective antipsychotic agent than chlorpromazine in a representative group of chronic schizophrenic patients,[10] as well as treatment-resistant schizophrenic patients.[11] Most earlier studies also found clozapine to be equal to or superior to typical antipsychotic drugs,[12] but there is some limited evidence to the contrary.[13] We recently have found that clozapine continues to produce improvement in treatment-resistant schizophrenic patients for at least the first 12 months of treatment.[14] Clozapine was found to be superior to chlorpromazine for both positive and negative symptoms at 6 weeks and longer. These results agree with retrospective, uncontrolled studies of Juul Povlsen et al,[15] Kuha and Meittenen,[16] and Lindström,[17] which include some patients treated for more than 10 years. Furthermore, clozapine does not elevate plasma PRL levels in humans.[18]

These four clinical advantages of clozapine: (1) fewer EPS, (2) no tardive dyskinesia (probably), (3) increased efficacy, and (4) no increase in plasma PRL levels in humans, constitute extraordinarily important clinical advantages that would ordinarily lead to the adoption of it or similar drugs as the primary treatment of schizophrenia. However, clozapine produces granulocytopenia in 1% of cases,[19] and even though this appears to be reversible if identified rapidly followed by immediate withdrawal of clozapine, this risk has limited its use. The clinical development of fluperlapine was stopped for the same reason. Melperone is the one typical antipsychotic drug for which no unusual safety risks have been identified. No controlled studies of the effect of melperone in treatment-resistant patients have been published. Other putative atypical drugs such as tiospirone and RMI-81582 have had limited clinical testing and have been withdrawn because of side effects unrelated to granulocytopenia.

Because there is a clear rationale for clozapine-like drugs with a better safety profile, it is critical to understand their mechanism of action. This can lead to a more rapid identification of candidate drugs for clinical testing. Furthermore, it could lead to an increased understanding of schizophrenia.[1] The four clinical advantages of clozapine might be due to the same chemical effect(s) or as many as four different features.[1] It seems most likely that one mechanism might be involved, but, as discussed below, this may have many factors contributing to it. It appears that low EPS and the probable lack of causation of tardive dyskinesia are based on the same mechanism. This feature also may be related to the lack of effect of clozapine on plasma PRL levels in humans. As will be discussed, the latter effect could be due to the ability of clozapine to increase DA release in the median eminence,[20] which contains the terminals of the tuberoinfundibular (TIDA) neurons that are critical to control of PRL secretion. Clozapine also increases DA release in other DA terminal areas.[21] The ability of clozapine to increase DA release may be the consequence of a number of aspects of its pharmacology, which could differ from region to region. The intriguing possibility that the enhanced antipsychotic efficacy of clozapine is also based, in part, on increased DA release will be discussed in detail subsequently. The importance of serotonin (5-HT) in the unique effects of clozapine will also be considered.

Selective Effects on Mesolimbic *vs* Mesostriatal Dopamine Neurons

The basis for neuroleptic-induced EPS has been thought to be blockade of D-2 DA receptors in the striatum.[22] D-2 receptors are those DA receptors that are negatively coupled (ie, inhibitory to adenylate cyclase). D-1 receptors are those DA receptors whose stimulation lead to an increase in adenylate cyclase activity.[23] Clozapine's affinity for the striatal D-2 receptor is 101 nm which is low compared with chlorpromazine (3.0 nm) and haloperidol (1.10 nm).[24] Nevertheless, the affinity of clozapine for the striatal D-2 receptor is in accord with its clinical potency as an antipsychotic drug.[25]

Clozapine produces a dose-dependent increase in rat striatal homovanillic acid (HVA), the major metabolite of DA, and an increase in tyrosine hydroxylase activity, the rate limiting step in DA synthesis.[26,3] It also antagonizes the cataleptogenic effect of prochlorperazine,[26] a most unusual effect for an antipsychotic drug. On this basis, Bartholini et al[26] proposed that clozapine produces a reversible blockade of DA receptors in the striatum; that is, one in which the release of DA from nerve terminals via feedback activation is able to partially overcome the effect of receptor blockade. The antiserotonergic effect of clozapine also may be relevant to this anticataleptogenic effect (see below). In vivo dialysis studies have established that clozapine, acutely and chronically, can stimulate DA release from the rat striatum and nucleus accumbens (Ichikawa and Meltzer, in preparation). The ability of clozapine to enhance DA turnover in the striatum was reported to increase after chronic administration,[27] but another study demonstrated the development of tolerance to this action comparable to that produced by typical neuroleptic drugs.[28] However, we have found no decrease of the effect of clozapine on DA release in the striatum by in vivo dialysis after 21 days administration of clozapine (Ichikawa and Meltzer, in preparation).

Because of the low EPS produced by clozapine, numerous investigators have studied the relative effect of clozapine on DA turnover in the striatum *vs* the nucleus accumbens. A greater effect of clozapine on DA release in the rabbit limbic system was found by Andén and Stock[29] and in the rat by Zivkovic et al.[30] No difference in DA release in these two brain regions in the rat was reported by Bartholini et al,[31] Westernik and Korf,[32] Stawarz et al,[33] Weisel and Sedvall,[34] Walters and Roth,[35] Wilk et al,[36] Waldmeier and Maitre,[37] and Maidment and Marsden.[38] Preliminary in vivo dialysis data suggest the nucleus accumbens is more sensitive to clozapine than the striatum (Ichikawa and Meltzer, in preparation). Species differences could account for the enhanced response in the accumbens reported by Andén and Stock.[29] The difference was marked only at the 5 mg/kg intravenous dose; the differences at 2.5 and 10 mg/kg were smaller. Zivkovic et al[30] also reported a greater effect of clozapine in the striatum; these authors measured DA turnover by assessing the specific activity of ^{3}H-DA formed from ^{3}H-tyrosine. The other studies assessed the rate of disappearance of DA after alpha-methylparatyrosine pretreatment,[37] DOPA accumulation after decarboxylase inhibition,[35] or percentage increase in HVA or dihydroxyphenylacetic acid (DOPAC). The latter may be less reliable because HVA concentrations may mainly result in intraneuronal DA metabolism. Waldmier and Maitre[37] required very high doses of clozapine to achieve any effect (100 mg/kg, orally). Thus, it may be that the biochemical effect of clozapine to increase DA turnover is greater in the limbic system than in the striatum. This issue will be more meaningfully studied by in vivo dialysis or voltammetry. Clinical data clearly suggest clozapine produces much less disruption of dopaminergic neurotransmission in the nigrostriatal pathway both acutely and chronically. Nevertheless, the ability of clozapine to block the symptoms of tardive dyskinesia strongly suggests it does affect the nigrostriatal pathway. The ability of clozapine to block 11-C–raclopride binding in the caudate–putamen of patients treated with clozapine is consistent with this conclusion.[39]

Effect of Chronic Administration on Dopamine Receptors

Chronic administration of haloperidol to rats increases the number of striatal DA receptors (Bmax)[40] and a shift to the left of the dose-response curve to the behavioral effects of DA agonists.[41] Most studies have found that clozapine causes no change in the Bmax of 3-H-spiperone binding in rat striatum and no supersensitivity to DA agonists[42–47]; however, two studies have reported increased stereotypy and Bmax.[48,49] The former studies appear more reliable. Treatment for up to 20 months with clozapine did not alter the Bmax of the binding of the DA agonist, 3-H-spiperone, the D-2 antagonist 3-H-N-propylapomorphine, or 3-H-piflutixol, under conditions in which it bound mainly to D-1 receptors, to mesolimbic receptor binding sites. In fact, no evidence was found to indicate that after 20 months treatment with haloperidol, sulpiride, or clozapine, DA receptor blockade persisted in the limbic system.[50] However, 9 to 12 months administration of clozapine did increase the Bmax of 3-H-piflutixol but not 3-H-spiperone or 3-H-N-propylapomorphine binding. No effect of chronic clozapine on adenylate cyclase activity or stereotyped behavior was found.[51] These results could be relevant to the failure of clozapine to produce tardive dyskinesia, but this is purely speculative because the evidence that links tardive dyskinesia to increased D-2 receptor sensitivity in the striatum is minimal.

Acute doses of clozapine have been reported to increase the firing rate of ventral tegmental (A10) but not nigrostriatal (A9) DA neurons in three studies.[52-54] However, Souto et al[55] found an increase in the firing rate of both the A9 and A10 DA neurons. The reasons for these discrepancies are unclear. As mentioned, in vivo dialysis suggests chronic clozapine administration increases DA release in both areas (Ichikawa and Meltzer, in preparation). In vivo voltammetry has revealed that acute administration of clozapine increases DA release in the nucleus accumbens but not in the striatum.[56,57] The reasons for these discrepancies are not immediately apparent.

Chronic administration of clozapine to the rat produces a suppression of firing rate of the A10 DA neurons but not the A9 DA neurons.[53,52] This appears to be due to so-called depolarization inactivation, because the silent DA neurons begin to fire after microiontophoretic application of the inhibitory neurotransmitter, GABA[52] or apomorphine.[54] In vivo voltametry also found selective decreases in DA release in the nucleus accumbens but not the striatum.[58] It has been suggested that the anticholinergic and/or anti-alpha$_1$-adrenergic properties of clozapine account for its selective effect on mesolimbic DA neurons.[52,59,60] Its serotonergic effects also may be important because chronic haloperidol plus the 5-HT$_2$ antagonist, ritanserin, produces the same effect (Bunney BS, personal communication, 1988). The issue of the temporal development of the biological effects of clozapine is very relevant to the time course of its action. Clozapine may act within the first week of administration to ameliorate positive and negative symptoms in some treatment-resistant patients,[11,14] but others take 3 to 12 months before responding.[14] It is likely that these differences are mediated by effects of clozapine on DA, 5-HT, and other neurotransmitters together with adaptive changes that occur over long periods, including changes in the release of DA and DA receptor sensitivity.

Neuroendocrine Effects of Clozapine on Tuberoinfundibular Dopamine Neurons

Clozapine produces a dose-related increase in PRL secretion in rats.[61,62] However, this increase lasts about half as long as that produced by equivalent doses of typical neuroleptics. Short-lived increases in plasma PRL concentration are also produced by other atypical antipsychotic drugs, such as melperone and fluperlapine.[20] This is not due to pharmacokinetic factors, because clozapine levels, as assessed by a radioreceptor assay, are persistently increased even after plasma PRL levels have decreased. The rapid decrease in plasma PRL levels after clozapine and other atypical antipsychotic drugs appears to be related to an increase in activity of the TIDA neurons.[20]

The mechanism(s) by which clozapine increases DA release from the TIDA neurons are complex. Neurotensin, a neuropeptide, can mimic the effects of clozapine on DA synthesis in TIDA neurons.[62] This effect of clozapine and neurotensin can be blocked by neurotensin antisera.[62] The clozapine-induced activation of TIDA neurons is also antagonized by the D-1 agonist SKF 38393 but not by the D-2 agonist quinpirole.[63] However, this effect is not produced by the potent D-1 antagonist SCH 23390,[63] nor does SCH 23390 block the effect of SKF 38393 on the clozapine-induced increase in DOPA accumulation (Berry, Meltzer, and Gudelsky, unpublished observation). We also have found that pretreatment with parachlorophenylalanine, an inhibitor of 5-HT synthesis, blocks the effect of clozapine on DA synthesis in the TIDA neurons. Thus, at least three factors might be involved in mediating the action of clozapine to increase DA synthesis and release in TIDA neurons: stimulation of neurotensin, an effect mediated via 5-HT, and possibly a DA-dependent mechanism.

A similar mechanism may be responsible for the lack of effect of clozapine on plasma PRL levels in humans. It suggests that clozapine may increase DA release in TIDA neurons in humans, as well as in rodents. As mentioned, there is in vivo dialysis evidence that clozapine increases DA release in the mesocortical, mesolimbic, and mesostriatal DA neurons[21] (Ichikawa and Meltzer, in preparation). It is possible that clozapine may do the same in humans. The ability to increase DA release in the frontal cortex may be related to its effects on negative symptoms (see below).

Clozapine and other atypical neuroleptic drugs increased plasma corticosterone levels in rats.[64] However, in humans, clozapine does not increase and appears to lower plasma cortisol. The basis for the increase in rodents is unknown. It may be related to its dopaminergic-serotonergic influence as it is shared by atypical antipsychotics. Increasing the release of 5-HT could account for increased release of corticotropin releasing hormone.

Effects on D-1 Mechanisms

Chronic clozapine administration may upregulate striatal D-1 receptors, and D-1 antagonism may contribute to its ability to increase DA release in the TIDA. SKF 38393 also blocked the ability of clozapine and fluperlapine to increase the release of DA in the striatum and prefrontal cortex.[21] Clozapine has a modest affinity for the D-1 receptor (146 nm with 3-H-SCH 23390 as a ligand[24]. This is much less than that of even haloperidol (91 nm), so this cannot be the basis for any unique action mediated through the D-1 mechanism. There is some evidence that acute or chronic administration of SCH 23390 does not produce depolarization inactivation of the A9 and A10 dopamine neurons as does clozapine,[65,66] but Goldstein and Litwin[67] reported that SCH 23390 at low doses (0.0125 to 0.05 mg/kg) increased the activity of A9 and A10 neurons, but chronic administration produced depolarization inactivation of the A10 DA neurons only. Andersen et al[68] reported that clozapine and other atypical antipsychotic drugs are more potent inhibitors of the binding of the D-1 antagonist 3-H-SCH 23390 to D-1 receptors in vivo than would be expected on the basis of their in vitro affinities. No such difference was noted for typical neuroleptics. Andersen and Braestrup[69] subsequently reported that clozapine and fluperlapine were more potent inhibitors of DA-stimulated adenylate cyclase than would be expected from their affinity for the 3-H-SCH 23390 binding site. They suggest clozapine-like drugs bind to the adenylate cyclase-coupled state of the D-1 receptor with high affinity. Other evidence in support of a D-1 mechanism of action of clozapine has been offered by Chipkin and Latranyi[70] and Altar et al.[71]

There is other evidence that argues against the importance of a D-1 dopaminergic mechanism. Meltzer et al[24] identified 20 typical and 18 atypical antipsychotic drugs and determined their Ki values for the rat striatal D-1 and D-2 and cortical 5-HT$_2$ receptor binding sites. Univariate analyses showed significantly lower D-2 but not 5-HT$_2$ or D-1 affinities. D-2 and 5-HT$_2$ affinities were significantly correlated for the atypical drugs (rho $= 0.78$, $N = 18$, $P = 0.0001$) but not for the typical drugs (rho $= 0.18$, $N = 20$, $P = 0.44$). Multivariate analysis showed that the atypical drugs could be discriminated from the typical drugs by the D-2 and 5-HT$_2$ affinities alone without significant contribution from the D-1 affinity. The D-2 affinity accounted for 66% of the variance, and the 5-HT$_2$ affinity accounted for 16%. A classification analysis based on the D-2, 5-HT$_2$, and D-1 affinities correctly discriminated 34 of 38 compounds. These results do not necessarily indicate that D-1 affinities are unimportant in vivo. They do suggest that clozapine-type antipsychotic drugs can be identified by their D-2 and 5-HT$_2$ affinities, together with a test such as the conditioned avoidance test which indicates antipsychotic activity. Adding other features, such as brief increases in PRL stimulation in rodents[64] or weak catalepsy in rodents, should lead to highly accurate identification of candidate atypical antipsychotic drugs with few false-positive results. It is unclear if drugs with relatively high affinty for the D-1 receptor such as SCH 23390 are antipsychotic. Clinical trials are awaited with great interest. However, even if such drugs are not effective, the D-1 component of clozapine action might still be important.

Clozapine and Serotonin

Clozapine has been found to have significant effects on serotonergic neurotransmission. Clozapine increases the concentration of 5-HT and 5-hydroxyindoleacetic acid (5-HIAA), the major metabolite of 5-HT, in rat brain.[72,73,3] In a more detailed study of the effect of clozapine on the metabolism of 5-HT in rat brain, Ruch et al[74] found that clozapine, but not four typical neuroleptics, at a dose of 80 mg/kg, but not 20 mg/kg, increased brain 5-HT and 5-HIAA concentrations. However, clozapine at this dose did not change whole brain 5-HT turnover as indicated by the change in brain 5-HT and 5-HIAA concentrations after administration of the tryptophan hydroxylase inhibitor, 6-fluorotryptophan. They also found no effect of clozapine, 80 mg/kg, on the rate of disappearance of 3-H-5-HT from the brainstem. It would be of interest to study the effect of clozapine on 5-HT turnover using contemporary methods in specific brain regions, for example, the hippocampus and striatum, before concluding that clozapine has no effect on 5-HT turnover. Clozapine, 80 mg/kg, but not haloperidol or loxapine, did increase the concentration of tryptophan and the accumulation of 3-H-tryptophan in both brainstem and limbic areas after intravenous 3-H-tryptophan. Ruch et al[74] suggested that the increase in 5-HT and 5-HIAA were due to increased 5-HT synthesis. The increase in 5-HT or 5-HIAA were no longer present after seven daily doses of clozapine. However, Stralendorff et al[75] found the effect of clozapine on brain 5-HT and 5-HIAA was enhanced after chronic treatment. No tolerance develops to the ability of clozapine to increase rat brain HVA concentrations.[27] Clozapine, 80 mg/kg, decreases plasma total tryptophan and increases plasma free tryptophan. However, typical neuroleptic drugs produced similar effects. Ruch et al[74] concluded that the effects on plasma tryptophan were not related to the effects on brain tryptophan. Nevertheless, they suggested increased brain 5-HT synthesis was related to increased brain tryptophan, perhaps due to an effect on the brain transport system for tryptophan. They concluded that these effects of clozapine on brain 5-HT synthesis were not likely to be related to its antipsychotic effect but perhaps to its sedative properties.

Ackenheil et al[73] and Banki[76] found an elevated concentration of 5-HIAA in the cerebrospinal fluid of clozapine-treated patients, but this was not replicated by Gerlach et al.[77] Ackenheil et al[73] also found increased 5-HIAA concentrations in urine after clozapine treatment. Banki[76] found elevated platelet 5-HT levels that persisted for at least 30 days. No correlation between clinical effectiveness and blood 5-HT or CSF 5-HIAA concentrations was found, but there was a weak relation to sedation.

The effect of clozapine on the 5-HT-sensitive adenylate cyclase of neonatal rat brain was studied by Enjalbert et al.[78] Clozapine was the most potent inhibitor of cyclic AMP production of seven neuroleptics tested. There are multiple 5-HT receptors linked to adenylate cyclase in brain,[79,80] most notably the 5-HT_{1A} receptor.[81] Studies of the effect of acute and chronic clozapine administration on specific adenylate cyclase-linked 5-HT receptors would be of interest.

The effect of atypical antipsychotic drugs on serotonin (5-HT) receptors also has been suggested to be relevant to their unique properties. Clozapine has been found to be a potent 5-HT antagonist in vivo. Thus, it blocks the hyperthermic effects of fenfluramine and 5-hydroxytryptophan,[82,83] the 5-HTP-induced head twitch in rats,[84] the quipazine-induced twitch of the mylohyoid muscle in the rodent,[85] and the 5-HT-related ability of low doses of LSD to potentiate apomorphine-induced hypermotility.[86] Clozapine also inhibited the binding of 3-H-5-HT to rat cortical synaptosomes with an IC_{50} of 2.8×10^{-7} [85] and blocked the discriminative stimulus in rats due to the 5-HT agonist, quipazine.[87] Clozapine, melperone, and setoperone, three atypical antipsychotic drugs, but not haloperidol or chlorpromazine, two typical antipsychotic drugs, produced a dose-dependent inhibition of the hyperthermic response to the $5-HT_2$ agonist MK-212.[88] None of the three drugs blocked the hypothermic response to the $5-HT_{1A}$ agonist, 8-OH-DPAT. The three atypical drugs, but not haloperidol or chlorpromazine, also blocked the increases in corticosterone produced by MK-212 but not 8-OH-DPAT. These results indicate that clozapine and other atypical drugs are $5-HT_2$ antagonists in vivo.

Rasmussen and Aghajanian[89] reported that clozapine plus four other antipsychotic drugs antagonized the effect of the 5-HT hallucinogen, 2,5-dimethoxy-4-methylamphetamine (DOM), to decrease spontaneous activity and increase the response to peripheral nerve stimulation of locus coeruleus neurons in anesthetized rats. The ED_{100}s for reversing the effects of DOM correlated with $5-HT_2$ receptor affinities. Clozapine also has been found to inhibit the increase in PRL and cortisol secretion after MK-212 or 5-HTP in chronically treated schizophrenic patients. Other antipsychotic drugs, for example, chlorpromazine and thioridazine, did not.[1] Sulpizio et al[82] and Lai et al[85] suggested that the antiserotonergic properties of clozapine, in relation to its antidopaminergic properties, might account for its lack of EPS as there is considerable evidence that 5-HT antagonists antagonize the ability of neuroleptic drugs to produce catalepsy.[90] Both Nash et al[88] and Rasmussen and Aghajanian[89] suggested that the atypical properties of clozapine may be related to its $5-HT_2$ receptor-blocking properties. Altar et al[91] compared the affinity of clozapine, six other atypical antipsychotic drugs, and three typical drugs (haloperidol, metoclopramide, and pimozide), for the $5-HT_2$ binding site in rat cortex and the D-2 site in rat caudate-putamen. The $5-HT_2$/D-2 ratio was notably larger for the typical drugs. They too suggested that an effect of the atypical antipsychotic drugs at $5-HT_2$ receptors may counteract the induction of EPS resulting from D-2 receptor blockade.

Clozapine has yet other effects on $5-HT_2$ receptors. Reynolds et al[92] and Lee and Tang[93] reported that chronic clozapine treatment downregulated $5-HT_2$ receptors in rat frontal cortex. We have found that a single dose of clozapine does the same for at least 7 days.[94] This effect is not unique to atypical neuroleptic drugs. Loxapine produces a similar pattern.

Clozapine also has been shown to affect 5-HT release by several mechanisms. Serotonin release can be modulated by 5-HT autoreceptors,[95] by noradrenergic receptors,[96] and by DA receptors, at least in the limbic system.[97] Serotonin release also is enhanced by feedback mechanisms secondary to blockade of postsynaptic 5-HT receptors. Drescher and Hetey[98] studied the ability of clozapine to block 5-HT autoreceptors in synaptosomes from rat nucleus accumbens. Clozapine inhibited this effect of 5-HT, as well as the ability of DA to block 5-HT release in this preparation. The action of clozapine on the presynaptic DA receptor mediating 5-HT release was relatively weak (EC_{50} 10 nm), compared with its effect on the 5-HT autoreceptor (EC_{50} 1.0 nm). Conversely, its effect on DA-induced inhibition of DA release (EC_{50} 0.5 nm) was more potent than its ability to block the effect of 5-HT on DA release (EC_{50} 7.0 nm). They concluded that the effect of clozapine on the 5-HT autoreceptor may be important for its antipsychotic action.

Dopaminergic-Serotonergic Interaction

How could increased dopaminergic activity occur in the mesolimbic system while at the same time decreased dopaminergic activity is present in the mesocortical dopaminergic system? Bannon and Roth[99] have suggested the cortical-subcortical DA interactions may be a factor. Lesions of the frontal cortex in rodents enhance the behavioral effects of indirect or direct DA agonists and diminish the ability of DA antagonists to induce catalepsy.[100,101] There is some evidence that the prefrontal cortex may be particularly important in this regard.[102,103,100] These findings suggest there may be an inhibitory efferent pathway from the prefrontal and other cortical pathways that regulates the dopaminergic output of the mesostriatal and mesolimbic DA neurons. Carter and Pycock[100] reported that prefrontal lesions increased subcortical DA turnover, but other studies that used larger frontal lesions did not observe this effect.[101,104] Behavioral interventions (eg, social isolation) have been reported to decrease subcortical DA turnover while increasing DA turnover in the prefrontal cortex.[105] Bannon and Roth[99] proposed that some symptoms of schizophrenia (ie, cognitive disturbances, attentional dysfunction, and "a diminution in affective and social behavior") could be related to the prefrontal disturbances in DA metabolism. We and others have suggested this decreased dopaminergic activity might underlie the negative symptoms of schizophrenia (ie, flat or inappropriate affect, withdrawal, lack of motivation, anhedonia, etc), which are important components of the deficit state.[106–108] We have proposed that the ability of a DA agonist such as L-DOPA, the precursor of DA, to activate schizophrenic patients might be related to correcting endogenous or neuroleptic-induced deficits in dopaminergic activity.[22,107]

A second way in which decreased dopaminergic activity in the mesolimbic and mesostriatal DA neurons and decreased activity in the frontal cortex could come about is via serotonergic-dopaminergic interactions. It is well established that the dorsal and median raphe serotonergic neurons have an inhibitory effect on the striatal DA neurons. Thus, lesions of the dorsal raphe or antiserotonergic drugs block the catalepsy due to DA antagonists.[109] Catalepsy is dependent on decreased dopaminergic activity in the striatum.[110] Nicolaou et al[111] demonstrated that ipsilateral lesions of the dorsal raphe produced increases in dihydroxyphenylacetic acid (DOPAC) and homovanillic acid (HVA), the major metabolites of DA, in the ipsilateral substantia nigra; a similar effect occurred in the striatum after lesion of the median raphe. Ipsilateral turning after apomorphine was noted in rats with dorsal raphe lesions. The reverse was true in rats with median raphe lesions. Nicolaou et al[111] interpreted these results as an indication that the dorsal and median raphe nuclei may exert a tonic inhibitory effect on DA metabolism in their respective areas of innervation.

Hervé et al[112] reported that electrolytic lesions of the dorsal raphe nucleus markedly increased the rate of DA use in the nucleus accumbens, had a smaller effect in the striatum, and no effect in the frontal cortex 4 days after the lesion. They concluded that dorsal raphe serotonergic neurons regulate mesolimbic but not mesocortical dopaminergic neurons. Subsequently, Hervé et al[113] reported that 5 days after an electrolytic lesion of the median raphe, DA use was decreased in the frontal cortex but increased in the nucleus accumbens. Both effects were no longer present 17 days after the lesion. Bilateral lesions of habenula produce selective acute increases in DA use in the prefrontal cortex, but have no such effect on the nucleus accumbens.[114] Thus, it is clear that DA cells projecting to the nucleus accumbens and prefrontal cortex are subject to differing serotonergic and other inputs. It could be that at some phases of schizophrenia, this type of effect (ie, 5-HT-mediated effect of the dorsal and median raphe nuclei and the habenula) leads to increased subcortical and decreased frontal cortical activity. The ability of clozapine to increase serotonergic activity by the mechanism described by Drescher and Hetey,[98] that is, blockade of the inhibitory effect of 5-HT and DA on 5-HT release might be most important in the frontal cortex, leading to increased DA release (opposite to the effect noted by Hervé et al[113] after median raphe lesions). Clozapine might decrease dopaminergic transmission in the nucleus accumbens by a variety of mechanisms: for example, increased release of 5-HT, which in turn leads to decreased DA release, or by blocking D-1 and D-2 receptors. Clozapine also blocks the firing of dorsal raphe neurons in the rat[115] and markedly downregulates 5-HT$_2$ receptors in the rodent frontal cortex.[93,94]

It is not possible to predict what treatment with clozapine might do to correct pathologic serotonergic influences on dopaminergic activity in the prefrontal cortex, nucleus accumbens, and striatum in schizophrenic patients. However, on the basis of the evidence reviewed here, it is possible to hypothesize that clozapine could correct 5-HT-mediated abnormalities leading to decreased dopaminergic activity in the prefrontal cortex while at the same time decreasing dopaminergic activity in the nucleus accumbens. This would mimic the effects of median raphe stimulation described above, or of dorsal raphe stimulation (decreased DA use in the nucleus accumbens only). There is considerable, albeit far from definitive, evidence for the role of 5-HT in schizophrenia.[116,117] It is beyond the scope of this chapter to consider this evidence here. Suffice it to say, clozapine and the other atypical neuroleptic drugs as a group, differ from the typical neuroleptics, mainly in regard to their relative D-2 and 5-HT$_2$ properties. This could mean that these drugs act to correct some abnormality that stems from a dysfunction in the relationship of the neuronal events mediated by these two receptors. However, whereas therapeutic benefit may stem from altering 5-HT$_2$ and D-2-mediated neuronal activity in a coordinated manner, it could be that this process ameliorates some defect in only one of these neurotransmitter systems or neither.

Conclusions and Summary

Clozapine, the prototype of an atypical antipsychotic drug, has been shown to have at least four major clinical advantages that may be shared, at least to some extent, by all atypical antipsychotic drugs: 1) minimal acute and subacute extrapyramidal symptoms; 2) no tardive dyskinesia; 3) no plasma prolactin increases in man; and 4) increased efficacy in treating positive and negative symptoms in treatment-resistant schizophrenic patients. It seems reasonable that all these effects may be based on the same mechanism which differentiates clozapine and other atypical antipsychotic drugs from typical drugs.

The evidence reviewed here suggests that the abilities of clozapine to block D-2 and 5-HT$_2$ receptors and to enhance DA and 5-HT release in a coordinated manner are the crucial characteristics that convey its unique clinical effects. This conclusion derives from the fact that it is these features, in relation to one another, that differentiate clozapine and other atypical antipsychotic drugs from the typical antipsychotic drugs. It would be far better to have data from patients to support this hypothesis. There are some data at hand,[1] but much more is needed.

It would seem that there is a possibility that all four clinical advantages of clozapine may be related to the influence of this dopaminergic-serotonergic complex on the nigrostriatal, mesolimbic, mesocortical, and TIDA neurons. Clozapine also has strong anticholinergic effects,[118] anti-alpha-adrenergic effects,[3,119] beta-adrenergic blocking properties,[120] ability to increase GABA turnover in the striatum and decrease it in the substantia nigra,[121] ability to enhance glutaminergic neurotransmission,[122] and effects on neurotensin concentrations in discrete brain nuclei.[123]

It is not possible to be sure if any of those effects independently contribute to the four clinical advantages of clozapine or whether they are related to the dopaminergic-serotonergic effects emphasized in this chapter. The hypothesis that one mechanism, however complex, is involved in all the unique features of clozapine, seems to have the greatest heuristic value at this time.

Acknowledgment. Supported, in part, by USPHS MH 41684, MH 41683, USPHS Research Career Scientist Award to HYM, MH 47808, and by the Cleveland and Sawyer Foundations. The assistance of Ms. Diane Mack in preparing this manuscript is gratefully acknowledged.

References

1. Meltzer HY: Clozapine: clinical advantages and biological mechanisms, in C Schulz, C Tamminga (eds): *Schizophrenia: A Scientific Focus.* New York, Oxford Press, 1989.
2. Berzewski H, Helmchen H, Hippius H, et al: Das Klinische werkungspektrum eines neuen dibenzdiazepin-derivates. *Arzneimittelforschung* 1969;19: 496–498.
3. Burki HR, Ruch W, Asper H: Effects of clozapine, thioridazine, perlapine and haloperidol on the metabolism of the biogenic amines in the brain of the rat. *Psychopharmacologia* 1975;41:27–33.
4. Angst J, Bente D, Berner P, et al: Das clinische Wirkungsbild von clozapine (untersuchung mit dem AMP-system). *Pharmakopsychiatrie* 1971;4:200–211.
5. Matz R, Rick W, Oh D, et al: Clozapine, a potential antipsychotic agent without extrapyramidal manifestations. *Curr Ther Res* 1954;16:687–695.
6. Bjerkenstedt L, Härnryd C, Grimm V, et al: A double-blind comparison of melperone and thiothixene in psychotic women using a new rating scale, the CPRS. *Arch Psychiatr Nervenkraz* 1978;226:157–172.
7. Woggon B, Angst J, Bartels M, et al: Antipsychotic efficacy of fluperlapine: an open multicenter trial. *Neuropsychobiology* 1984;11:116–120.
8. Young MA, Meltzer HY, Fang VS: RMI-81,582: a novel antipsychotic drug. *Psychopharmacology* 1980;67:101–106.
9. Meltzer HY, Luchins DJ: Effect of clozapine in severe tardive dyskinesia: a case report. *J Clin Psychopharmacology* 1984;4:316–322.
10. Cleghorn J, Honigfeld, G, Abuzzahab FS, et al: The risks and benefits of clozapine versus chlorpromazine. *J Clin Psychopharmacol* 1987;7:377–384.
11. Kane J, Honigfeld G, Singer J, et al: Clozapine for the treatment-resistant schizophrenic: a double-blind comparison versus chlorpromazine/benztropine. *Arch Gen Psychiatry* 1988;45:789–796.
12. Honigfeld G, Patin J, Singer J: Clozapine: antipsychotic activity in treatment-resistant schizophrenics. *Adv Therapy* 1984;1:77–97.
13. van Praag HM, Korf J, Dols, L: Clozapine versus perphenazine: the value of the biochemical mode of action of neuroleptics in predicting their therapeutic activity. *Br J Psychiatry* 1976;129:547–555.
14. Meltzer HY, Bastani B, Kwon K, et al: A prospective study of clozapine in treatment resistant schizophrenic patients: I: Preliminary report. *Psychopharmacology,* in press.

15. Juul Polvsen V, Noring V, Fog R, et al: Tolerability and therapeutic effect of clozapine: a retrospective investigation of 216 patients treated with clozapine for up to 12 years. *Acta Psychiatr Scand* 1985;71:176–185.

16. Kuha S, Meittenen E: Long-term effect of clozapine in schizophrenia: a retrospective study of 108 chronic schizophrenics treated with clozapine for up to 7 years. *Nord Psychiatr Tidskr* 1986;40:225–230.

17. Lindström LH: The effect of long-term treatment with clozapine in schizophrenia: a retrospective study in 96 patients treated with clozapine for up to 13 years. *Acta Psychiatr Scand* 1988;77:524–529.

18. Meltzer HY, Goode DJ, Schyve PM, et al: Effect of clozapine on human serum prolactin levels. *Am J Psychiatry* 1979;136:1550–1555.

19. Amsler HA, Teerenhovi L, Barth E, et al: Agranulocytosis in patients treated with clozapine. A study of the Finnish epidemic. *Acta Psychiat Scand* 1977;56:241–248.

20. Koenig JI, Gudelsky GA, Meltzer HY: Stimulation of corticosterone and β-endorphin secretion by selective 5-HT receptor subtype activation. *Eur J Pharmacol* 1987;137:1–8.

21. Imperato A, Angelucci L: Effects of the atypical neuroleptics clozapine and fluperlapine on the in vivo dopamine release in the dorsal striatum and in the prefrontal cortex. Abstracts of the XVI CINP Congress, Munich, 1988. *Psychopharmacol* 1988; 96 (suppl 1): 79.

22. Meltzer HY, Stahl SM: The dopamine hypothesis of schizophrenia: a review. *Schiz Bull* 1976;2:19–76.

23. Kebabian JW, Calne DB: Multiple receptors for dopamine. *Nature* 1979; 277:93–96.

24. Meltzer HY, Matsubara S, Lee J-C: Classification of typical and atypical antipsychotic drugs on the basis of dopamine D-1, D-2, and serotonin$_2$ pk$_i$ values. *J. Pharm. Exp. Therap*, in press.

25. Seeman P, Lee T, Chau-wong M, et al: Antipsychotic drug doses and neuroleptic/dopamine receptors. *Nature* 1976;261:717–718.

26. Bartholini G, Haefely W, Jalfre M, et al: Effect of clozapine on cerebral catecholaminergic neurone systems. *Br J Pharmacol* 1972;46:736–740.

27. Burki HR, Ruch W, Asper H, et al: Effect of single and repeated administration of clozapine on the metabolism of dopamine and noradrenaline in the brain of the rat. *Eur J Pharmacol* 1974;27:180–190.

28. Waldmeier PC, Maitre L: Clozapine: reduction of the initial dopamine turnover increase by repeated treatment. *Eur J Pharmacol* 1976;38:197–203.

29. Andén NE, Stock G: Effect of clozapine on the turnover of dopamine in the corpus striatum and in the limbic system. *J Pharmacy Pharmacol* 1973;25: 346–348.

30. Zivkovic G, Guidotti A, Revuelta A, et al: Effect of thioridazine, clozapine, and other antipsychotics in the kinetic state of tyrosine hydroxylase and on the turnover state of dopamine in striatum and nucleus accumbens. *J Pharmacol Exp Ther* 1975;194:37–46.

31. Bartholini G, Keller HH, Pletscher A: Drug-induced changes of dopamine turnover in striatum and limbic system of the rat. *J Pharm Pharmacol* 1975;27:439–442.

32. Westernik BHC, Korf J: Influence of drugs on striatal and limbic homovanillic acid concentration in the rat brain. *Eur J Pharmacol* 1975;33:31–40.

33. Stawarz RJ, Hill H, Robinson SE, et al: On the significance of the increase in homovanillic acid (HVA) caused by antipsychotic drugs in corpus striatum and limbic forebrain. *Psychopharmacologia (Berl)* 1975;43:125–130.

34. Weisel FA, Sedvall G: Effects of antipsychotic drugs on homovanillic acid levels in striatum and olfactory tubercle of the rat. *Eur J Pharmacol* 1975;30:364–367.

35. Walters JR, Roth RH: Dopaminergic neurons: an in vivo system of measuring drug interactions with presynaptic receptors. *Naunyn-Schmeideberg's Arch Pharmacol* 1976;296:5–14.

36. Wilk S, Watson E, Stanley ME: Differential sensitivity of two dopaminergic structures in rat brain to haloperidol and to clozapine. *J Pharmacol Exp Ther* 1975;195:265–270.

37. Waldmeier PC, Maitre L: On the relevance of preferential increases of meso-limbic versus striatal dopamine turnover for the prediction of antipsychotic activity of psychotropic drugs. *J Neurochem* 1976;27:589–587.

38. Maidment NT, Marsden C: Acute administration of clozapine, thioridazine and metoclopramide increases extracellular DOPAC and decreases extracellular 5-HIAA, measured in the nucleus accumbens and striatum of the rat using in vivo voltammetry. *Neuropharmacology* 1987;26:187–193.

39. Fardé L, Wiesel F-A, Halldin C, et al: Central D2-dopamine receptor occupancy in schizophrenic patients treated with antipsychotic drugs. *Arch Gen Psychiatry* 1988;45:71–76.

40. Burt DR, Creese I. Snyder SH: Antischizophrenic drugs. Chronic treatment elevates dopamine receptor binding in brain. *Science* 1976;196:326–328.

41. Tarsy D, Baldessarini RJ: Behavioral supersensitivity to apomorphine following chronic treatment with drugs which interfere with the synaptic function of catecholamines. *Neuropharmacology* 1974;13:927–940.

42. Sayers AC, Burke AR, Ruch W, et al: Neuroleptic-induced hypersensitivity of striatal dopamine receptors in the rat as a model of tardive dyskinesia: effect of clozapine, haloperidol, loxapine, and chlorpromazine. *Psychopharmacology* 1975;41:97–104.

43. Gnegy M, Uzunov P, Costa E: Participation of an endogenous Ca^{++}-binding protein activator in the development of drug-induced supersensitivity of striatal dopamine receptors. *J Pharmacol Exp Ther* 1977;202:558–564.

44. Kobayashi RM, Fields JZ, Hrusck RE, et al: Brain neurotransmitter receptors and chronic antipsychotic drug treatment: a model for tardive dyskinesia, in Usdin E (ed): *Animal Models in Psychiatry*. New York, Pergamon Press, 1978, pp 405–409.

45. Racagni G, Bruno F, Bugatti A, et al: Behavioral and biochemical correlates after haloperidol and clozapine long-term treatment, in Catabeni G, Racagni G, Spano PF, Costa E (eds): *Long-term Effects of Neuroleptics. Adv Biochem Psychopharmacol* 1980;24:45–52.

46. Seeger TF, Thal L, Gardner EL: Behavioral and biochemical aspects of neuroleptic-induced dopaminergic supersensitivity. Studies with chronic clozapine and haloperidol. *Psychopharmacology* 1982;76:182–187.

47. Rupniak NMJ, Kilpatrick G, Hall MD, et al: Differential alterations in striatal dopamine receptor sensitivity induced by repeated administration of clinically equivalent doses of haloperidol, sulpiride or clozapine in rats. *Psychopharmacology* 1984;84:512–519.

48. Smith RC, Davis JM: Behavioral evidence for supersensitivity after chronic administration of haloperidol. *Life Sci* 1976;19:725–732.
49. Allikmets LH, Zarkovsky AM, Nurk AM: Changes in catalepsy and receptor sensitivity following chronic neuroleptic treatment. *Eur J Pharmacol* 1981;75:145–147.
50. Rupniak NMJ, Hall MD, Kelly E, et al; Mesolimbic dopamine function is not altered during continuous or chronic tratment of rats with typical or atypical neuroleptic drugs. *J Neural Transmission* 1985;62:249–266.
51. Rupniak NMJ, Hall MD, Mann S, et al: Chronic treatment with clozapine unlike haloperidol, does not induce changes in striatal D-2 receptor function in the rat. *Biochem Pharmacol* 1985;34:2755–2763.
52. Chiodo LA, Bunney BS: Typical and atypical neuroleptics differential effects of chronic administration on the activity of A9 and A10 midbrain dopaminergic neurons. *J. Neurosci* 1983;3:1607–1619.
53. White FJ, Wang RY: Differential effects of classical and atypical antipsychotic drugs on A9 and A10 dopamine cells. *Science* 1983;221:1054–1057.
54. Hand TH, Hu X-T, Wang RY: Differential effects of acute clozapine and haloperidol on the activity of ventral tegmental (A10) and nigrostriatal (A9) dopamine neurons. *Brain Res* 1987;415:257–269.
55. Souto M, Monti JM, Althier H: Effect of clozapine on the activity of central dopaminergic and noradrenergic neurons. *Pharmacol Biochem Behavior* 1979;10:5–9.
56. Huff R, Adams RN: Dopamine release in nucleus accumbens and striatum by clozapine: simultaneous monitoring by in vivo electrochemistry. *Neuropharmacology* 1980;19:587–590.
57. Lane RF, Blaha CD: Electrochemistry in vivo: application to CNS pharmacology. *Ann NY Acad Sci* 1986;473:50–69.
58. Blaha CD, Lane RF: Chronic treatment with classical and atypical antipsychotic drugs differentially decrease dopamine release in striatum and nucleus accumbens in vivo. *Neurosci Lett* 1987;78:188–204.
59. Chiodo LA, Bunney BS: Possible mechanisms by which repeated clozapine administration differentially affects the activity of two subpopulations of midbrain dopamine neurons. *J Neuroscience* 1985;5:2539–2544.
60. Lane RF, Blaha CD, Rivet JM: Selective inhibition of mesolimbic dopamine release following chronic administration of clozapine: involvement of alpha$_1$-noradrenergic receptor demonstrated by in vivo voltammetry. *Brain Res* 1988;460:398–401.
61. Meltzer HY, Daniels S, Fang VS: Clozapine increases rat serum prolactin levels. *Life Sci* 1975;17:339–342.
62. Gudelsky GA, Berry SA, Meltzer HY: Neurotensin activates tuberoinfundibular dopamine neurons and increases serum corticosterone concentrations. *Neuroendocrinology* 1989;49:604–609.
63. Gudelsky GA, Meltzer HY: Activation of tuberoinfundibular dopamine neurons following the acute administration of atypical antipsychotics. *Neuropsychopharmacology* 1989;2:45–51.
64. Gudelsky GA, Nash JF, Koenig JI, et al: Neuroendocrine effects of typical and atypical antipsychotics in the rat. *Psychopharmacol Bull* 1987;23:483–486.

65. Kabzinski AM, Szewczak MR, Cornfeldt ML, et al: Differential effects of dopamine agonists and antagonists on the spontaneous electrical activity of A9 and A10 dopamine neurons. *Neurosci Abstr* 1987;13:908.
66. Esposito E, Bunney BS: Effect of acute and chronic treatment with SCH 23390 on the spontaneous activity of midbrain dopamine neurons. *Neurosci Abs* 1988;14:931.
67. Goldstein JM, Litwin LC: Spontaneous activity of A9 and A10 dopamine neurons after acute and chronic administration of the selective dopamine D-1 receptor antagonist SCH 23390. *Eur J Pharmacol* 1988;155:175–180.
68. Andersen PH, Nielsen EB, Gronvald FC, et al: Some atypical neuroleptics inhibit [3-H]SCH-23390 binding in vivo. *Eur J Pharmacol* 1986;120:143–144.
69. Andersen PH, Braestrup C: Evidence for different states of the dopamine D-1 receptor: clozapine and fluperlapine may preferentially label an adenylate cyclase-coupled state of the D-1 receptor. *J. Neurochemistry* 1986;47:1830–1831.
70. Chipkin RE, Latranyi MB: Similarity of clozapine and SCH 23390 in reserpinized rats suggest a common mechanism of action. *Eur J Pharmacol* 1987;136:371–375.
71. Altar CA, Boyar WC, Wasley A, et al: Dopamine neurochemical profile of atypical antipsychotics resembles that of D-1 antagonists. *Naunyn-Schmiedeberg's Arch Pharmacol* 1988;338:162–168.
72. Maj J, Sowinska H, Boran L, et al: The central action of clozapine. *Pol J Pharmacol Pharm* 1974;26:425–435.
73. Ackenheil M, Beckmann H, Greil W, et al: Antipsychotic efficacy of clozapine in correlation to changes in catecholamine metabolism in man. *Adv Biochem Psychopharm* 1974;9:647–658.
74. Ruch W, Asper H, Bürki HR: Effect of clozapine on the metabolism of serotonin in rat brain. *Psychopharmacologia (Berl)* 1976;46:103–109.
75. Stralendorff B, Ackenheil M, Zimmerman J: Akute und chronishe werkung von clozapine, haloperidol und sulpirid auf den stoffwechsel giogener amine in rattenhirn. *Arzneim Forsch* 1976;26:1096–1098.
76. Banki CM: Alterations of cerebrospinal fluid 5-hydroxyindoleacetic acid, and total blood serotonin content during clozapine treatment. *Psychopharmacology 1978;56:195–198.*
77. Gerlach J, Thorsen K, Fog R: Extrapyramidal reactions and amine metabolites in cerebrospinal fluid during haloperidol and clozapine treatment of schizophrenic patient. *Psychopharmacologica (Berl)* 1975;40:341–350.
78. Enjalbert A, Hamon M, Bourgoin S, et al: Postsynaptic serotonin-sensitive adenylate cyclase in the central nervous system. II. Comparison with dopamine- and isoproterenol-sensitive adenylate cyclases in rat brain. *Mol Pharmacol* 1978;14:11–23.
79. Green JP, Maayani S: Nomenclature, classification and notation of receptors: 5-hydroxytryptamine receptors and binding sties as examples, in Black JW, Jenkinson DH, Gerskowitch VP (eds): *Perspective on Receptor Classification.* New York, Alan R. Liss Inc., 1987; pp 237–267.
80. Conn PJ, Sanders-Bush E: Central serotonin receptors: effector symptoms, physiological roles and regulation. *Psychopharmacology* 1987;92: 267–277.

81. Devivo M, Maayani S: Characterization of the 5-hydroxytryptamine receptor-mediated inhibition of forskolin-stimulated adenylate cyclase activity in guinea pig and rat hippocampal membranes. *J Pharmacol Exp Ther* 1986; 238:248–253.

82. Sulpizio A, Fowler FJ, Macko E: Antagonism of fenfluramine-induced hyperthermia: a measure of central serotonin inhibition. *Life Sci* 1978;22:1439–1446.

83. Fjalland B: Neuroleptic influence on hyperthermia induced by 5-hydroxytryptophan and p-methoxyamphetamine in MAOI-pretreated rabbits. *Psychopharmacology* 1979;63:113–117.

84. Maj J, Baran L, Bigajska BK, et al: The influence of neuroleptics on the behavioral effect of 5-hydroxytryptophan. *Pol J Pharmacol Pharm* 1978; 30:431–440.

85. Lai H, Carino MA, Horita A: Antiserotonin properties of neuroleptic drug, in HI Yamamura, RW Olsen, E Usdin (eds): *Psychopharmacology and Biochemistry or Neurotransmitter Receptor*. New York, Elsevier–North Holland, 1980; pp 347–353.

86. Fink H, Morgenstern R, Oelssner W: Clozapine—a serotonin antagonist? *Pharmacology Biochem Behavior* 1984;20:513–517.

87. Friedman RL, Sanders-Bush E, Barrett RL: Clozapine blocks descriptive and discriminative stimulus effects of quipazine. *Eur J Pharmacol* 1985;106:191–193.

88. Nash JF, Meltzer HY, Gudelsky GA: Antagonism of serotonin receptor mediacted neuroendocrine and temperature responses by atypical neuroleptics in the rat. *Eur J Pharmacol* 1988;151:463–469.

89. Rasmussen K, Aghajanian GK: Potency of antipsychotics in reversing the effects of a hallucinogenic drug on locus coeruleus neurons correlates with $5-HT_2$ binding affinity. *Neuropsychopharmacology* 1988;1:101–107.

90. Waldmeier PC, Delini-Atula AA: Serotonin-dopamine interactions in the nigrostriatal system. *Eur J Pharmacol* 1979;55:363–373.

91. Altar CA, Wasley AM, Neale RF, et al: Typical and atypical antipsychotic occupancy of D2 and S_2 receptors: an autoradiographic analysis in rat brain. *Brain Res Bull* 1986;16:517–525.

92. Reynolds GP, Garrett NJ, Rupniak N, et al: Chronic clozapine treatment of rats downregulates cortical $5-HT_2$ receptors. *Eur J Pharmacol* 1983;89:325–326.

93. Lee T, Tang SW: Loxapine and clozapine decrease serotonin (S_2) but do not elevate dopamine (D_2 receptor numbers in the rat brain). *Psychiatry Res* 1984;12:277–285.

94. Matsubara S, Meltzer HY: Acute effects of neuroleptics on $5-HT_2$ receptor density in rat cerebral cortex. *Life Science*, in press.

95. Moret C: Pharmacology of the serotonin autoreceptor, in AR Green (ed): *Neuropharmacology of Serotonin*. Oxford, Oxford Press, 1985, pp 21–49.

96. Gothert M: Role of autoreceptors in the function of the peripheral and central nervous system. *Drug Res* 1985;35:1909–1916.

97. Hetey L, Drescher K, Oelssner W: Different influence of antipsychotics and serotonin antagonists on presynaptic receptors modulating the synaptosomal release of dopamine and serotonin. *Wiss Z Humboldt–Univ Berl* 1982; 31:487–489.

98. Drescher K, Hetey L: Influence of antipsychotics and serotonin antagonists on presynaptic receptors modulating the release of serotonin in synaptosomes of the nucleus accumbens of rats. *Neuropharmacology* 1988;27:31–36.

99. Bannon MJ, Roth RH: Pharmacology of mesocortical dopamine neurons. *Pharmacol Res* 1983;35:53–68.

100. Carter CJ, Pycock CJ: Behavioral and biochemical effects of dopamine and noradrenaline depletion within the medial prefrontal cortex of the rat. *Brain Res* 1980;192:163–176.

101. Scatton B, Worms P, Lloyd KG, et al: Cortical modulation of striatal function. *Brain Res* 1982;232:331–343.

102. Pycock CJ, Carter CJ, Kerwin RW: Effect of 6-hydroxydopamine lesions of the medial prefrontal cortex on neurotransmitter systems in subcortical sites in the rat. *J Neurochem* 1980;34:91–99.

103. Pycock CJ, Kerwin RW, Carter CJ: Effects of lesion of cortical dopamine terminals on subcortical dopamine receptors in rats. *Nature (Lomd)* 1980;286:74–77.

104. Scatton B: Effect of repeated treatment with neuroleptics on dopamine metabolism in cell bodies and terminals in dopaminergic systems in the rat brain, in Cattabeni F, Racagni G, Spano PF, Costa E (eds): *Advances in Biochemical Psychopharmacology*. New York, Raven Press, 1980, pp 31–36.

105. Blanc G, Hervé D, Simon H, et al: Response to stress of mesocorticofrontal dopaminergic neurons in rats after long-term isolation. *Nature* 1980;284:265–267.

106. Meltzer HY: Biochemical studies in schizophrenia, in L Bellak (ed): *Disorders of the Schizophrenic Syndrome*. New York, Basic Books, Inc., 1979, pp 45–149.

107. Meltzer HY: Dopamine and negative symptoms in schizophrenia: critique of the type I–type II hypothesis, in M Alpert (ed): *Controversies in Schizophrenia: Changes and Constancies*. New York, Guilford Press, 1985, pp 110–136.

108. Mackay AVP: Positive and negative schizophrenic symptoms and the role of dopamine. *Br J Psychiatry* 1980;137:379–383.

109. Costall B, Kelly DM, Naylor RJ: Nomifensine: a potent dopaminergic agonist of antiparkinson potential. *Psychopharmacol (Berl)* 1975;41:153–164.

110. Sanberg PR, Bunsey MD Giordano M, et al: The catalepsy test: its ups and downs. *Behavioral Neurosci* 1988;102:748–759.

111. Nicolaou NM, Garcia-Munoz M, Arbuthrott GW, et al: Interactions between serotonergic and dopaminergic systems in rat brain demonstrated by small unilateral lesions of the raphe nuclei. *Eur J Pharmacol* 1979;57:295–305.

112. Hervé D, Simon H, Blanc G, et al: Increased utilization of dopamine in the nucleus accumbens but not in the cerebral cortex after dorsal raphé lesion in the rat. *Neurosci Lett* 1979;75:127–133.

113. Hervé D, Simon H, Blanc G, et al: Opposite changes in dopamine utilization in the nucleus accumbens and the frontal cortex after electrolytic lesion of the median raphe in the rat. *Brain Res* 1981;216:422–428.

114. Lisoprawski A, Hervé D, Blanc G, et al: Selective activation of the mesocortical frontal dopaminergic neurons induced by lesion of the habenula in the rat. *Brain Res* 1980;183:229–234.

115. Gallager DW, Aghaganian GK: Effect of antipsychotic drugs on the firing of dorsal raphé cells. I. Role of adrenergic system. *Eur J Pharmacol* 1976;39:341–355.
116. Stahl SM, Wets K: Indoleamines and schizophrenia, in Henn FA, DeLisi LE (eds): *Handbook of Schizophrenia*. Elsevier, Elsevier Science Publishing BV 1987, pp 257–296.
117. Bleich A, Brown S, Kahn R, et al: The role of serotonin in schizophrenia. *Schiz Bull* 1988;14:297.
118. Racagni G, Cheney DL, Trabucchi M, et al: In vivo actions of clozapine and haloperidol on the turnover rate of acetylcholine in rat striatum. *J Pharmacol Exp Ther* 1976;196:323–332.
119. Cohen BM, Lipinski JF: In vivo potencies of antipsychotic drugs in blocking alpha₁ noradrenergic and dopamine D-2 receptors: implications for drug mechanisms of action. *Life Sci* 1986;39:2571–2580.
120. Gross G, Schümann HJ: Effect of long-term treatment with atypical neuroleptic drugs on beta adrenoceptor binding in rat cerebral cortex and myocardium. *Naunyn-Schmiedeberg's Arch Pharmacol* 1982;321:271–275.
121. Maggi A, Cattebeni F, Bruno F, et al: Haloperidol and clozapine: specificity of action on GABA in the nigrostria system. *Brain Res* 1977;133:382–385.
122. Schmidt WJ: Intrastriatal injection of DL-2-amino-5-phosphonovaleric acid (AP-5) induces sniffing stereotypy that is antagonized by haloperidol and clozapine. *Psychopharmacology* 1986;90:123–130.
123. Kilts CD, Anderson CM, Bissette G, et al: Differential effects of antipsychotic drugs on the neurotensin concentration of discrete rat brain nuclei. *Biochem Pharmacol* 1988;37:1547–1554.

12
Psychopharmacologic Treatment of Schizophrenia

JOHN M. KANE

The introduction of pharmacologic treatments for schizophrenia remains one of the major advances of twentieth century medicine. Despite the availability and efficacy of these compounds the treatment of schizophrenia continues to pose numerous challenges to clinicians, not only because of its prevalence, severity, and complexity, but also because its treatment requires an integration of a variety of different prospectives (eg, biological, psychological, and psychosocial).[1] Other chapters in this book have reviewed data relating to phenomenologic, genetic, neuroanatomic, psychophysiologic, and psychosocial aspects of this illness, providing extensive documentation of both its complexity and its probable heterogeneity.

Any clinician treating patients with schizophrenia is confronted with an ongoing need to integrate and assimilate new information, while continuing to consider the potential implications of new findings in a variety of areas as they may impact on the planning of specific strategies. In addition, schizophrenia is an illness with enormous variation in mode of onset, premorbid adjustment, phenomenology, and social and environmental factors, all of which may influence treatment response and ultimate level of adaptation. Even within subjects there can be considerable variation in psychopathology and treatment response over time.

This chapter attempts to summarize some aspects of our current approach to the psychopharmacologic treatment of schizophrenia, to emphasize recent developments, and to indicate areas where further clinical observation and research are necessary.

General Principles of Pharmacotherapy

Treatment of Acute Episode

In discussing the acute treatment of schizophrenia, we are generally referring to that phase of the illness that includes obvious signs and symptoms with substantial behavioral dysfunction, as well as the consequent psychosocial and vocational disability. Although the mode of onset of an acute episode varies enormously, usually an acute exacerbation is manifested by an increase in positive symptoms such as hallucinations, delusions, thought disorder, and behavioral dysregulation. It is also possible that an increase in negative symptoms, such as extreme withdrawal or even catatonia, may also occur. Even within an episode the form and content of symptoms may change over time and it is particularly important for clinicians to recognize that the clinical presentation of a schizophrenic illness largely involves subjective experiences that the individual may or may not be able to describe reliably or consistently. It may be particularly difficult to date the onset of subtle prodromal symptoms that may represent gradual changes in behavior and can sometimes be attributed to situational circumstances or stressful life events.

What Type of Neuroleptic Medication?

Antipsychotic (or neuroleptic) medications remain the primary treatment modality for an acute episode or an acute exacerbation of a schizophrenic illness. The therapeutic efficacy of these medications has been demonstrated in numerous double-blind, placebo-controlled trials; however, a considerable subgroup of schizophrenic patients (even during a first episode of the illness) derive little if any benefit from drug treatment. This should not be surprising given the assumed heterogeneity of the illness. In fact, we are fortunate to have a treatment that is as effective as it is in such a large proportion of patients.

It is likely that heterogeneity in drug responses is influenced by a variety of biologic (eg, genetic, neurochemical, or neuroanatomical) factors, as well as psychological, psychosocial, and environmental influences. It is likely that any further advance in our understanding of any of these areas could ultimately lead to an improvement in our treatment efficacy or specificity. There are a variety of pharmacologic factors that should be considered by a clinician in planning treatment for an individual experiencing an acute episode.

Although we have been using antipsychotic compounds for more than 30 years and have seen the introduction of different chemical classes, there are at present no convincing data that among those medications currently marketed in the United States any one is more effective either in schizophrenia in general or in specific subtypes of the disorder.[2,3] (Clozapine may be an exception to this statement and will be discussed subsequently.) We should not, however, dismiss the possibility that differences may exist between different classes of drugs or that one subgroup of patients may be more responsive to a particular type of medication than another. It is important to recognize that very few studies provide generalizable data on differential treatment response to specific agents. Almost all of the available data are based on comparisons of overall or group mean response rate contrasting one drug *vs* another. If we randomly assign patients to drug A or drug B and observe a 70 to 80% response rate with each drug, this does not necessarily enable us to conclude that any given individual would respond equally well to either drug. Unfortunately, there are remarkably few studies looking at the interchangeability of neuroleptic drugs, despite the obvious clinical importance of this issue.[4] For example, if a given individual fails to respond to a standard course of an antipsychotic drug given an adequate dose for an adequate duration, what is the next logical treatment alternative? Despite some anecdotal experience that some patients who show a poor response to one drug might benefit from another drug, it is difficult to establish a cause and effect relationship in a single case because other considerations besides the change in medication (eg, additional time on any treatment) could also contribute to improvement. Although clinicians certainly follow various strategies in the treatment of such patients (changing drugs, increasing dose, or waiting an additional period of time), sufficient research has not been conducted to provide adequate guidelines.

The preclinical observations that many antipsychotic drugs do differ in their relative affinities for specific brain receptors[5,6] (particularly the dopamine receptors which may mediate therapeutic response) also support the possibility that drugs may vary in their spectrum of therapeutic activity as they vary in their spectrum of adverse effects. It is also important to note, however, that the milligram potency of various antipsychotic drugs has been suggested to correlate with receptor affinity in theoretically relevant binding assays.[5]

Many mental health professionals continue to believe that sedating drugs (eg, chlorpromazine) are more appropriate in treating highly excited or agitated patients than are nonsedating or high-potency drugs (eg, haloperidol, fluphenazine, trifluoperazine). This relationship has never been established and there are numerous investigations suggesting that high- and low-potency drugs are equally effective for both types of patients.

Despite the assumed equivalence of different classes of antipsychotics, there are factors that the clinician should consider when using a particular agent. First of all, if a given individual has a history of responding to a specific antipsychotic agent (or if an ill family member has responded well to a particular agent), then this should be considered strongly as the first treatment of choice. By the same token, if a patient provides a history of adverse reactions to specific drugs, then this should enter into the clinician's consideration. For those patients in whom compliance and medication taking has been a problem during the maintenance phase of treatment, consideration of preparing for the use of long-acting injectable neuroleptics should be a factor. Therefore, using fluphenazine or haloperidol orally during the acute treatment phase may be advantageous.

Dosage

There are still insufficient data regarding dose-response curves for anti-psychotic drugs (the related issue of drug blood levels will be discussed subsequently). Unfortunately, many studies of drug efficacy have not used fixed doses. When flexible doses are used, the clinician adjusts the dose based on clinical response. As a result it may be difficult to establish a dose-response relationship if, for example, a patient receiving a given dose of an antipsychotic drug shows little improvement for 10 days, the clinician may decide to increase the dose and subsequent improvement might then be attributed to the higher dose when in fact the same degree of improvement may have occurred merely by allowing more time on the original dose. In those studies that have compared relatively high doses (defined as those in excess of 2,000 mg chlorpromazine or equivalent) as compared with standard dose treatment, there is little evidence of statistically significant advantages for the high dose.[7] This certainly does not preclude the possibility that for some individuals a higher dose may be helpful, but it would suggest that these individuals represent a small subgroup, and it calls for better means of identifying appropriate candidates for high-dose treatment rather than applying it to all patients who fail to respond to an initial course of medication. Overall, the literature suggests that doses of 400 to 600 mg/day of chlorpromazine or equivalent should be sufficient for the average patient.

There clearly has been a tendency since the introduction of the so-called high-potency drugs to use larger and larger doses, because apart from the neurologic or parkinsonian side effects these compounds are very well tolerated when given in high doses. It is my belief that this practice should be discouraged unless it is clearly established that such doses are necessary to produce a therapeutic response in a given individual. Even within the spectrum considered as "standard" or even "low" doses, there is increasing evidence that doses far less than previously used may be effective when using high-potency compounds. For example, Van Putten et al[8] contrasted the effects of three different doses of haloperidol (5, 10, or 20 mg daily) during a 4-week trial in 76 newly admitted drug-free male schizophrenic patients. After 1 week of treatment, those individuals receiving 5 mg/day were not doing as well as those in the intermediate- or high-dose groups. By the end of the second week, however, patients given 5 mg/day had improved clinical ratings by almost as much as those receiving the higher doses. In addition, patients receiving the highest (20 mg) dose experienced substantially more akinesia and were rated as worse than previously on the "withdrawal-retardation" scores. After 3 weeks of treatment the group taking 5 mg had improved as much as the group taking 10 mg, whereas the patients receiving the highest dose did score better on the overall clinical ratings, dropped out of treatment more frequently, and had significantly higher adverse effects ratings. Overall, the 20-mg treatment did produce superior antipsychotic efficacy, but at the price of an increase in akinesia or akathisia and a substantially higher dropout rate.

McEvoy et al[9] have reported on research with the "neuroleptic threshold" approach in newly admitted schizophrenic patients. These investigators begin with 2 mg/day of haloperidol, and doses are increased by 2 mg every other day until a mild hypokinesia-rigidity occurs (or to a maximum of 10 mg/day). The mean dose at which the neuroleptic threshold was achieved was 3.2 ± 2 mg daily. The investigators reported that 82% of their patients who had had five or fewer previous hospitalizations achieved at least a moderate degree of therapeutic benefit during the 3 weeks of treatment with these small doses. This is in contrast to those patients with more than five previous hospitalizations, where only 33% showed such response.

Clearly these studies are suggestive in indicating that doses lower than those frequently used may be sufficient for the acute treatment of a schizophrenic episode. Baldessarini et al,[10] in reviewing multiple studies on dose and treatment efficacy, concluded that doses below 250 mg/day of chlorpromazine equivalents tended not to be adequate for many patients, but that 500 to 700 mg/day appeared to be optimal, with higher doses more likely to generate adverse effects.

It is also important to recognize that dose equivalence among antipsychotic drugs has not been well established. Chlorpromazine has frequently been the standard against which equivalent doses are explored, but unfortunately, the customary method of determining dose equivalencies are crude and unsystematic. The usual method has involved a double-blind clinical trial contrasting two antipsychotic medications, with the clinician adjusting dose according to clinical response. At the completion of the trial, a comparison is made regarding the dosage ranges used, and a conversion ratio between the two compounds is suggested. In addition, in some cases results from drug-placebo comparisons are pooled to identify the clinically "effective" dosage range for a particular compound. There are a variety of pitfalls in assuming the validity of these results, and it is also important to consider the possibility that conversion ratios that may be appropriate at the low end of the dosage spectrum may not apply at the higher end. Another report by Baldessarini et al[11] suggests that clinicians are using dissimilar dosing practices with high-potency compounds as compared with low-potency antipsychotics. These workers[11] compared the findings of a survey of 110 private hospital inpatients with the dosing practices reported in a survey of nearly 16,000 Veterans Administration patients. Doses of high-potency drugs above the daily equivalent of 1 g of chlorpromazine accounted for more than 40% of all prescriptions. The mean chlorpromazine equivalent dose of the two most potent antipsychotic agents (haloperidol and fluphenazine) was 3.54 times as high as the mean dose prescribed of chlorpromazine or thioridazine.

As these authors suggested, the sedative and autonomic effects of low-potency drugs may limit their use in the higher dose range, whereas it is feasible for clinicians to increase doses of high-potency antipsychotic drugs without substantial increase in immediate adverse effects.

A factor that might contribute to the use of higher doses is the increasing pressure that clinicians are experiencing to reduce length of hospital stay to comply with efforts at cost containment. The problem, however, is that the use of "rapid neuroleptization" and/or high-dose treatment has not been shown to reduce the time required for these drugs to exert their therapeutic effect or to improve clinical outcome in general. Although it is apparent that the time course of antipsychotic drug response is unpredictable, with a degree of clinical improvement occurring rapidly in some patients and more slowly in others, it is our clinical experience and impression from reviewing the literature that in many cases 4 to 6 weeks (or even longer) is necessary to begin to see the full therapeutic benefit. As indicated previously, we would benefit from more research indicating at what point a clinician should consider alternative strategies when a patient is not responding adequately.

Drug Blood Levels

Soon after the recognition of enormous individual variability in absorption and metabolism of antipsychotic drugs and the availability of assays to measure levels of these compounds in blood, there was considerable interest in attempting to explore the relationship between blood levels and clinical response. It was assumed that this strategy would go a long way toward explaining the wide variability in drug response seen among patients with schizophrenia. To a major extent these efforts have not been rewarding, but blood levels may have some use in specific clinical situations. Clearly, there have been major advances in the methodology available to measure minute amounts of antipsychotic compounds in clinical specimens (eg, plasma, cerebrospinal fluid, and red blood cells). It is unfortunate, however, that despite the increasingly sophisticated technology, flaws in the design and methodology of clinical trials have frequently limited the importance and generalizibility of the findings. Many studies have suffered from prognostic and diagnostic heterogeneity. It is important to consider the types of patients who are included in such a study. If for example, individuals who have proven unresponsive to antipsychotic treatment, either fully or partially, are included in such studies, the ability to find meaningful correlations may be limited severely. It is also important to allow for the development of a steady state blood level after fixed-dose treatment to be able to relate blood levels to clinical response. If dosage adjustment is based on clinical response, then those patients who are (for whatever reason) poor responders to antipsychotic drugs regardless of dose or blood level may end up with the highest blood levels. It is possible then that this might be interpreted as negating the value of blood levels or suggesting that high blood levels are in fact antitherapeutic. It is also important to recognize that the length of time in a trial is critical because, as discussed, many patients with schizophrenia require several weeks to achieve full therapeutic benefit from pharmacotherapy. Those studies that have examined the relationship between blood level and clinical response after relatively brief periods of time (eg, 14 days) may be measuring one aspect of clinical effect such as reduction in psychomotor agitation or excitement, whereas other aspects of psychopathology may not have improved within the same time frame.

Although many of the studies conducted to date have not been ideal, there is a mounting body of evidence suggesting that in the case of haloperidol there may be a curvilinear relationship between blood level and clinical response or a putative "therapeutic window."[12–14] Although these findings are intriguing, considerable further work should be conducted before a therapeutic window can be definitely established. One of the current problems is that many of the studies that have suggested an upper limit to therapeutic blood level have had relatively few patients in that category. In addition, hardly any attempts have been made at randomly assigning those patients whose blood level is out of the therapeutic range to a dosage necessary to manipulate the blood level into the putative therapeutic range, with an appropriate control group remaining at their current blood level to control for continued time on drug. Until this is done in a systematic replicable fashion it will be difficult to draw firm conclusions.

These considerations are also important in the context of the previous discussion regarding high-dose or megadose treatment. If patients were identified on the basis of unusually low blood levels given the amount of medication prescribed, then these individuals might be ideal candidates for a high-dose or megadose treatment strategy (assuming the low blood level is not due to noncompliance in medication taking). On the other hand, if studies using substantial dosage increases do involve a very heterogeneous group of drug responders and nonresponders, then the likelihood of seeing a desired clinical effect may be reduced considerably.

It is also important to consider the possibility that those patients showing a poor clinical response at the higher end of the blood level range are in fact experiencing behaviorally manifest adverse effects that could alter or impede therapeutic response. Although investigators have suggested that an increase in side effects does not account for the lack of beneficial effect at higher blood levels, I believe that this question requires further study as behaviorally manifest adverse effects can frequently be difficult to distinguish from psychopathology, and a patient in the midst of an acute psychotic episode may not be able to articulate adequately subjective feelings and sensations in a way that would facilitate a differential diagnosis.

At present the overall use of measuring blood levels of antipsychotic compounds is far from clear, but the available data should encourage clinicians and investigators to recognize the potential problems of using doses that are too high as well as the importance of careful clinical evaluation and research methodology.

Extrapyramidal Side Effects

Among the most common and troublesome side effects are those involving extrapyramidal movement disorders, including dystonia, parkinsonism, akathisia, tardive dyskinesia, and tardive dystonia. Estimates of the incidence of these reactions vary considerably from less than 5% to more than 90% of neuroleptic-treated patients. The relationship that exists between neuroleptic dosage and drug-induced extrapyramidal side effects (EPS) is not a simple one. Given the fact that not all patients have the same vulnerability to developing EPS, and not all neuroleptics have the same propensity to produce EPS, this should not be surprising. In addition, the dose-response relationship as well as the time of onset and duration of the adverse effect are not necessarily the same in dystonias, akathisia, and akinesia. In addition, bioavailability, prior neuroleptic exposure, age, sex, and other manifestations of CNS dysfunction, as well as possibly even genetic factors, may play an important role in the incidence and intensity of EPS.

Drug-induced dystonia, akathisia, and pseudoparkinsonism clearly can occur early in treatment, but there is a frequent misconception that complete tolerance to these effects develops over time and that they do not remain a problem in long-term or maintenance treatment. This is clearly not the case. Those studies reporting results of substantial dose reduction during the maintenance phase of antipsychotic drug treatment suggest the impact of this strategy on continued manifestations of EPS.[15]

The prophylactic use of antiparkinsonian drugs remains controversial and is clearly more of an issue when high-potency antipsychotic agents are used. In my view the advantages of instituting prophylactic antiparkinsonian treatment include the potential avoidance of frightening neurologic reactions (acute dystonia), as well as the prevention of akathisia or akinesia, which can mimic psychopathology and result in an inappropriate increase in psychotropic medication. It is also quite likely that patients who do experience adverse reactions during the acute phase of antipsychotic drug treatment are more prone to develop subsequent noncompliance. The disadvantages of using prophylactic antiparkinsonian medications include the possibility that it is not necessary, given the fact that not all patients will develop these adverse effects, as well as the potential for increasing the degree of anticholinergic toxicity.

The clinician should attempt to discontinue antiparkinsonian drugs, if they are being administered, after the first 1 or 2 months of acute treatment. However, discontinuation should be followed by careful examination for the reemergence of EPS, which can often be subtle. If these adverse effects do emerge, then reducing the dose of the antipsychotic drug may be appropriate. A major problem, however, remains the lack of recognition of EPS in many clinical settings.

The chronic and potentially persistent adverse neurological effects associated with neuroleptic drugs such as tardive dyskinesia and tardive dystonia remain a major concern. Epidemiological data suggest that neuroleptic treatment is an important etiological factor in the development of involuntary movements, although individual vulnerability varies considerably, and some patients may exhibit abnormal movements unrelated to neuroleptic exposure.

Data from an ongoing prospective study of tardive dyskinesia development suggests an incidence of 4% per year with antipsychotic drug exposure for at least the first 5 to 6 years of drug treatment.[16] The majority of these cases were rated as mild and did not increase in severity during the 2- to 3-year follow-up period, despite the fact that many patients continue to receive neuroleptics. Data from other follow-up studies also suggest that tardive dyskinesia is not generally progressive despite the continued administration of antipsychotic drugs.[17,18] Improvement in abnormal involuntary movements appears to be more likely, however, if antipsychotic drugs can be discontinued, particularly soon after the first evidence of tardive dyskinesia emerges.

There is a small subgroup of patients who develop a very severe and progressive form of tardive dyskinesia, and at present we are unable to identify those risk factors that account for this variability in vulnerability. This would emphasize the need for caution in the use of antipsychotic drugs in general. The single most frequently implicated risk factor for the development of tardive dyskinesia is age, although the normal aging process in itself does not appear to produce a substantial degree of abnormal involuntary movements. Increasing age among drug-treated patients appears to increase not only the risk of developing tardive dyskinesia but also its severity and likelihood of persistence. At present there are no proven safe and effective treatments for this condition. Although antipsychotic drug dosage reduction and, particularly, discontinuation can have a definite beneficial effect, complete drug discontinuation is frequently not feasible.

Although antipsychotic drugs may symptomatically improve a variety of conditions, they should not be used when equally effective and safer treatments are available, as for example, in patients with affective or anxiety disorders.

Predictors of Response and Role of Alternative Treatments

Given the considerable variability in antipsychotic medication responsiveness, repeated attempts have been made to explore potential predictors of therapeutic response. There are a variety of suggestions in the literature which include variables ranging from premorbid social adjust-ment to ventricular brain ratio; however, there are no well-established predictors of antipsychotic drug response during an acute episode or ex-acerbation with useful degrees of sensitivity or specificity. At the present time, unless there is a specific contraindication, any patient presenting with a schizophrenic illness who warrants pharmacologic treatment should receive a trial of antipsychotic medication. At the same time there have been some suggestions that a subgroup of patients with schizophre-nia may respond to lithium, electroconvulsive therapy (ECT), or may at times improve without somatic treatment.

Although it is hoped that at some point future research will provide evidence on which to base recommendations for a particular alternative somatic therapy, at present the recommendation with regard to antipsy-chotic drugs would conclude that they are the most effective treatment for the largest proportion of patients with this illness.

Strategies for Managing Antipsychotic Drug Nonresponders

Despite the fact that antipsychotic drugs are the treatment of first choice for an acute schizophrenic episode, it is clear that a substantial number of individuals derive little if any benefit from these agents. The treatment of such individuals continues to present a major clinical dilemma. It is frequently in this context that clinicians will explore the use of various antipsychotic drug classes, megadoses, high doses of parenteral medica-tion, concomitant lithium, propranolol, carbamazepine, ECT, and experi-mental compounds.

Although the literature is replete with anecdotal reports describing pa-tients who have benefitted from such strategies, there are few systematic and well-controlled studies suggesting any more than occasional benefit. It is certainly reasonable for the clinician to conduct a ''therapeutic trial'' of some alternative treatment strategies in patients who fail to respond to an adequate course of antipsychotics, but there should also be a point where we may have to recognize and accept our inability to help some patients given the current state of our knowledge.

In the context of treating refractory patients, it is particularly important to identify and document target symptoms as well as response within a reasonable time frame. In my experience in reviewing the treatment of many such patients, frequently an inadequate trial is used or there is lack of adequate follow-up and evaluation necessary to justify the continuation of a specific treatment.

The role of blood levels in this context is still far from established but may be helpful in identifying patients who are idiosyncratic metabolizers. Apart from this possibility we are not aware of data sufficient to establish any rational basis for determining the next appropriate treatment. For example, no comparisons have been conducted of ECT, lithium, and other alternative treatments in this context.

Clozapine for the Treatment-Refractory Patient

Clozapine belongs to the chemical class of dibenzodiazepines related chemically to the antipsychotic drug, loxapine. Clozapine's pharmacologic characteristics are somewhat different from loxapine and other available antipsychotic agents. Unlike "typical" neuroleptics, clozapine produces very slight and short-lived elevations in serum prolactin in patients receiving therapeutic doses.[19] Clozapine produces very little in the way of extrapyramidal side effects; it does not induce dystonia, and the incidence of akinesia or akathisia appears to be very low. There are very few cases of "dyskinesia" reported worldwide, and the nature of these cases is not entirely clear.

Several controlled clinical trials had been conducted with clozapine in the 1970s suggesting that it was an efficacious antipsychotic drug.[20] However, in 1975, granulocytopenia developed in 16 patients in Finland and agranulocytosis developed in 13 of these patients, with 8 fatalities resulting from secondary infection.[21] Based on the current experience with the drug, there have been more than 100 cases of agranulocytosis worldwide, and further development of this compound was curtailed in many countries in the late 1970s. Overall estimates continue to support the impression that the risk of agranulocytosis with clozapine exceeds that associated with other antipsychotic drugs. Currently based on a life-table method of calculating risk, data in the United States indicate a 2% cumulative incidence of agranulocytosis after 52 weeks of clozapine treatment.[22] Results of several of the previously mentioned clinical trials not only suggest that clozapine was an efficacious antipsychotic drug, but also that it may offer some advantage for patients who had failed to respond to other available neuroleptic drugs. Given this potential added benefit from clozapine, while at the same time considering the apparent increased risk of serious adverse effects, a multicenter trial was initiated in the United States to determine if in fact clozapine offered an advantage over other neuroleptics in carefully selected treatment-refractory patients.[23]

Two hundred sixty-eight treatment-refractory inpatients selected at 16 different hospitals participated in the clozapine vs chlorpromazine and benztropine comparison. There were high overall completion rates for both clozapine- and chlorpromazine-treated patients (88 and 87%, respectively). Clozapine proved to be superior to chlorpromazine on all of the major efficacy measures [Brief Psychiatric Rating Scale (BPRS) total score, BPRS cluster of four key psychotic items, Clinical Global Impression (CGI) scale].

Before the initiation of the study, a priori criteria were developed to categorize patients as "improved" or "unimproved." The criteria for defining a patient as improved included a reduction greater than 20% from baseline in the BPRS total score plus either a posttreatment CGI scale score of 3 (mild) or less or a posttreatment BPRS total score of 35 or lower. When these criteria were applied to all of those patients who completed at least 1 week of the double-blind trial, it was found that only 4% of the chlorpromazine-treated patients had improved in comparison to 30% of the clozapine-treated patients ($P < 0.001$). These results provided the most cogent evidence of clozapine's superiority.

Clozapine-Induced Agranulocytosis

Agranulocytosis is the most serious side effect of clozapine. If undetected it can be fatal and requires immediate drug discontinuation. Agranulocytosis is defined as a white blood cell count of less than 2,000 cells/m^3 with less than 500 cells/m^3 of polymorphonuclear leukocytes. Erythrocyte and platelet values are normal. The natural history of clozapine-induced agranulocytosis is fairly consistent. Most cases have occurred within the first 6 months of treatment, although infrequently cases have developed as long as 15 months after beginning the compound. The mode of onset is usually gradual with the white blood cell count declining and "shifting to the right" over a period of several weeks. There are cases, however, that have developed suddenly and, therefore, it is most prudent to require frequent (weekly) white blood cell monitoring. Recovery occurs within 7 to 21 days after discontinuing clozapine, unless secondary infection develops. No cases of aplastic anemia have occurred with clozapine.

The mechanism by which clozapine produces agranulocytosis is not clearly known. Possible mechanisms include a drug-induced autoimmune reaction to granulocytes, either circulating or in the bone marrow, or drug-mediated toxicity in granulocyte production or survival. The pattern of agranulocytosis developing with clozapine is consistent with either an immune or toxic mechanism, but currently available evidence suggests the former. At the present time, weekly white blood cell counts are recommended on an indefinite basis for patients receiving this drug. Detailed reviews of the clinical management of clozapine are available.[24]

Pharmacologic Treatment of Negative Symptoms

To consider the effect of medications on negative symptoms it is necessary to discuss the definition of the target symptoms or syndrome and other entities that should be considered in the differential diagnosis.

As numerous investigators have emphasized, schizophrenia is associated with a variety of psychopathologic phenomena, none of which are consistently present or pathognomonic. Clinical trials have frequently used measures of outcome that focus on a relatively narrow range of "psychotic" signs and symptoms, such as delusions, hallucinations, and thought disorder, whereas some of the most profound disabilities that we observe with schizophrenia involve impairments in such areas as drive, motivation, pleasure capacity, and spontaneity. Although most clinicians easily recognize this aspect of the illness, there are a variety of causes of these potential "deficits" that must be considered in planning and assessing the impact of various treatment strategies. It is also important to recognize that so-called negative symptoms may be seen in a variety of nonschizophrenic conditions.

Behaviorally manifested adverse effects of neuroleptics such as akinesia may be associated with blunted affect, diminished spontaneity, and/or psychomotor retardation. These effects can persist well into the maintenance phase of treatment, and it should not be assumed that tolerance develops to this aspect of neuroleptic adverse effects.

Secondly, the presence of a mood disorder also may complicate the assessment of negative symptoms, and patients with schizophrenia may experience various forms of dysphoria. Specifically, postpsychotic depression has been described frequently in patients with this illness. The dysphoria experienced by patients may vary from relatively "endogenomorphic" presentations with vegetative signs and symptoms of depression to that dysphoria associated with extreme and chronic demoralization. Clearly, many patients with schizophrenia have good reason to be demoralized, and it is important to consider this phenomenon in the differential diagnosis. An assumption is made that a positive experience and positive environmental manipulations might be capable of elevating dysphoria in this context, whereas endogenomorphic depression would not be amenable to such influences.

Several studies have been conducted using antidepressant drugs in the treatment of those depressions occurring in the context of a schizophrenic illness. The most methodologically sophisticated study has been conducted by Siris et al,[25] and it suggests that imipramine is an effective treatment for patients with postpsychotic depression. Interestingly, Siris et al[26] also evaluated improvement in "negative" symptom areas and found that one half of the patients who met the criteria for postpsychotic depression also satisfied the criteria for negative symptoms. In addition to being rated as more severely ill on global measures, the negative-symptom patients tended to worry more and to experience more phobic anxiety, but there is little evidence that they were more depressed. None of the criterion items for negative symptoms improved with statistical significance in the imipramine-treated group as compared with the placebo-controlled group; however, improvement in three other symptom areas referable to depression (psychomotor agitation, self-reproach, and negative self-evaluation) did improve more in the imipramine-treated group to a significant degree.

There has been some concern that the use of antidepressant medications in patients with schizophrenia could produce an exacerbation of psychotic signs and symptoms, but in general this does not appear to be the case.[27,28] When such treatment is used, patients should be observed closely and the antidepressant should be given with a neuroleptic.

With regard to neuroleptic effects on negative symptoms, a major area of confusion has been the evaluation of the impact of neuroleptics and the potential for different degrees of responsiveness of a particular target sign or symptom depending upon the phase of illness that a given patient is experiencing and whether or not clinically significant positive symptoms are also apparent. During an acute psychotic exacerbation many patients experience not only an increase in delusions, hallucinations, and thought disorder, but also an increase in emotional withdrawal, blunted affect, or psychomotor retardation. The extent to which these negative symptoms represent a secondary response to the positive symptoms or are different manifestations of the same underlying pathophysiologic process is not clear.[29] In either case the negative symptoms that occur in this context can improve substantially (along with positive symptoms) in response to neuroleptic drug treatment.[30]

On the other hand, those negative symptoms that are present after the resolution of positive symptoms may represent a different aspect of the schizophrenic illness that might be considered a more enduring or persistent "deficit" state or more purely negative symptoms. The extent to which these manifestations of the illness are indicative of a potentially different or specific subtype of the schizophrenic syndrome is of enormous practical and heuristic interest.[31] It is this particular aspect of negative symptomatology that represents the major treatment challenge for mental health professionals, as a great deal of the disability associated with chronic schizophrenia revolves around diminished drive, impaired affect, and social withdrawal.

In general, most clinical trials of different neuroleptics or neuroleptic classes have not shown significant superiority of one drug or drug class over another in the treatment of positive or negative symptoms. Several investigators have suggested that the diphenylbutylpiperidines (pimozide, clopimozide, fluspirilene, and penfluridol) are superior in the treatment of negative symptoms as compared with other neuroleptics and also have suggested that this might be due to their effects as calcium-channel blockers.[32–34] Although it is unlikely that this class of compounds has unique properties with regard to calcium-channel antagonism, those clinical trials addressing their impact on negative symptoms are suggestive. However, the overall impression is not one of substantial difference from other drugs consistently shown across several measures. When there are differences they tend to favor this class of drugs, which may suggest some advantages for some patients. A major concern in these and other studies remains the issue of dose equivalency and whether or not one group is experiencing more extrapyramidal side effects than another. Even when attempts are made to rate parkinsonian side effects, subtle differences between groups can influence behavioral ratings but not necessarily be apparent on direct ratings of extrapyramidal side effects.

Maintenance Treatment

The "acute" phase in the treatment of schizophrenia involves an attempt to alleviate the signs and symptoms associated with an acute relapse or exacerbation. The therapeutic response that is obtained during this treatment phase will to some extent determine the rationale and expectations of subsequent continuation or maintenance treatment. In some cases continued neuroleptic treatment is truly prophylactic, with the goal being the prevention of a new episode. In other cases where patients have failed to achieve a complete remission of psychopathology, continued drug treatment may be viewed as controlling or suppressing ongoing manifestations of the illness rather than preventing a new episode.

Maintenance antipsychotic drug treatment has proven to be of enormous value in reducing the risk of psychotic relapse and rehospitalization. Numerous double-blind, placebo-controlled clinical trials have been conducted to provide evidence of this conclusion.[35,36] In the past 10 years a new generation of clinical trials have been conducted that have been much more sophisticated. They have focused not only on rates of relapse and rehospitalization, but on other factors relevant to assessing the overall benefits and risks of maintenance drug treatment.[37]

The desire to reduce adverse effects, particularly tardive dyskinesia and behaviorally manifested parkinsonian side effects, has led to an increasing interest in attempting to identify minimum dosage requirements for the long-term treatment of schizophrenia. Dosage reduction strategies have been encouraging in suggesting that compliance in medication taking can be increased and adverse effects can be reduced, while relapse rates may not increase substantially.[38-41] Clearly, clinical judgment and careful supervision is necessary to assure the maximum benefits and minimal risks associated with this type of treatment.

The possibility that some patients may not require continuous medication has fostered research on so-called "intermittent" or "targeted" strategies that go well beyond earlier suggestions of "drug holidays" in supporting the possibility that some individuals may do well without antipsychotic drugs for substantial periods of time, and that a full-blown psychotic relapse could be prevented by identifying early or prodromal signs of exacerbation and reinstituting medication promptly.

This type of strategy is a partial outgrowth of observations made by Herz and Melville[42] that many patients experience relatively characteristic signs or symptoms during the early stages of relapse, and that if the

TABLE 12.1. Relapse rate after drug discontinuation among patients in long-term remission.

Investigator	N	Time in remission (yr)	Length of followup off drug (mo)	Relapse rate (%)
Hogarty et al, 1976[49]	41	2–3	12	65
Johnson, 1976[50]	23	1–2	6	53
Dencker, et al, 1980[51]	32	2	24	94
Cheung, 1981[48]	30	3–5	18	62
Johnson, 1979[52]	60	1–4	18	80
Wistedt, 1981[53]	14	1/2	12	100

(From Kane.[1])

clinician and families are knowledgeable regarding this pattern, this can facilitate early recognition and reinstitution of drug treatment when appropriate. One assumption underlying this strategy is that lengthy interruptions in drug administration may minimize the risk of adverse effects. Although this is clearly the case for some adverse effects (eg, drug-induced parkinsonism, cognitive and neuroendocrine effects), the impact of this strategy on the incidence of tardive dyskinesia has yet to be fully established.[43]

Ideally, we would like to have methods that would enable us to identify specific patients who are best suited for a particular strategy on the basis of their propensity to relapse within a relatively short time after neuroleptic drug discontinuation.[44] The work of Lieberman et al[45] using response to methylphenidate infusions as a potential predictor of relapse is a logical extension of early work by Janowsky et al[46] and Angrist et al.[47] Lieberman's results suggest that those patients experiencing a transient exacerbation of psychotic signs and symptoms after 0.5 mg/km of intravenous methylphenidate will relapse sooner (after antipsychotic drug withdrawal) than patients not responding to methylphenidate. This strategy does not necessarily identify patients who can be maintained medication free on an indefinite basis, but in our experience this remains a very small subgroup. Even for those patients who have been in remission for a substantial length of time on neuroleptic drugs, the risk of relapse after drug discontinuation appears to be considerable[48–53] (Table 12.1).

Summary

Antipsychotic medication continues to be the mainstay of treatment in both the acute and chronic phases of a schizophrenic illness. We continue to have limited information as to the most appropriate treatments for individuals who fail to respond to an adequate course of antipsychotic medication. There are a variety of studies that suggest that antipsychotic drug blood levels may have some usefulness in certain situations, but more data are necessary before their application can be recommended on a routine basis. The atypical antipsychotic agent, clozapine, appears to hold some promise for a subgroup of refractory patients; however, an apparent increased risk of agranulocytosis must be considered in the indications for using this compound.

In recent years there has been increased emphasis on improving the potential benefits of long-term neuroleptic treatment and minimizing risks by attempting to establish minimum effective dose requirements for all phases of treatment. More sophisticated and comprehensive assessment measures have been applied in long-term treatment trials, enabling us to be more specific about treatment goals and treatment evaluation.

Extrapyramidal side effects continue to be a major clinical problem in the use of antipsychotic drugs; their diagnosis is complicated by their potential to mimic aspects of schizophrenic psychopathology, and clinical recognition continues to be a problem. Tardive dyskinesia remains one of the most common and serious long-term adverse effects associated with antipsychotic drugs. New data in recent years suggest that tardive dyskinesia is frequently not progressive, and may in fact improve if dosage reduction can be used among those patients who continue to require antipsychotic drug treatment.

In general, although not all patients respond to antipsychotic drugs to the desired extent, we have no predictors that would enable us to identify nonresponders before an adequate trial. Therefore, a course of antipsychotic medication remains indicated for patients with a diagnosis of schizophrenia or schizophreniform illness, unless there is a clear contraindication to the use of this class of agents.

References

1. Kane JM: Treatment of schizophrenia. *Schizophr Bull* 1987;13:147–171.
2. Davis JM, Schaffer CB, Killian GA, et al: Important issues in the drug treatment of schizophrenia. *Schizophr Bull* 1980;6:70–87.
3. Klein DF, Davis JM: *Diagnosis and Drug Treatment of Psychiatric Disorders.* Baltimore, Williams & Wilkins, 1969.
4. Gardos G: Are antipsychotic drugs interchangeable? *J Nerv Ment Dis* 1978;159:343–348.
5. Creese I, Burt DR, Snyder SH: Dopamine receptor binding predicts clinical and pharmacological potencies of antischizophrenic drugs. *Science* 1976;192:481–483.
6. Richelson E: Neuroleptic affinities for human brain receptors and their use in predicting adverse effects. *J Clin Psychiatry* 1985;45:331–336.
7. Davis JM, Barder J, Kane JM: Antipsychotic drugs, in Kaplan HI, Sadock BJ (eds): *Comprehensive Textbook of Psychiatry,* ed 5. Baltimore, Williams & Wilkins, 1989, pp. 1591–1626.
8. Van Putten T, Marder SR, Mintz J: The therapeutic index of haloperidol in

newly admitted schizophrenic patients. *Psychopharmacol Bull* 1987;23:201–205.

9. McEvoy J, Stiller RL, Farr R: Plasma haloperidol levels drawn at neuroleptic threshold doses: A pilot study. *J Clin Psychopharmacol* 1986;6:133–138.

10. Baldessarini RJ, Cohen BM, Teicher MH: Significance of neuroleptic dose and plasma level in the pharmacological treatment of psychoses. *Arch Gen Psychiatry* 1988;45:79–91.

11. Baldessarini R, Katz B, Cotton P: Dissimilar dosing with high-potency and low-potency neuroleptics. *Am J Psychiatry* 1984;141:748–752.

12. Smith RC, Baumgartner R, Shvartsburd A, et al: Comparative efficacy of red cell and plasma haloperidol as predictors of clinical response in schizophrenia. *Psychopharmacology* 1985;85:449–455.

13. Mavroidis ML, Kanter DR, Hirschowitz J, et al: Clinical response and plasma haloperidol levels in schizophrenia. *Psychopharmacology* 1983;81:354–356.

14. Van Putten T, Marder SR, May PR, et al: Plasma levels of haloperidol and clinical response. *Psychopharmacol Bull* 1985;21:69–72.

15. Marder SR, Van Putten T, Mintz J, et al: Costs and benefits of two doses of fluphenazine. *Arch Gen Psychiatry* 1984;41:1025–1029.

16. Kane JM, Woerner M, Borenstein M, et al: Integrating incidence and prevalence of tardive dyskinesia. *Psychopharmacol Bull* 1986;22:254–258.

17. Gardos G, Perenyi A, Cole JO, et al: Tardive dyskinesia: changes after three years. *J Clin Psychopharmacol* 1983;3:315–318.

18. Casey DE: Tardive dyskinesia: what is the natural history? *Int Drug Ther Newslett* 1983;18:13–16.

19. Kane JM, Cooper TB, Sachar EJ, et al: Clozapine: plasma levels and prolactin response. *Psychopharmacology* 1981;73:184–187.

20. Honigfeld G, Patin J, Singer J: Clozapine: antipsychotic activity in treatment-resistant schizophrenics. *Adv Ther* 1984;1:77–97.

21. Giffith RW, Saameli K: Clozapine and agranulocytosis. *Lancet* 1975;ii:657.

22. Lieberman JA, Johns CA, Kane JM, et al: Clozapine-induced agranulocytosis: noncross-reactivity with other psychotropic drugs. *J Clin Psychiatry* 1988;49:271–277.

23. Kane J, Honigfeld G, Singer J, et al: Clozapine for the treatment-resistant schizophrenic. *Arch Gen Psychiatry* 1988;45:789–796.

24. Lieberman JA, Kane J, Johns C: Clozapine: guidelines for clinical management. Submitted, *J Clin Psychiatry.*

25. Siris SG, Morgan V, Vagerstrom R, et al: Adjunctive imipramine in the treatment of postpsychotic depression: a controlled trial. *Arch Gen Psychiatry* 1987;44:533–539.

26. Siris SG, Adan F, Cohen M, et al: Targeted treatment of depression-like symptoms in schizophrenia. *Psychopharmacol Bull* 1987;23:85–89.

27. Brenner R, Shopsin B: The use of monoamine oxidase inhibitors in schizophrenia. *Biol Psychiatry* 1980;15:633–647.

28. Prusoff BA, Williams DH, Weissman MM, et al: Treatment of secondary depression in schizophrenia. *Arch Gen Psychiatry* 1979;36:569–575.

29. Carpenter WT Jr: Thoughts on the treatment of schizophrenia. *Schizophr Bull* 1986;12:527–539.

30. Goldberg SC: Negative and deficit symptoms in schizophrenia do respond to neuroleptics. *Schizophr Bull* 1985;11:453–456.

31. Crow TJ: Molecular pathology of schizophrenia: more than one disease process? *Br Med J* 1980;280:66–86.
32. Kolivakis T, Azian H, Kingstone E: A double-blind comparison of pimozide and chlorpromazine in the maintenance of chronic schizophrenic patients. *Curr Ther Res* 1974;16:998–1004.
33. Haas S, Beckmann H: Pimozide versus haloperidol in acute schizophrenia: a double-blind controlled study. *Pharmacopsychiatry* 1982;15:70–74.
34. Lapierre WD: A controlled study of penfluridol in the treatment of chronic schizophrenia. *Am J Psychiatry* 1978;135:956–959.
35. Davis JM: Overview: maintenance therapy in psychiatry: I. Schizophrenia. *Am J Psychiatry* 1975;132:1237–1245.
36. Kane JM, Lieberman JA: Maintenance pharmacotherapy in schizophrenia, in Meltzer HY (ed): *Psychopharmacology, The Third Generation of Progress: The Emergence of Molecular Biology and Biological Psychiatry.* New York, Raven Press, 1988.
37. Kane J (ed): *Drug Maintenance Strategies in Schizophrenia.* Washington, DC, American Psychiatry Press, 1984.
38. Kane JM, Rifkin A, Woerner M, et al: Low-dose neuroleptic treatment of outpatient schizophrenics: I. Preliminary results for relapse rates. *Arch Gen Psychiatry* 1983;40:893–896.
39. Marder SR, Van Putten T, Mintz J, et al: Costs and benefits of two doses of fluphenazine. *Arch Gen Psychiatry* 1984;41:1025–1029.
40. Marder SR, Van Putten T, Mintz J, et al: Low- and conventional-dose maintenance therapy with fluphenazine decanoate: two-year outcome. *Arch Gen Psychiatry* 1987;44:518–521.
41. Hogarty GE, McEvoy JP, Munetz M, et al: Dose of fluphenazine, familial expressed emotion, and outcome in schizophrenia: Results of a two-year controlled study. *Arch Gen Psychiatry* 1988;45:797–805.
42. Herz MI, Melville C: Relapse in schizophrenia. *Am J Psychiatry* 1980;137:801–805.
43. Degkwitz R, Binsack HF, Herkert H, et al: Zum problem der persistierenten extrapyramidalen hyperkinesen nach langfristiger anwendung von neuroleptika. *Nervenarzt* 1967;38:170–174.
44. Lieberman JA, Kane JM (eds): *Predictors of Relapse in Schizophrenia.* Washington DC, American Psychiatric Press, 1986.
45. Lieberman JA, Kane JM, Sarantakos S, et al: Prediction of relapse in schizophrenia. *Arch Gen Psychiatry* 1987;44:597–603.
46. Janowsky DS, El-Yousef K, Davis JM, et al: Provocations of schizophrenic symptoms by intravenous administration of methylphenidate. *Arch Gen Psychiatry* 1973;28:185–191.
47. Angrist B, Rotrosen J, Gershon SL: Responses to apomorphine, amphetamine and neuroleptics in schizophrenic subjects. *Psychopharmacology* 1980;67:31–38.
48. Cheung HK: Schizophrenics fully remitted on neuroleptics for 3–5 years: to stop or continue drugs? *Br J Psychiatry* 1981;138:490–494.
49. Hogarty GE, Ulrich RF, Mussare F, et al: Drug discontinuation among long-term successfully maintained schizophrenic outpatients. *Dis Nerv Sys* 1976;37:494–500.
50. Johnson DAW: The duration of maintenance therapy in chronic schizophrenia. *Acta Psychiatr Scand* 1976;53:298–301.

51. Dencker SJ, Lepp M, Malm U: Do schizophrenics well-adapted in the community need neuroleptics? A depot neuroleptic withdrawal study. *Acta Psychiatr Scand* 1980;279:64–76.
52. Johnson DAW: Further observations on the duration of depot neuroleptic maintenance therapy in schizophrenia. *Br J Psychiatry* 1979;135:524–530.
53. Wistedt B: A depot neuroleptic withdrawal study: a controlled study of the clinical effects of the withdrawal of depot fluphenazine decanoate and depot flupenthixol decanoate in chronic schizophrenic patients. *Acta Psychiatr Scand* 1981;64:65–84.

Part III
Delivery Systems for Managing Schizophrenic Patients

13
Current Perspectives in the United States on the Chronically Mentally Ill

JOHN A. TALBOTT

The current situation of the chronically mentally ill in the United States is believed by most experts to be suboptimal. Hundreds of chronically mentally ill persons are homeless in each of our major urban centers, thousands are now imprisoned in our overcrowded correctional system, and more than half a million are housed but not treated in our "new" institution—the nursing home.

How did this happen, in the world's richest country, with such an abundance of good ideas and innovative programs? In this chapter, I attempt to answer this question by reviewing the history leading up to our deinstitutionalization effort, the problems that have ensued since it began in 1955, proposed and attempted solutions to the problems, and some thoughts about the future.

Historical Background

As with so many other areas, the current problems of the chronically mentally ill can only be fully appreciated through an understanding of the historical background underlying the situation.

State Mental Hospitals

America was discovered in 1492 and the United States colonized by the British beginning in 1620. Early documents from the colonies demonstrate striking examples of inhumanity toward some mentally ill persons.[1] Whereas most localities established institutions for the poor and needy (almshouses), the idle and disorderly (workhouses), and rogues and vagabonds (jails), clearly none of these was suitable for the care and treatment of the severely and chronically mentally ill, although they were frequently housed there.[2]

In 1752, the first separate unit for the mentally ill in a general hospital was established at the Pennsylvania Hospital in Philadelphia; in 1773, the first "public" hospital for the mentally ill opened in Williamsburg, Virginia; and in 1821, a private hospital, the Bloomingdale Asylum, modeled after the Tuke Retreat, opened.[3] Up to this point, care and treatment of the mentally ill tended to be haphazard, depending on availability and accessibility, as well as highly variable, depending on locale.

During the 19th century, however, individual states, starting with Massachusetts and New York, began to build state mental hospitals to care for and treat the mentally ill. An indefatigable reformer, Dorothea Dix, successfully led a lengthy fight to establish state mental hospitals in every state, arguing that the localities could not adequately care for this population.[2,3]

State hospitals continued to dominate the landscape of American psychiatry for the remainder of the 19th and most of the 20th centuries, although they were beset by criticism, scandals, and problems throughout.[4] At their height, in 1955, they housed fully 558,992 persons.[5]

Alternatives to State Hospitals

Starting in 1855, with the Farm at St. Anne, a number of alternative programs were established in the United States. During the next 100 years these included (Fig. 13.1) everything from aftercare to travelling clinics and from day hospitals to halfway houses.[6]

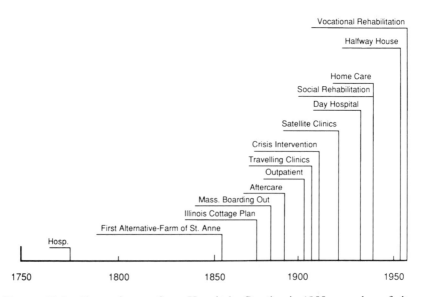

FIGURE 13.1. Alternatives to State Hospitals. Starting in 1855 a number of alternative programs to state hospitals were established in the United States.

In addition, nonstate hospital alternatives, primarily general hospital units and psychopathic hospitals associated with universities (such as the Boston Psychopathic Hospital and the Payne Whitney Psychiatric Clinic of New York City), were established.[7]

Finally, almost every level of American government (federal, state, county, and city) had facilities that it either funded and operated directly or financed through contracts. This included: Federal Public Health, Armed Forces, and Veteran's Administration facilities; State Mental Hospitals, Children's Hospitals, and Alcohol and Drug Abuse Facilities; and County and City Hospitals and Clinics.

The Onset of Deinstitutionalization

In 1955, after more than a century of growth, the census in state hospitals reached its peak of almost 560,000 persons (Fig. 13.2).[5] It has steadily decreased in the past 34 years until it stands now at almost 110,000—an 80% reduction!

The reasons behind this extraordinary reversal in decades of increasing state hospital populations are many and their interaction complex. They include forces that were philosophical, technological, economic, and legal.[8]

Philosophical Reasons

In 1939, Albert Deutch published *Shame of the States*, documenting the horrors of state institutions.[9] Subsequently, two events during World War

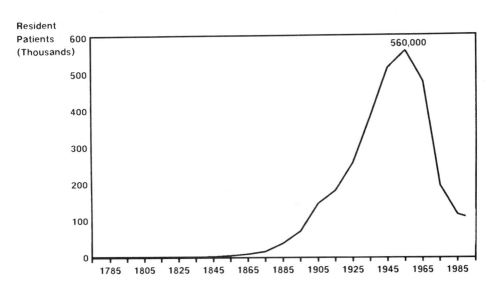

FIGURE 13.2. State Hospital Population. After a peak in 1955, deinstitutionalization resulted in an 80% decrease over the next three decades.

II had an important influence on later developments. First, at one point the number of persons rejected from military services for mental disorders exceeded the *entire number* of inductees. Second, some persons seeking exemption from service on the basis of religious/conscientious objection were assigned to work in mental hospitals and were shocked by what they saw.

After the war, in 1946, the US Congress adopted a National Mental Health Act that supported research, training, and assistance to individual states for prevention and treatment. Then in 1953, the President of the American Psychiatric Association called for an examination of state hospitals in his presidential address. During the same period, American psychiatrists began to consider the innovations occurring in the United Kingdom, such as the "open door," and community and social psychiatry took hold.

This philosophy of treating people as much as possible "in the community" rather than in "institutions" was translated into action through a World Health Organization (WHO) Committee Report in 1954, the first state legislation for community mental health services in New York in 1954, and, eventually, at the federal level in the Community Mental Health Centers Act of 1965 (Table 13.1).

TABLE 13.1. Community Mental Health Center antecedents.

		Regulations	
WHO Committee (1954)	New York State (1954)	CMHC (1965)	CMHC Amendment (1975)
	Inpatient	Inpatient	Inpatient
Outpatient	Outpatient	Outpatient	Outpatient
Partial hospital		Partial hospital	Partial hospital
		Emergency (24 hr)	Emergency (24 hr)
Community education	Consultation & education	Consultation & education	Consultation & education
		Diagnostic	
		Precare & aftercare	Screening patients for courts & agencies prior to state hospital
			Follow-up care
Rehabilitation	Rehabilitation	Rehabilitation	
Research		Research & evaluation	Transitional housing
			Services for elderly
			Services for children
			Services for alcoholics
			Services for drug problems

WHO = World Health Organization; CMHC = Community Mental Health Center.

Technology

The year 1955 was not only the year that state hospital censuses turned around, it was also the year chlorpromazine was introduced into those systems for the first time.[10] Many saw the two events causally.[10]

Economics

Traditionally, the states had assumed the burden of funding the care and treatment of the severely and chronically mentally ill through state tax levies. However, three new and large federal initiatives altered that necessity, allowing states to begin to shift the burden to largely a federal responsibility, especially if care was provided "in the community."[11]

These three new massive national programs were: Medicare, providing health care for the elderly regardless of income, in 1965; Medicaid, covering health care for the poor, in 1966; and Social Security Insurance/Social Security Disability Insurance (SSI/SSDI), entitling both those disabled for mental or physical reasons who had worked before and those who had not, with social services including money for housing, in 1973.

Legal/Legislative Forces

A fourth influence was wielded by civil liberties lawyers through the courts, state regulations, and state legislatures in the 1960s and 1970s.[12] Some of these initiatives were directed to rehabilitation programs (eg, Souder vs Brennan) intended to end involuntary servitude among long-stay patients. Some were to give patients the Right To Refuse Treatment; however, most were directed at stopping treatment in hospitals through attempts to abolish involuntary commitment itself, to stop involuntary commitment without treatment (the so-called Right To Treatment issue), or to discharge patients or treat them from the start in Less Restrictive Alternatives.

Problems of Deinstitutionalization

Since 1955, there have been many problems encountered by the chronically mentally ill as well as the service systems seeking to help them. Surely the most obvious is the fact that although many persons receive better care "in the community" than they did in far distant state institutions, many do not. Indeed, it is the lack of any real treatment, rehabilitation, and care for those now housed in nursing homes, jails, or community residences coupled with the lack of anything for those both homeless and mentally ill that is the most visible negative consequence of our deinstitutionalization process. In addition, because the auspices of responsibility for care were transferred from a definable entity, the hospital, to an intangible one, the community, the net result for many was the loss of responsibility for care. This, coupled with shorter lengths of stay, led to a situation many referred to as the "revolving door."[13]

To dig beneath these more visible problems to the root causes, however, I will use a survey of psychiatrists, conducted in conjunction with the President's Commission on Mental Health, that detailed most of the underlying issues.[14] Although there were many issues mentioned in this survey, I have arbitrarily divided them into four large categories: treatment and services, external forces, professional concerns, and research issues.

Treatment and Services

Depopulation Rather Than Deinstitutionalization

Deinstitutionalization is intended to imply movement of both patients and services from institutional to community auspices. In our case we experienced largely the depopulation of state hospitals. The rapidity of the process, lack of planning, paucity of community facilities, and inadequacy of shifts in funding all contributed to the disaster.

Continuum of Community Care Facilities

This depopulation movement revealed the necessity for a continuum of programs, including inpatient and outpatient care, quarterway and halfway houses, day hospitals, chronic care, and a variety of living opportunities, such as group homes, foster care, domiciliary care, and self-care.

Adequate Numbers of Facilities and Programs

In addition, the past 34-years experience has revealed how few such programs we have to care for the deinstitutionalized and never-institutionalized mentally ill.

Continuity of Care

The fragmentation of services provided by each separate level of government has led to extreme difficulty in ensuring continuity of care by one caregiver, one mental health care team, or even one program.

Responsibility for Care

Deinstitutionalization demonstrated, as nothing before had, that no single person, team, or program was responsible any longer for any one patient, group of patients, or the mentally ill as a whole.

Involvement of Families

In the wake of American deinstitutionalization, many families became the primary caregivers, a role for which they were not trained, equipped, or recompensed. In addition, the residue of blame for the illnesses of their offspring often tainted professional relationships. Positive cooperative collaboration was all too infrequent.

Mental Hospitals

Even with their depopulation, state facilities were shown to be inadequate in providing quality psychiatric treatment, rehabilitation, and care. In addition, their mixed and sometimes confused roles as providers of: (1) acute care, (2) chronic care, (3) geriatric care, (4) aftercare, and (5) asylum or custodial care compounded their poor functioning.

Community Care

In addition to the lack of an adequate range, number, and funding for such programs, there were revealed to be inadequate professional consultation, staffing, and follow-up.

New Approaches to Care

Newer approaches to care, such as assertive outreach and case management, were more successful than traditional sitting and waiting for patients to enter offices or programs.

Models for Service Delivery

Finally, the movement demonstrated the paucity of models of comprehensive, coordinated, and continuous treatment as well as rehabilitation and care for the population.

External Forces

Adequate Funding

As deinstitutionalization in America proceeded, the inadequacy of funding for institutional, community, asylum, and home-care became apparent.

Flexible Financing

However, even more obvious was the inefficiency of the financing system. Money was administered and distributed by separate federal, state, and local agencies, often with different definitions of their recipients and with the net result of both overlapping services and gaps in service.

Unification of Funding

Deinstitutionalization also demonstrated the degree to which funding was fragmented in such a way that channels of money moved down in a parallel, uncoordinated way from federal to state to local levels. Hence, patients and caregivers scrambled to put together the various funding streams rather than have them available to patients in a single "package."

Discrimination in Funding

In addition, there was overt discrimination, with certain housing, educational, and medical money going to pay for the physically but not the mentally ill or handicapped.

Adequate Nonmedical, Nonpsychiatric Services

Deinstitutionalization also revealed the paucity of care, rehabilitation, and supportive services, including housing, socialization, vocational, employment, transportation, and homemaking services.

Public Attitudes

Deinstitutionalization demonstrated the low public opinion of those suffering from mental illness, lower than almost any other "have not" group, such as the mentally retarded, drug abusers, and prisoners.

Advocacy

Deinstitutionalization also revealed how little visibility, political strength, and public sympathy was afforded the chronically mentally ill and how much citizen advocacy and celebrity attention was needed.

Legal Problems

Finally, the host of problems raised by increasing encroachments of the law on services provided to the severely and chronically mentally ill became clearer as the movement progressed. These included the: inability of families to obtain treatment for their afflicted relatives; inability to provide effective treatment; inability for providers to exchange information; inability to provide the most therapeutic setting instead of the least restrictive setting; inability to live in any area; and inability to achieve a "right to treatment in the community."

Professional Issues

Attitudinal Problems

Those working in the field are not immune from attitudinal biases. Indeed, many also harbor unrealistic expectations for the population coupled with according to them a lower status than other patients, who may be seen as more "interesting" or "better teaching material."

The Role of Psychiatrists

Deinstitutionalization in America also brought about the realization that in many sectors of public psychiatry, psychiatrists served only as writers of prescriptions and were not involved with comprehensive treatment planning, service delivery, and outcome evaluation.

Suitable Training

In many professions, including psychiatry, training was reductionistic along either biological or psychological lines, with little integration or application of known modern rehabilitative and community programs. In addition, exposure to a comprehensive range of high quality services for the chronically ill was unusual.

Research and Evaluation

Services Research

In the aftermath of deinstitutionalization it became clear that few service system experiments had been held and much more research was needed.

Effective Programs

In addition, there were few descriptions of programs whose effectiveness had been measured against other programs.

Optimal Treatment

No guidelines existed for determination of which patients with what disorders and correlated disabilities should be treated with which modalities of treatment in what settings.

Research on Chronicity

Likewise, there is little understanding of what produces and what maintains chronicity.

Resistance

Resistance of patients, families, and professionals became more pronounced with deinstitutionalization, and little was known about how to counter it.

Further Epidemiology

In addition, whereas something was known about the dimensions of the population and its subgroups, more needed to be known about its parameters and characteristics to better design responsive service systems with defined boundaries.

Long-Term Medication

The cost benefits of long-term medication, whether tardive dyskinesia or kidney effects, were also believed to require further exploration from financial, family burden, and societal impact points of view.

Financing and Cost Benefit Studies

Underlying many of the above are issues of efficiency and effectiveness to ensure optimal cost-effective, yet outcome-oriented, treatment programs.

Attempted and Proposed Solutions

In many respects, the solutions flow from the problems, as illustrated in Table 13.2. However, putting the individual solutions together in a comprehensive package necessitates further refinement.

Organizational Responses

The American Psychiatric Association's Report on the Chronically Ill

In 1978, after 3 years of study, the American Psychiatric Association (APA), issued its first report on the problem: *The Chronic Mentally Ill: Problems, Solutions, and Recommendations for a Public Policy.*[15] This report spelled out the details of the consequences of the deinstitutionalization process in the United States and made specific recommendations, summarized below, constituting part of the President's Commission on Mental Health Report.[16] These recommendations were later incorporated in *Towards A Public Policy on the Chronic Mentally Ill,*[17] as well as implemented as the Mental Health Systems Act,[18] also referred to below.

The APA's Second Report—Homeless Mentally Ill

However, only 6 years after its first report, the APA issued a second, addressed to the problem of the deluge of severely and chronically mentally ill patients now flooding the streets of America. This report, although completely new in approach, focus, and data, reinforced the recommendations made in the first.[19]

TABLE 13.2. Solutions to the problems engendered by deinstitutionalization.

Problems	Solutions
Treatment and Services	
Depopulation	Deinstitutionalization
No continuum	Continuum of facilities
Inadequate numbers	Adequate numbers
Discontinuity	Continuity of care
No responsibility	Responsibility
Families not involved	Involve families
Poor mental hospital	Improve mental hospitals
Inadequate community care	Adequate community care
Traditional care	Innovative care
Few service delivery models	Develop new models
External Forces	
Inadequate funding	Adequate funding
Inflexible financing	Flexible financing
Fragmented funding	Unify funding
Discrimination in funding	Equality in funding
Inadequate housing, rehab, etc	Adequate housing, rehab
Bad public attitudes	Improve public attitudes
Little advocacy	Improve advocacy
Legal barriers	Alter laws
Professional issues	
Negative attitudes	Alter attitudes
Psychiatric role limitations	Expand role
Unsuitable training	Alter training
Research and evaluation	
Inadequate services research	Increase services research
Little effectiveness research	Increase effectiveness research
Little treatment research	Increase treatment research
Little chronicity research	Increase chronicity research
Little about resistance	Learn more re:resistance
Little epidemiology	More epidemiology
Inadequate long-term drug therapy research	More long-term drug therapy research
Few financing studies	More financing studies

Derived, with permission, from Talbott, J.A., Kaplan, S.R. (eds.): Psychiatric Administration: A Comprehensive Text for the Clinician/Executive. Grune and Stratton, 1982.

The National Alliance for the Mentally Ill

In 1979, a group of family members met in Madison, Wisconsin and founded the National Alliance for the Mentally Ill (NAMI).[20]

Governmental Initiatives

The Community Mental Health Center Amendment

In 1975, the Community Mental Health Center Act was amended for the first time (Table 13.1) to try to fill some of the gaps revealed in its first 10 years. Transitional housing and services for children and the elderly as well as alcoholics and drug abusers were added.

The National Institute of Mental Health Community Support Program

In 1977, the National Institute of Mental Health (NIMH) inaugurated the Community Support Program calling for additional services: identification of the population; assistance applying for entitlements; crisis stabilization; psychosocial rehabilitation; supportive services; medical and mental health care; backup to families; involvement of the community; protection of patient rights; and case management.[21]

Chronic Mental Patient Plan (NIMH)

In 1978, the President's (Carter) Commission on Mental Health issued its final report,[15] portions of which used the APA's report.[14] Shortly thereafter, the NIMH issued a plan called "Towards a Public Policy on the Chronic Mentally Ill."[16] Both called for sweeping improvements in funding and research for the population. Indeed, a new federal act, the Mental Health Systems Act,[17] held the promise of implementing all these recommendations. However, months after it was enacted, it was made moot by the new President's (Reagan) elimination of all special funding to individual states and lumping them into "block grants."

The McKinney Homeless Act

In 1987, the US Congress, in part responding to the APA's second report on the homeless mentally ill,[18] passed a bill designed to provide assistance to states to deal with this most visible negative consequence of America's deinstitutionalization process—the homeless.[21]

Financing Initiatives

Managed Care Systems

Since Henry Kaiser established health care systems for his employees in World War II, there have been health maintenance organizations (HMOs) that seek to prevent more costly inpatient care through screening, prevention, and treatment in less costly outpatient settings. During the Nixon Administration (1969 to 1974), Congress passed a bill encouraging such new organized care systems. Unfortunately, few offered much psychiatric care at all, and those which did, tended to exclude the severely and chronically mentally ill.[22]

Corporate Psychiatry

During the past decade in particular, we have seen the arrival of corporate health care—the buying of private or university (and a few public) psychiatric hospitals by for-profit chains (not unlike McDonald's).[23] The effect on the chronically mentally ill and deinstitutionalization is not direct, although it is ironic that they are revitalizing and expanding institutions not emptying them, and they are suspected of "creaming off" better-paying patients, leaving the more chronic and disabled to others.

Prospective Pricing

In another attempt to control costs, the US Congress in 1984[24] changed its practice of paying for the elderly in hospitals (Medicare) from after-the-fact costs incurred for each patient to before-the-fact pricing by diagnosis, so-called diagnosis-related groups (DRGs). Although most psychiatric patients were exempted, those not so were treated for shorter periods (ie, their lengths of hospital stay decreased). Patients with psychotic illnesses were expected to have an average length of stay of only 10.6 days per episode.

National Health Insurance

Although the concept of national health insurance has been seriously discussed in almost every recent Democratic administration (Roosevelt, Truman, Kennedy, and Carter), it has never been enacted in any form. Another common goal, catastrophic insurance, which could be structured to cover severe and chronic mental illnesses, has been enacted in 1988 for the elderly, but without provision for mental illnesses.

Service Experiments

The Mendota Program

One of the best conducted, researched, and disseminated comprehensive programs for the chronically mentally ill took place at the Mendota Mental Health Center in Madison, Wisconsin, by Leonard Stein and Mary Ann Test.[25] At present, Dr. Stein is director of the mental health services in an entire county (Dane) that receives a predetermined amount of dollars per resident (eg, capitation) and must provide all necessary services within the system. Results of this bigger program can be expected soon.

Other Capitation Programs

There are several other such experiments now underway in New York State (in Monroe and Livingston Counties) and Arizona (Pima County), whose results will not be known for some time.[26]

The Robert Wood Johnson Foundation Project

Starting with the premise that improved services could be provided through administrative and fiscal coordination and unification at the local government level, nine cities are participating in an experiment to attempt just that, as well as to increase housing opportunities for the chronically mentally ill.[27] The program is running from 1987 to 1992, and the full evaluation will appear shortly thereafter.

A Comprehensive Entitlement

Finally, one idea that is currently a mere proposal involves taking all federal money directed toward the chronically mentally ill and placing it in one big new mental health entitlement for the population.[28] If, then, appropriate state and city/county money was added, the comprehensive needs of the population might well be met.

The Future

Speculation about the future is always risky despite our continuing drive to do so.[29] If it were true that the most accurate predictor of tomorrow's weather is today's, then we in the United States are in serious trouble.

For despite 34 years of attempting to bring about community care for the severely and chronically mentally ill who once inhabited our nation's state mental hospitals, we are still far short of the goal. Indeed, whereas it is apparent (despite the bulk of this chapter) that many persons were helped by deinstitutionalization, a sizeable few have been badly hurt.

Of our 1.7 to 3 million persons with chronic mental illness, up to a quarter million may be homeless, up to three quarters of a million may be in often inadequate "community residences," and up to a million may be in nursing homes, where no specific psychiatric treatment or care is offered.[18,30]

What is most amazing is America's lack of shame over the casualties of this social experiment, which failed, in my opinion, not because it was bad, but because it was ill or not planned, hastily carried out, and unconnected with necessary preliminary administrative and financing shifts.

When I am asked how deinstitutionalization has worked in the United States, I reply that I do not know, because I have not seen it carried out— all I've seen is depopulation of our public institutions, "detreatmentization" of thousands of severely and chronically mentally ill persons, and transinstitutionalization of many of the state hospital's inhabitants to nursing homes, jails, or community mini-institutions.

What the future holds will depend on the several exciting administrative and financing experiments now taking place, on the research, both basic and applied, regarding this population, and on a willingness of our nation to finance humane comprehensive, largely community-based treatment, rehabilitation, and care until a definitive treatment, preventive methodology, or cure is discovered.

Summary

In this chapter I attempted to demonstrate current perspectives on the chronically mentally ill in the United States through an examination of the history leading up to our deinstitutionalization effort, the problems that have ensued since it began in 1955, proposed and attempted solutions to the problems, and some thoughts about the future.

The background to deinstitutionalization in the United States involves our historical dependence on state mental hospitals since the 19th century, the subsequent development of alternatives to those institutions since 1855, and the four forces that drove the process of deinstitutionalization in the United States in 1955. These forces include: philosophy (treatment in the community); technology (introduction of chlorpromazine); law (patients' civil liberties); and economics (Federal funding for the mentally ill).

The problems created by deinstitutionalization involve neglect and harm to many of those de- or not institutionalized; individuals who now find themselves receiving inferior or no care in jails, nursing homes, or living on the streets themselves. I have detailed the problems as they pertain to: treatment and services (depopulation rather than deinstitutionalization, lack of adequate numbers, the need for a continuum of community care facilities, and inadequacy of care in mental hospitals and the community); external forces (inadequate, inefficient, and fragmented funding, inadequate nonmedical and nonpsychiatric services, and low public opinion of the mentally ill); professional issues (inadequate training and limited role of psychiatrists); and research and evaluation (inadequacy of services research and research on chronicity and lack of assessment of program efficacy and cost benefits of long-term medication).

I then summarized the attempts to address or redress the situation. These include: responses from the American Psychiatric Association (reports on the Chronically Ill and Homeless Mentally Ill); other organizational responses (NAMI); governmental initiatives (CMHC Amendment, NIMH Community Support Program and Chronic Mental Health Plan, and McKinney Homeless Act); financing initiatives (managed care systems, corporate psychiatry, prospective pricing, and national health insurance); and service experiments (capitation programs, Robert Wood Johnson Foundation Project, and a comprehensive entitlement).

Finally, I speculate about the future, which I see as bleak given America's inability to feel a sense of outrage about the scandalous conditions that exist for our mentally ill in hospitals and substandard community residences that are attempting to provide treatment and care, not to mention the thousands now in need of treatment, rehabilitation, and care who reside in nursing homes, jails, and on the streets themselves. This inability translates directly into the ineffectiveness to date of various remedies. Perhaps, however, the few innovative initiatives and experiments cited that are now underway can be translated into broader action, once they are scientifically evaluated and disseminated.

References

1. Deutsch A: *The Mentally Ill in America: A History of Their Care and Treatment from Colonial Times,* ed 2. New York, Columbia University Press, 1949.
2. Rothman DJ: *The Discovery of the Asylum: Social Order and Disorder in the New Republic.* Boston, Little Brown, 1971.
3. Dain N: From colonial America to bicentennial America: two centuries of vicissitudes in the institutional care of mental patients. *Bull NY Acad Med* 1976;52:1179–1196.
4. Talbott JA: *The Death of the Asylum: A Critical Study of State Hospital Management, Services, and Care.* New York, Grune & Stratton, 1978.
5. Meyer NG: Provisional Patient Movement and Administrative Data State and County Psychiatric Inpatient Services, July 1, 1974 to June 30, 1975, Mental Health Statistical Note no. 132. Rockville, MD, US Department of Health, Education and Welfare, 1976.
6. Talbott JA: Twentieth century developments in American community psychiatry. *Psych Quart* 1982;54:207–219.
7. Hurd HM (ed): *The Institutional Care of the Insane in the United States and Canada.* Baltimore, MD, Johns Hopkins Press, 1946 (vol 1).
8. Talbott JA: Deinstitutionalization: avoiding the disasters of the past. *Hosp Commun Psych* 1979;30:621–624.
9. Deutsch A: *Shame of the States.* Garden City, NY, Doubleday, 1937.
10. Brill H, Patton RE: Analysis of population reduction in New York State mental hospitals during the first four years of large-scale therapy with psychotropic drugs. *Am J Psych* 1959;116:495–509.
11. Scull AT: *Decarceration: Community Treatment and the Deviant: A Radical View.* Englewood Cliffs, NJ, Prentice–Hall, 1977.
12. Stone AA: *Mental Health and Law: A System in Transition.* Rockville, MD, National Institute of Mental Health, 1975.
13. Talbott JA (ed): What are the problems of the chronic mental patient—a report of a survey of psychiatrists' concerns, in *The Chronic Mental Patient: Problems, Solutions, and Recommendations for a Public Policy.* Washington, DC, The American Psychiatric Association, 1978.
14. Talbott JA (ed): *The Chronic Mental Patient: Problems, Solutions and Recommendations for A Public Policy.* Washington, DC, The American Psychiatric Association, 1978.
15. President's Commission on Mental Health: *Report of the President's Commission on Mental Health.* Washington, DC, US Government Printing Office, 1978.
16. Toward A National Plan for the Chronically Mentally Ill: Report to the Secretary by the Department of Health and Human Services Steering Committee on the Chronically Mentally Ill (DHHS publication no. (ADM) 81-1077). Rockville, MD, Department of Health & Human Services, 1981.
17. Public Law 96-398, Mental Health Systems Act, 1980.
18. Lamb HR (ed): *The Homeless Mentally Ill: A Task Force Report of the American Psychiatric Association.* Washington, DC, The American Psychiatric Association, 1984.

19. Sokas P: Rapidly growing NAMI becomes influencial advocate for mentally ill. *Hosp Commun Psych* 1986;37:88–89.
20. Sharfstein S, Turner JE, Clark H: Financing issues in the delivery of services to the chronically mentally ill and disabled, in *The Chronic Mental Patient: Problems, Solutions, and Recommendations for a Public Policy.* Washington, DC, The American Psychiatric Association, 1978, pp 137–150.
21. Public Law 100-77, July 1987.
22. Bittker MD: Health maintenance organizations and prepaid psychiatry, in *The New Economics and Psychiatric Care.* Washington, DC, The American Psychiatric Association, 1985, pp 119–129.
23. Levenson AI: Issues surrounding the ownership of private psychiatric hospitals by investor-owned hospital chains. *Hosp Commun Psych* 1983;34:1127–1131.
24. Public Law 98-21, 1984.
25. Stein L, Test MA: A state hospital-initiated community program, in *The Chronic Mentally Ill: Treatment, Programs, Systems.* New York, Human Sciences Press, 1981, pp 160–174.
26. Lehman AF, Possidente S, Hawker F: The quality of life of chronic patients in a state hospital and in community residences. *Hosp Commun Psych* 1986;37:901–907.
27. Aiken LH, Somers SA, Shore M: Private foundations in health affairs: a case study of the development of a national initiative for the chronically mentally ill. *American Psychologist* 1986;41:1290–1295.
28. Talbott JA, Sharfstein S: A proposal for future funding of chronic and episodic mental illness. *Hosp Commun Psych* 1986;37:1126–1130.
29. Talbott JA (ed): *Our Patients' Future in a Changing World.* Washington, DC, The American Psychiatric Press, Inc., 1986.
30. Goldman HH, Manderscheid RW: Epidemiology of chronic mental disorder, in *The Chronic Mental Patient/II.* Washington, DC, The American Psychiatric Press, Inc., 1987, pp 41–63.

14
Policy on Chronic Mental Illness in Canada: Current Status and Future Directions

Gaston P. Harnois

Canada has a population of 26 million people living in 10 provinces; 80% of the population lives within 100 k of the US border. It is estimated that 0.9% of Canadians have or have had schizophrenia, with men being at somewhat higher risk overall than women (1% *vs* 0.7%, respectively).[1] New cases requiring hospitalization occur at a rate of about 0.05% nationwide.[2] Like most countries in the West, Canada has transferred a large number of schizophrenic patients from institutional settings into the community in recent years. It is estimated that there is one hospitalized schizophrenic patient for every four living in the community.[3] However, funding for community programs for schizophrenics continues to be considerably below that allocated for institutional care in Canada.[3]

Studies of outcome of schizophrenic patients followed over time [4,5] indicate that about one fourth recover after a single schizophrenic episode and do not experience a recurrence. For another fourth of schizophrenics, a favorable outcome is likely, whereas about 20% have an outcome rated "intermediate." The remainder of the patients (about 30%) have an unfavorable outcome and require extensive care for the rest of their lives to achieve an acceptable existence. These severely disabled patients make up about 0.3% of the Canadian population. Another measure of morbidity due to schizophrenia is the time lost from employment due to the severity of the disorder. In one outcome study, patients reported that 28% of the potential work time from their first hospitalization to final follow-up was lost due to their illness.[5] This finding translates into more than 56,000 "lost person years" each year for schizophrenic patients in Canada.[3,5]

General Background on Health Care in Canada

Under the Canadian Constitution, the provinces have the primary responsibility for health and social services. National health goals are clearly defined in the Canadian Constitution: the primary objective of Canadian health care policy is to protect, promote, and restore the physical and mental well-being of residents of Canada and to facilitate reasonable access to health services without financial or other barriers.

Canadians can achieve further improvements in their well-being through combining lifestyles that emphasize collective action against the social, environmental, and occupational causes of disease. The Canadian Government published, in 1986, a major orientation paper called "Achieving Health for All"[6] in which it can be seen that there is developing what amounts to a national health policy encompassing both health services and health promotion.

In mental health, the main areas of federal[7] responsibilities are: regulation related to the prevention of disorders that are essentially neurological; some regulatory, research, informational, and related aspects of the protection and advancement of human rights; prevention of crime; collection, analysis and publication of statistics; and programs designed to maximize employment and meet the information, training, and income security needs of the unemployed and immigrants.

The federal government has been quite active in the promotion of health and the prevention of alcoholism and drug addiction.[7] Support of mental health research comes from three agencies: the National Health Research and Development Program; the Social Sciences and Humanities Research Council; and the Medical Research Council. This support is far from being proportional to the percentage of the cost of mental health within the overall health system. Unlike the US Government, the Canadian Government does not have a system of national health institutes such as the U.S. National Institute of Mental Health (NIMH).

Presently, the federal government finances approximately 40% of the costs of the two national programs, namely: Medicare and hospitalization.[7] It has set the five basic criteria to which all provincial plans must adhere: public administration, comprehensiveness, universality, portability, and accessibility.

Since 1977 the federal government has moved from a position of open-handed cost sharing to one of block funding, which is broadly called established programs financing (EPF); this has allowed the Federal Government to limit sharply its contribution to the rapidly expanding provincial health services. As in the United States, this gives rise to considerable debate between the provinces and the federal government.

Since the beginning of the universal hospitalization and medical coverage program, mental health services in psychiatric hospitals have been excluded from cost-sharing programs and left entirely under the responsibility of the provinces. Allegedly, this has been done to respect fully provincial jurisdiction; in fact, the reality seems to be that the national government did not want to undertake the financing of provincial psychiatric hospitals, which were left considerably underfunded as compared with general hospitals' departments of psychiatry, which are covered by Medicare.

As the federal policy document notes, this exclusion has "encouraged the continued administrative and philosophical separation of psychiatric hospitals from other health services."[7] In the Province of Quebec, where a single administrative structure exists since 1972 to cover both psychiatric and general hospitals, there is still a considerable disparity in staff/patient ratios and budgets between the two types of hospitals.

Many observers believe that the federal government could better use its considerable leverage power, given its taxation authority, to influence particular aspects of provincial mental health programs. Nonetheless, the federal government is showing renewed concern for mental health issues, and observers believe that it will become increasingly present, mostly in the area of mental health promotion as opposed to the actual delivery of mental health services. In its most recent publications, "Mental Health for Canadians: Striking a Balance,"[8] the Federal Government addresses three mental health challenges: to reduce inequalities through a better understanding of risk factors, a better coordination of policies, and an increase in public participation; to increase prevention through research, the teaching of stress management skills, and a focus on environmental factors; and to enhance coping through the commitment of a greater share of resources to community development as well as to support interdisciplinary actions.

The federal government has created an advisory committee on mental health, which broadly consists of representatives of provincial governments at the underdeputy ministerial level, together with their federal counterpart. Although they recognize the need to share information, many provinces believe that the two-tiered system of federal and provincial decision-making process leads to duplication of services, increased bureaucracy, and unnecessary costs.

The Care of Schizophrenic Patients in Canada

It cannot be said that there is a mental health policy for Canada; all provinces have legislation dealing with compulsory treatment, and most provinces have regulations outlining in greater or lesser details the organization of mental health services within their boundaries. The same, of course, is applicable to schizophrenia, the most prevalent form of psychosis in our country.

Like other developed countries, Canada has been influenced by developments in psychiatry over the past 35 years. Discoveries in psychopharmacology, advances in community psychiatry[9,10] (with a strong influence from the French model based on sectorization),[11,12] increasing concern over the rights of the mentally ill, deinstitutionalization programs,[13] and experimentation in social reinsertion[14] all have had a profound effect.[15] Models vary from one province to another.

Illustrating the current status of care of schizophrenic patients in Canada are the results of a follow-up study of schizophrenic patients done in four Canadian provincial locations by Dr. Brenda Wattie,[16] who was then Director of the Mental Health Division at Health & Welfare Canada in 1985; the situation has not changed substantially since the report was published.

As shown in Table 14.1, there has been an overall reduction of 75% in the rated bed capacity in operating institutions from 1964 to 1979 in all Canadian provinces.[17] Even though they give a clear indication of trends, these figures have to be interpreted cautiously because in many provinces the decrease is accounted for through a change in the categorization of beds rather than through their closing down (eg, many beds formerly labelled "psychiatric" are now called "nursing home beds").

In Canada as elsewhere, the various deinstitutionalization programs have not all met with marked success. The issue is now understood to be extremely complex; multisectorial interventions requiring multiagency cooperation tend to be the exception rather than the rule.

As the Canadian system is universal and publicly financed, individuals do not pay directly the hospital or the physician; there is, for all intent, a single system which avoids the disadvantages of a two-tiered service system such as is found in the United States. It would appear that the community mental health programs are more often used by welfare clients and suffer from a lesser quality of staffing, as opposed to services that can be obtained privately by middle or upper class citizens in the United States who can carry an adequate level of health care insurance and who are not normally seen in community mental health centers.

TABLE 14.1. Rated bed capacity in operating institutions per capita decrease 1964–1979 by province.

	1964	1968	1972	1976	1978–79	Percentage decrease 1964–79
Newfoundland	1.7	3.4	1.7	1.0	0.9	47.0
Prince Edward Island	3.7	1.8	2.6	2.5	2.0	45.9
Nova Scotia	4.0	3.6	2.3	1.8	1.0	75.0
New Brunswick	2.7	2.6	2.6	2.2	1.5	44.4
Quebec	3.6	3.7	3.2	0.9	0.6	83.3
Ontario	3.6	3.5	2.5	2.0	1.0	72.2
Manitoba	3.8	3.2	2.6	2.3	1.1	71.0
Saskatchewan	4.0	3.2	2.2	2.2	2.7	82.5
Alberta	3.9	3.9	3.0	2.6	0.8	79.5
British Columbia	3.7	3.4	2.8	2.1	1.4	62.2
Canada	3.6	3.4	2.7	1.7	0.9	75.0

Derived, with permission, from reference 17.
Bed capacity per 1,000 population.

Follow-up Study of Schizophrenic Patients

Design

The study undertaken by Wattie aims at the follow-up of schizophrenic patients in four Canadian locations: "It was hoped to investigate any interactional relationships between the group of patient outcomes on the one hand, and personalized circumstances and variation in treatment and ongoing care received by the patient on the other."[16]

The data have been reported according to four systems rather than four provinces. This is because each system cannot purport to be representative of all services given in any given province; however, they attempt to describe the "systemic" nature of service delivery issues and are believed to be representative of what goes on in Canada. The sample includes two western provinces, a central province, and one maritime province. The Province of Quebec, with its specific French cultural background, was not part of the study and will be presented in some detail later.

System 1 (Alberta) is an urban area of medium size drawing on a patient catchment population of approximately 300,000. Rural dwellers comprised 19.6% of the patient sample. This is a prosperous area and the longest driving distance to the metropolitan area is approximately 2 hours. There is no local psychiatric hospital, and the general hospital has a 30-bed unit. There is a psychiatric hospital 60 miles away from the metropolis.

System 2 (Saskatchewan) is in a university city of 135,000 people with three general hospitals, two of which have psychiatric units totaling 54 beds. The total catchment area is 240,000 persons; there is a strongly community-based mental health and psychiatric program with little use of a single psychiatric hospital 80 miles away.

System 3 (Ontario) has two medium-sized towns and surrounding rural area with a catchment population of approximately 200,000. Each town has a general hospital with a psychiatric unit of respectively 21 and 18 beds; long-term psychiatric patients are sent to a large psychiatric hospital approximately 250 miles away.

System 4 (Nova Scotia) is in a metropolitan area serving a population of approximately 280,000 people, including the surrounding rural area. There were sizeable pockets of unemployment during the study. There are two psychiatric hospitals of 700 and 176 beds, respectively, as well as 80 beds in the psychiatric units of general hospitals.

As shown in Table 14.1, there has been a dramatic decrease in patient days per 1,000 population in psychiatric hospitals of provinces included in the study.[17] The study only covers adult schizophrenic patients who have received psychiatric treatment in the past 10 years, but not less than 18 months before the study was carried out. The use of strict diagnostic criteria for schizophrenia resulted in many cases being eliminated; the total final cohort was 182 patients. The information obtained from these patients is described in Table 14.2.

The report reviews a number of studies dealing with measures of patient outcomes, and notes that a patient's ability to stay out of the hospital is to be rejected as an index of success because hospitalization tends to be a function of a patient's social circumstance rather than the state of his mental health.[16] Also, the report adheres to the notion mentioned by Turner and Gartrell[18] to the effect that patients from a lower class background are more likely to become long-term patients, and that "at least for men, social class position and time spent in hospital are reliably associated." It also notes the relationship between marital status and length of hospitalization.

The report accepts the idea of Bland et al[19] who reported on a 10-year follow-up of patients in Alberta, where it was found that prognostic indi-

TABLE 14.2. Information obtained from interprovincial study of 182 patients.

Personal information	Housing and living condition	Components of treatment & care	Functional outcomes
Sex	Urban/rural	Referral source	Work performance
Age	Nature of housing	Professionals	or domestic
Marital status	Status of housing	involved in	competence
Household	Length of residence	assessment	measures
income	Status of furnishings	diagnosis	Personal care
Family	Co-residents	Length of time since	measures
members in	Status of	diagnosis	Personal
contact*	neighborhood	Mode of therapy	independence
	Crowding	Primary Therapist	measures
	Television	Treatment setting	Physical activity
	Telephone	Time in hospital	measures
	Yard	Current supervision	Socialization
	Accessibility of	Rehabilitation	measures
	stores	planning	Presence/absence of
	Accessibility of	Vocational	symptoms
	recreation	assistance	Present problems
	Transportation	Maintenance	Present satisfaction
		agency	Personal confidence
		Professionals	
		engaged in	
		maintenance	
		Resource person	
		named by patient	
		Current medication	
		levels and	
		administration	
		Patient-expressed	
		satisfaction	

*Criterion of being in contact with patient at least once a month.
Derived, with permission, from Wattie.[16]

cators failed to predict more than 25% of the outcome. It also accepts the notion described by Strauss and Carpenter[20] to the effect that "outcome is not a single process or phenomenon but is comprised of several semi-independent processes best conceptualized as open-linked systems, the major ones being social relations, employment, relief of symptoms and duration of hospitalization." Carpenter further noted that although they are interrelated, each system has its own determinants and mechanisms.[20]

Results

With respect to gender, it is noted that 54.2% of male patients and 28.8% of female patients were below the age of 30 (Table 14.3); later, the situation reversed, with 25.7% of males and 42.5% of females found over the age of 40.[16,21] Female schizophrenic patients are considerably more likely to have ever been married by a ratio of 2.5 to 1 (Table 14.4). By comparison with 55% of male patients, 79% of female patients lived in a household where other relatives lived. In general, female patients lived in situations where household incomes were higher than those of male patients. "These gender differences suggest that the female schizophrenic patient has a later age of onset and is more likely to be protected by family members, including a spouse, from poverty and poor living conditions than is the male patient."[16,21]

The main sources of referral to psychiatry were, on the one hand, the family, self and friends and, on the other hand, the general practitioner. From Systems 1 to 4, the percentages of self, family and friend referrals were, respectively, 64.7%, 40.5%, 56.3%, and 9.1%. General practitioner referrals were, respectively, 19.6%, 43.2%, 20.8%, and 59.1%. "Direct access to psychiatric care by patient and family was the major pathway to care overall and inversely related to proportion of medical referrals in the same location. As expected, the general practitioner is the major professional referrant in all systems."[16]

Across the four systems, 98.9% of cases receive chemotherapy, whereas milieu therapy and electroconvulsive therapy (ECT) are much less fashionable, although remaining constant in Systems 1 and 2.[16] The primary therapists are psychiatrists for 43.3% of patients, nurses for 40.4%, and general practitioners for 16% (in System 3 only).

Bed utilization is greater in general hospitals as opposed to psychiatric

TABLE 14.3. Percentages of male and female patients by age groups.

Count percentage	<20	20–29	30–39	40–49	50+	All ages
Male	2.75	51.38	20.18	18.35	7.3	100.00
Female	5.48	23.29	28.77	19.18	23.3	100.00
Both sexes	5.48	40.11	23.63	18.68	13.7	100.00

Derived, with permission, from Wattie.[16, 21]

TABLE 14.4. Marital status of male and female patients.

Count row percentage	Married and common-law	Ever married	Divorced/separated/ widowed	Now single	Always single	Totals
Males	18		13		78	109
	16.5%		11.9%		71.6%	100%
		31		91		
		28.4%		83.5%		
Females	37		14		22	73
	50.7%		19.2%		30.1%	100%
		51		36		
		69.9%		49.3%		
Totals	55		27		100	182
	30.2%		14.8%		54.9%	100%
		82		127		
		45.1%		69.8%		

Derived, with permission, from Wattie.[16, 21]

hospitals in all but System 4; a low rate of psychiatric bed utilization in System 2 reflects the attrition of psychiatric hospitals in the Province of Saskatchewan.

There is a wide variation in the descriptive use of rehabilitation conferences as well as in the identified names of professionals having taken part in rehabilitation conferences.[16] The psychiatrist was mentioned most often; there were wide variations by systems in the use of psychiatrists, occupational therapists, and social workers; the latter profession was rated surprisingly low, given its obvious usual involvement in discharge planning. There were intersystemic differences in vocational assistance to the patients, ranging from a proportion of 41% of the cases assisted in System 4 to 20% of cases in System 1.

System 3 makes most use of community mental health centers and there exist substantially more nursing home programs in System 2 (Table 14.5). Concerning professionals recorded as maintaining care in the community (Table 14.6), physicians dominate with 61.2%, followed by nurses with 26.8%.

There was an attempt to measure the degree of homogeneity of the systems by measuring a number of variables, such as type of agency or professional maintaining contact, level of medication, presence or absence of input by a nonpsychiatric medical specialist, and so on. Wattie notes that where health agencies and physicians are involved in post treatment contact, the patients are less likely to be medicated, are not so heavily medicated, and are more likely to take medication orally and on their own responsibility as opposed to injection by another.[16]

"A cluster effect of less functional patients being conferenced, being more often hospitalized, being seen by nonphysicians and being heavily

TABLE 14.5. Agencies maintaining on-going care.

Agency	Location 1	2	3 (%)	4	Whole group
Outpatient clinic	14.4	18.1	8.8	44.9	16.0
General practitioner	13.5	5.6	19.5	14.3	15.0
Psychiatrist's office	36.0	47.2	12.9	16.3	25.1
Total	64.0	70.8	41.2	75.5	56.1
Community mental health clinic or center	28.8	13.9	56.7	12.2	37.1
Social agency	0.0	4.2	1.0	2.0	1.4
Nursing program	0.9	11.1	0.0	0.0	2.1
Other	6.3	0.0	1.0	10.2	3.3
All agencies	100.0	100.0	100.0	100.0	100.0
Total Number Recorded	139	89	200	55	483

Derived, with permission, from Wattie.[16]
Percentages of mentions for 3 episodes.

TABLE 14.6. Professionals maintaining on-going care.

Professional	Location 1	2	3 (%)	4	Whole group	with totals by disciplines
Psychiatrist	40.0	60.8	26.1	46.2	36.8	
General practitioner	14.8	6.9	31.0	37.2	24.4	
Total physicians						61.2
Psychologist	3.2	2.0	0.6	1.3		1.5
Mental health social worker	12.3	3.9	5.8	9.0	7.4	
Community agency social worker	5.8	3.9	1.2	0.0	2.5	
Total social workers						9.9
Mental health clinic nurse	8.4	16.7	33.3	6.4	22.1	
Public health nurse	13.5	5.9	1.4	0.0	4.7	
Total nurses						26.8
Vocational counsellor	1.9	0.0	0.6	0.0		0.7
All professionals	100.0	100.0	100.0	100.0	100.0	
Total number recorded	306	89	200	55	483	

Derived, with permission, from Wattie.[16]
2 recorded, up to 3 episodes.

medicated seems to have been operating."[16] The inference from these two analyses is that "a system of care does indeed 'hang together' to form a recognizable integrated entity. This entity, 'the system,' may resemble other systems in greater or lesser degree, but is probably unique in time and place, owing something to history and sociocultural environment, something to legislation and financial support, something to particular personalities whose bent and enthusiasm may have marked local or regional practices."

Families and friends are named as the first crisis resource by a patient to the tune of 41.9% (Table 14.7). The low utilization of psychiatrists in System 2 as a crisis resource is interpreted by Wattie as a sign that these professionals do not make their patients "overdependent." In addition, patients in System 2 were the least medicated overall.

The study also reveals an association between a favorable outcome and a group of variables broadly called "accessibility variables," including such things as the use of a telephone and accessibility to transport services, shops, and recreational activities.[16] The data therefore suggest a "complex of variables" that allow one to predict a more favorable issue. They are: the patient is now, or has been married; the patient is female; and the patient has good access to the outside world. Other indicators of favorable outcome are: the patient and/or spouse rents an apartment or owns a house; the patient's sociological class background is high; the patient's income level is high; and the patient has children in regular contact.

TABLE 14.7. Professionals and others named as crisis resource by patient.

| | Location | | | | |
| | | | | | Whole group |
Professional/other	1	2	3 (%)	4	
Psychiatrist	23.6	15.0	18.9	44.0	22.5
General practitioner	13.9	5.0	12.2	4.0	10.6
Total physicians					33.1
Psychologist	1.4	0.0	0.0	0.0	0.4
Social worker	8.3	5.0	6.6	4.0	6.6
Nurse	5.5	12.5	23.5	4.0	13.7
Family/friend	41.6	62.5	32.2	44.0	41.9
Vocational Counsellor Occupational Therapist, etc	5.5	0.0	6.6	0.0	4.4
Total named	100.0	100.0	100.0	100.0	100.0
Total number recorded	72	40	90	25	227

Derived, with permission, from Wattie.[16]
Percentage of mentions.

Even though not all data and tables written by Wattie have been included in the present text, the study clearly suggests that schizophrenic patients in System 2 have had the most favorable outcome.[16] "This cannot be ascribed to independent variables originating in patient demography, socioeconomic circumstances or pathology," but seems to arise from the total system of care offered in System 2. The system variables that differentiated System 2 were: less hospitalization in total bed days; shorter individual periods in the hospital; and greater use of the general, as opposed to psychiatric, hospital. Also, in System 2 Wattie found: lower levels of current medication; more lodging in single rooms; less rehabilitation conferencing; more direct involvement by the psychiatrist throughout; and that the psychiatrist is more likely to maintain contact in the community.

Among the particular features of System 2 are the facts that psychiatrists, through a continuity of care agreement: remain responsible for patients who are readmitted; are involved in the regular monitoring of ambulatory patients; and supervise the medication. Patients also are offered better than average lodging conditions.[16] It would therefore appear that the maintenance of a close link between the patient and the psychiatrist is one of the cornerstones of the success achieved in System 2; this is a provincially supported system strongly directed toward minimizing hospital stays and maintenance of the patient in the community. However, systematic involvement of psychiatrists in terms of responsibility for the patient from the beginning to the end of the community reintegration process is one of its key aspects. Wattie also suggests that the data, according to which less functional (and less rewarding) patients may be directed from medical professionals and facilities to social workers and social agencies, should be examined at the local program level.

The Mental Health Policy of Quebec

With its 6.5 million people, the Province of Quebec is the only Canadian province to have decided to move ahead and to propose a formal mental health policy. Direct costs of mental illness account for approximately 18% of the overall health budget of the province, inclusive of mental retardation; the indirect costs are much less known.

Lifetime prevalence of serious mental health problems is 15 to 20%; the prevalence of anxiety and depression in the adult population is of the order of 12%.[22] We also know that at this point in time, 10,000 patients live in psychiatric hospitals, 5,000 live in so-called "intermediary resources," and 15,000 patients live with their families.[23]

Using a grid developed by New York State,[24] which was applied to all psychiatric inpatients in 1985, an inquiry revealed that 15% of patients in psychiatric hospitals could leave and live an autonomous life with a systematic program of support. Furthermore, an additional 30% could be transferred to a community resource, which would require a greater degree of supervision and a more systematic program of social reinsertion. It is also noted that 50% of psychiatric hospital patients with a length of stay in excess of 3 years are schizophrenics, and 23% suffer from other types of nonorganic psychoses. To a lesser extent, these problems are also found in departments of psychiatry of general hospitals where there is also a high prevalence of problems related to alcoholism as well as problems of a neurotic nature.

The Committee mandated by the Minister of Health and Social Services to draft a mental health policy[25] quickly came to the conclusion that there were four actors on the mental health scene: the person, his or her family and relatives, mental health workers and professionals, and the community.

Priority Areas to be Addressed

After listening to representatives from all four groups, our Committee came up with seven priorities that the mental health policy should address. They are[25]:

1. Difficulties in approaching the person globally, in full respect of his life trajectory and according to a biopsychosocial orientation.
2. Need to give much more importance to the potential of the person.
3. Lack of complementarity as well as inequality of access.
4. Too little importance is given to community initiatives.
5. Lack of access to services near one's living milieu; too few services in prevention and rehabilitation.
6. Lack of links between different networks and sectors.
7. Lack of efforts in training and research.

Mental Health: Operational Definition

The Committee wrote a lengthy chapter on an operational definition of "mental health," that is, one which decision makers could act upon.[25] Suffice it to say that a triaxial definition of mental illness was retained, with biological, psychodevelopmental, and environmental components. The Committee was of the opinion that the mental health of a person can be gauged according to his or her capacity to use emotions in a manner appropriate to one's actions (affective component), to establish judgments that will allow one's actions to be adapted to circumstances (cognitive component), and to interact more significantly with one's environment (relational component).

We chose to restrict the use of the word "field" of mental health to persons living in difficult mental health situations.[25] We chose to use the word "domain" of mental health to talk of largely social phenomena and other realities that have an influence on groups, and, ultimately, on the health of the population in general.

After writing a chapter on the responsibility of the State in mental health, our Committee proposed a frame of reference which has basically the following two broad objectives.[25] First, in the field of mental health, allow each person whose mental health is either disturbed, or threatened to become so, to receive a response which is adapted to his or her needs. Second, in the domain of mental health, increase efforts to foster the maintenance or the maximum development of the mental health of the whole population. We then proposed two broad principles to achieve these objectives, namely: the priority of the person and the respect to which he or she is entitled; and equity or fairness as a fundamental preoccupation of all of our actions in mental health.

Orientation to Services

The Committee then retained seven specific orientations:[25]

1. Recourse to a global approach, integrating biological, psychological, and social dimensions of the mental health of an individual in the full respect of his or her rights.
2. The needs of the person as the main criterion to determine services to be offered, insisting on the maximum development of the individual and the contribution of his milieu.
3. The development of a partnership involving the contribution of the person, the family (including significant others), as well as mental health workers and the community.
4. The promotion of a community approach that favors principally the finding of solutions close to the milieu of life of the individual and the adjustment to the specific characteristics of local communities.
5. Priority to be given to the maintenance and the reintegration in the natural milieu, keeping in mind the following requirements: the availability of a response that is adaptive, a decent quality of life, and appropriate support.
6. Development of intersectorial cooperation, that is, of all sectors that have an influence on the mental health of individuals.
7. Aiming at interventions that are of highest quality, giving preference to those whose efficacy has been proven.

Recommendations

Although the policy document aims to cover the broad area of mental health, many of the recommendations were drafted having the most seriously handicapped patients in mind, that is, schizophrenics. Broadly summarized are recommendations for the involved actors (the patient, the family, the mental health worker, and the community).[25]

For the *person* (the patient) we retained four themes. First is the sensitization of the individual and his near relatives through a provincewide campaign of information. Second is a rapid response, which has to be given through the availability of a minimum range of services available to all the population. Third, continuity and coordination appeared to be the two most important elements of an adequate follow-up of persons suffering from severe mental problems. To bring this about, the Committee recommends that there be an obligation to develop an individualized service plan for all chronically mentally ill individuals. The plan is basically a tool that should also involve the person; it needs to be flexible and the person should be able to carry it with him. Finally, the respect of rights of persons will be fostered through the creation, on a regional or provincial basis, of a function of advocacy which should be exercised by ombudspersons. The services of the ombudsperson will be available to people in institutions as well as in the community.

For the *family*, it is recommended that we do away with the notion that the family is the cause of the mental illness of one of its members.[25] Because patients often return to their family, we propose that the family be considered as a significant actor; to this effect, the family should be fully informed by mental health workers, and receive the appropriate support which should make them capable of involving themselves in the care of one of their members. A specific recommendation aims at creating rapidly a respite program for those who have to look after a severely mentally ill individual.

In support of *mental health workers,* which includes everyone that works for and with the mentally ill, the Committee recognizes that human resources are our main wealth and tool. To improve the capacity of our mental health resources, we made specific recommendations concerning training and research.

We recommend that the continuing education budgets available be increased by 30;pc per year for the next 3 years, and that the training should largely take place where the patients are, that is, in the community.[25] We also recommend that during the next 2 years, the basic curriculum of general practitioners and nurses be reviewed to increase substantially their mental health components. We recommend that 15% of the health research budget be allocated to mental health research.

With respect to the *community,* the report proposes that the "legitimacy" of community and self-help groups be officially recognized. While respecting their autonomy, the government should support groups that work for the promotion and defense of the rights of the mentally ill. Community groups that provide services to the mentally ill should be eligible to receive up to 90% of their operating budget from the government.

Organization of Services

An important chapter deals with the organization of services.[25] Because the focus of the policy is the maintenance of the chronically mentally ill as close as possible to his milieu, many of the recommendations deal with the organization of services in the community. We recommend that the budgets available to community resources be doubled initially and that the government considers granting up to 90;pc of the costs of services given by them. We later identified the minimum range of services which should be available to all citizens. They include the following: information concerning available services as well as activities in prevention; crisis intervention as well as emergency care; services of orientation and reference on a permanent basis; and adequate long- and short-term treatment. Other services that should be provided are: those in the areas of rehabilitation and social reinsertion; adequate lodging and, where needed, a respite program for families and next-of-kins, as well as the availability of psychosocial interventions; and finally, support and befriending to persons in need of services dealing with work, education and leisure.

Concerning the planning of services, we believe that it should take place at the regional level, and for the metropolitan area of Montreal this should take place at the subregional level; we also believe that the four types of actors identified should be represented in the planning process.[25] Specific recommendations are made toward internetwork cooperation within the health sector and toward intersectorial cooperation involving such different sectors as education, justice, labor, manpower, minimum wage, housing, leisure, and municipal affairs.

There is an important chapter on deinstitutionalization, and criteria, or requirements, for successful deinstitutionalization are identified. They are the following four[24]: (1) crisis intervention 24 hours a day, (2) appropriate medication when required, (3) intervention with significant others, and (4) continuity in service availability.

After having said that deinstitutionalization should not have reducing costs as a primary objective, our Committee recommended that special efforts be made to identify the social impact as well as the economic impact of deinstitutionalization on the milieu.[25]

The report ends by regrouping all recommendations into a plan of action which is scaled over three phases, which might take approximately five years.[24] The policy document has been widely debated in the media, as well as on the occasion of a parliamentary commission which was held for two and a half weeks in Quebec's National Assembly.

Conclusions

It is our belief that the mere fact of being able to bring about a public debate on mental health is in itself a major step toward the necessary mobilization of the various actors toward the reaching of common goals. The very fact that the government is interested and is going forward toward the formulation of a systematic policy means that it is firmly committed to reaching these goals and to making available the necessary means that will be required, both financial and administrative.

It is also interesting to note that this mental health policy is formulated in the absence of an overall health policy. It is believed by most observers that the government will want, sooner or later, to bring about a formal overall health policy, and that the then existing mental health policy will be one of its key components.

Summary

Distinctive features of the health care system in Canada include, generally, a single-tier system of care based on a universal health care insurance plan. The primary responsibility of health care rests with the 10 Canadian provinces who contribute 60% of the cost of hospitalization and medical care (including psychiatric treatment), whereas the Federal contribution amounts to approximately 40%. However, with respect to hospitalization in psychiatry, the Federal contribution only applies to general hospitals and excludes mental hospitals, which must be paid for totally by the provinces. This creates a disparity between the levels of care offered in the two types of hospitals.

In a review of results of a four-province follow-up study of adult schizophrenics, a positive outcome was reflected by less hospitalizations, shorter hospitalizations, more hospitalizations in a general *vs* a psychiatric hospital, and less use of medication. Where health agencies and physicians were more involved, less medication was used and most of that was prescribed orally. Favorable outcome variables were marriage, children, adequate housing and income, and being female, as well as accessibility of telephones, shopping, and transportation. Independent of other variables, those patients who were followed by psychiatrists, who remained continuously involved throughout hospitalization as well as in ambulatory care, showed a better outcome.

Quebec is the only province in Canada with a formal mental health policy. In this policy, there are four designated actors: the patient, the family, the mental health worker, and the community. Seven mental health priorities have been delineated and include the need for: a global approach to the person along biopsychosocial lines; more attention to recognizing the potential of the person; reducing inequality of access to care; creating community initiatives; accessibility to services; community linkages; and emphasis on training and research.

The policy stresses that the priority of the person's needs, not those of the system, should be primary. The family should not be scapegoated and should be a significant part of the rehabilitation for which the family needs information and support as well as respite programs. For mental health professionals, the recommendations involve an increase in continuing education budgets by 30% with this training taking place in the community. Mental health research should receive 15% of the health research budget. Finally, the minimum range of services that should be available are information, crisis intervention, maintenance, long- and short-term treatment, rehabilitation, lodging and respite care along with psychosocial intervention, and befriending for work, support and recreation.

References

1. Statistics Canada: *Mental Health Statistics, vol. 1. Institutional admissions and separations* 1978 (1981).
2. Statistics Canada: *Mental Health Statistics, vol. II. Patients on books of institutions* 1976 (1979).
3. Bland RC: Long-term mental illness in Canada: an epidemiological perspective on schizophrenia and affective disorders. *Can J Psychiatry* 1984;29:242–246.
4. World Health Organization: *Schizophrenia. An International Follow-up Study.* New York, John Wiley & Sons, 1979.
5. Bland RC, Orn H: 14-year outcome in early schizophrenia. *Acta Psychiatr Scand* 1978;58:327–338.
6. Epp J: *Achieving Health for All: A Framework for Health Promotion, by the Minister of National Health and Welfare,* Canada, Health and Welfare, 1986, p 13.
7. Discussion Paper on Mental Health Policy, Working Group on Mental Health Policy, Health Services and Promotion Branch, Health and Welfare Canada, Draft, October 9, 1987.
8. Minister of Supply and Services Canada: Mental health for Canadians: striking a balance. Cat H39-128/1988E, ISBN 0-662-16347-8.
9. Castel R: La psychiatrie dans notre societe. *L'Evolution Psychiatrique* 1984;49(3):719–730.
10. Doyle M: Some French findings. *Nursing Mirror* 1981;153(9):29–30.
11. Lebovici S: La readaptation des malades mentaux: nouvelles structures et sectorisation. *Readaptation* 1979;261:7–10.
12. World Health Organization: *Health legislation: European Program.* Copenhagen, WHO Regional Office for Europe, 1981.
13. Leighton A: *Caring for the Mentally Ill People.* Cambridge, Cambridge University Press, 1982, pp 134–156.
14. Harnois GP: Challenges to the reintegration of the mentally ill in Quebec, Canada. *Int J Mental Health* 1987;15(4):6–15.
15. Cooper B: Social class and prognosis in schizophrenia. *Br J Prevent Soc Med* 1961;125:17–30.
16. Wattie BJS: *Follow-up of Study of Schizophrenic Patients in Four Canadian Provincial Locations,* Canada, Health and Welfare February 1985.
17. Statistics Canada: *Mental Health Statistics, vol III.* Catalogue 83-205, 1960, 1965, 1970-75, 1978-79.
18. Turner RJ, Gartrell JW: Social factors in psychiatric outcome: toward the resolution of interpretive controversies. *Am Sociol Rev* 1978;43:368–382.

19. Bland RC, Parker JH, Orn H: Prognosis in schizophrenia: prognostic predictors and outcome. *Arch Gen Psychiatry* 1976;33:949–954.
20. Strauss JS, Carpenter WT: The prediction of outcome in schizophrenia. *Arch Gen Psychiatry* 1972;27:729–746.
21. Wattie BJS, Kedward HB: Gender differences in living conditions found among male and female schizophrenic patients on a follow-up study. *Int J Soc Psychiatry* 1985; 31: 205–216.
22. Murphy JM, Leighton AH: Control and Prevention of Depression and Anxiety in a General Population: A Position Statement. Prepared for the Comite de la politique de sante mentale du Quebec, at the request of its President, Dr. Gaston P. Harnois. November 14, 1986, p 12.
23. Roberge P: La clientele psychiatrique vue a travers le Locs: quelques elements de description critique. Ministere de la Sante et des Services sociaux, 1986, 50 pages.
24. Bureau of Programme Evaluation: *Level of Care Survey*. Albany, NY, Office of Mental Health, 1982.
25. Pour Un Partenariat Elargi: Projet de Politique de Sante Mentale Pour le Quebec. Prepared by the Comite de la politique de sante mentale, presided by Dr. Gaston P. Harnois. October 1987, p 185.

15
Psychiatric Reform in Italy: Implications for the Treatment of Long-Term Schizophrenic Patients

MICHELE TANSELLA

Models of Community Psychiatry: Complementary or Alternative Community Services

In the past 2 decades mental health care has seen a gradual move from hospital to community care. More patients are now being treated, whenever possible, in ambulatory facilities rather than in remote bedcare institutions. However, this shift is proceeding at different speeds in various countries. In some of them the process appears to be slow, involving mainly nonpsychotic patients.

It has been noted that where a *complementary* model of community care is adopted new outpatient and community services are being added to the old, hospital-based system of care instead of replacing it.[1] According to this model the new services provide secondary or supplementary care to that provided by the hospital, which remains in a first-rank position within the system, and obviously a reduction in the use of hospitalization is not a common outcome. On the contrary, case register studies have demonstrated that an extension of community services made according to this organizational model leads to an *increase* in the number of admissions,[2] particularly for elderly people,[3] or to "a shift in the focus of attention toward a different and much less severely disturbed category of patients"[2] (p 30).

A rather different model has been introduced in Italy by the 1978 psychiatric reform.[4,5] The Italian legislation has been defined as "the most comprehensive community-oriented Mental Health Act in the Western industrialized world."[6] Its major provisions have been reported elsewhere.[7]

One of the distinctive features of the Italian model of community psychiatry is that community services are considered and planned as *alternatives* to the old system of care. These services, each designed for a catchment area of about 100,000 to 150,000 inhabitants, are public and are part of the National Health Service (NHS) introduced in Italy in 1978. They include outpatient facilities, day and residential training centres, and residential accommodations in hostels and sheltered workshops as well as inpatient units in general hospitals. Old long-term patients continue to be treated in mental hospitals, whose front doors have been closed without encouraging an abrupt increase in the trend of deinstitutionalization, which started in Italy in 1963.[7] The number of patients in mental hospitals, however, is progressively decreasing.

In the Italian model great emphasis is placed on ensuring that these alternative community services provide early diagnosis, prompt treatment, continuity of care, and long-term support for both the patients and their families, as well as on ensuring an integration between the various facilities and services within the geographically based system of care. Hospital psychiatry is considered to complement community care and not vice versa (the so-called "community priority"). The distinctive features of the Italian model of community care are summarized in Table 15.1.

It is worthwhile noting that in Italy the phasing out of the mental hospital is being achieved gradually, initially through a block on first admissions (since May 1978) and subsequently on all admissions (since January 1982). The reform aims at *preventing* the institutionalization of new patients, rather than speeding up the process of deinstitutionalization. It is therefore a very different model from the American community mental health experience, where an abrupt deinstitutionalization occurred.[8] Mechanic and Aiken[9] argued that Community Mental Health Centers in the United States have failed to meet the needs of the chronically ill, by serving instead large numbers of new patients with less severe problems. The Italian model, however, stresses the importance of providing care and support to all groups of patients in the at-risk population, establishing a close liaison with other medical and social community services, particularly with general practitioners.[10] Special attention is therefore given to new long-term patients treated in the community; the aim of care provided for them is to reverse the long accepted practice of isolating them in large institutions and to promote their integration in the community,

---

TABLE 15.1. Distinctive features of the Italian model of community psychiatry.

1. The phasing out of mental hospitals is intended to be a gradual process (by means of a block on admissions rather than an abrupt deinstitutionalization of chronic patients).
2. New services are designed to be alternative, rather than complementary or additional to mental hospitals.
3. It is hospital psychiatry which is considered complementary to community care, and not vice versa.
4. Integration is intended between the various facilities within the geographically based system of care, the same team providing domiciliary, outpatient and inpatient care. This approach facilitates continuity of care and long-term support.
5. There is special emphasis on multidisciplinary teamwork, domiciliary visits, and crisis intervention, and on easy access to the community mental health centers.

Reprinted with permission from Tansella and Zimmerman-Tansella.[1]

offering them an environment that is socially stimulating, while avoiding their exposure to great social pressures. On the other hand, the old long-term patients who are discharged from state hospitals according to rehabilitation programmes agreed on by the community services team, remain under the responsibility of the public, geographically based community service. This service is an integrated and comprehensive system of care also able to provide short spells of inpatient treatment in general hospital psychiatric units when necessary.

Implementation of the Italian Reform: Some Quantitative Evidence

National statistics and local register data have been used to provide quantitative evidence of the implementation of the Italian reform.[7] The available data show that there is a marked regional variation in service provision (with compliance, innovation, and well-structured community services in Northern and Central Italy and little or no reform in psychiatric services in Southern Italy), as well as a globally inadequate provision of alternative structures. The reasons for such a variable picture are social as well as political and reflect long-lasting differences in the tradition and background of the provision of psychiatric care in North-Central Italy as compared with the developing South. Thus, the North/South differences reported in the provision of psychiatric as well as of other health services are but a further aspect of one of the most crucial and difficult political/economic issues in Italy this century. Nevertheless, the evidence suggests that, where adequate community psychiatric services have been set up, they function successfully, providing comprehensive care for all types of psychiatric patients living in a delimited area, without backup from the state mental hospital.

The national suicide rate in Italy had risen since 1978,[11] a feature common to all European countries except Greece and the United Kingdom.[12] The analysis of regional data showed no evidence that the closure of mental hospital beds was related to the suicide rate, although the provision of general hospital psychiatric beds was negatively correlated with the pre-postreform change in the trend in the suicide rate; that is, regions that are well provided for (in terms of such beds) are also regions in which there has been a postreform decrease, or less of an increase, in the suicide rate.[11,13]

To explain the globally inadequate provision of alternative structures, it is worthwhile mentioning that the available data show that, paradoxically, in Italy the bulk of the resources devoted to psychiatric care (expenditure as well as personnel, especially psychiatric nurses) continue to be expended on state and private mental hospitals, even though these institutions provide care for a contracting population of patients.[7] This appears to be the price paid in the transitory phase of the process of moving from a hospital-based to a community-based system of care. While we need to build up rapidly the new system (the community services), we still have to support the old one (the mental hospitals with the old long-term patients still residing there).

Treating Patients With Schizophrenic Psychosis in an Area With a Community-Based System of Care

The South-Verona Experience

The Institute of Psychiatry of the University of Verona (in a city of 260,000 inhabitants located in Northern Italy) since 1978 has developed a community-based system of care, the South-Verona Community Psychiatric Service (CPS). This is a well-integrated, comprehensive service, which comprises various facilities including: a general hospital inpatient unit (15 beds), outpatient services, a mental health centre providing day-care and rehabilitation programmes, unstaffed apartments, and a supervised hostel (8 beds) for long-term patients. The CPS is responsible for providing psychiatric care to the residents in South-Verona, an area of 75,000 inhabitants that includes part of the city of Verona and three small neighbouring communities. Our model of care stresses multidisciplinary teamwork, extensive home support and home visiting, long-term continuous care, and social support. Normalization and patient autonomy are predominant goals of the South-Verona CPS. Great attention is also paid to reviewing patients in community care at regular intervals in ad hoc meetings, in which all the professionals of the district team take an active part. The structure of the service and the style of working has been described in detail elsewhere.[1,14]

The South-Verona area has been monitored since January 1979 by a Psychiatric Case Register (PCR)[15] and by an epidemiological/evaluative research team. The case register collects information from all public and private psychiatric units and services of the Province of Verona. Contacts with psychiatrists, psychologists, psychiatric nurses, and social workers are included. General practitioners, psychiatrists, and psychologists in private practice do not report data to the register. In the South-Verona PCR diagnoses are recorded according to an 11-fold classification system, giving collapsed ICD-9 categories. One of these categories includes schizophrenia and other nonaffective functional psychoses.

The aim of the following description is to summarize the results of studies conducted on patients with a diagnosis of schizophrenic psychosis, that is, a group of patients with a high risk of undergoing long-term treatment.

Descriptive Statistics

Figure 15.1 shows annual prevalence figures of schizophrenia and related disorders in South-Verona from 1979 to 1986. These figures, which show a small increasing trend in recent years, are lower than those reported in other case register areas (Table 15.2). The reasons for such differences are still unknown. Possible explanations are: first, the sociodemographic characteristics of South-Verona, an integrated area of a relatively small town (it is well-known that schizophrenia is more common in certain central districts of large towns and in socially isolated areas); and second, the low rates of long stay among patients existing in our area as a consequence of the process of deinstitutionalization which occurred in the last 2 decades.

The hypothesis that the low rates of schizophrenic disorders found in South-Verona as compared with other European case register areas may be due to different diagnostic criteria is not supported by the results of two studies recently completed in our unit. In the first study 103 cases were randomly selected from the Groningen (The Netherlands), Nottingham (UK) and South-Verona registers, and six raters were involved in coding these cases according to ICD-9. A substantial interrater reliability was found in the step of coding diagnostic descriptions according to ICD as well as in the step of grouping these codes in broad diagnostic categories.[16] In the second study three psychiatrists (two from South-Verona and one from Aarhus, Denmark) independently completed the Present State Examination (PSE) syndrome checklist for a consecutive series of patients admitted to our hospital unit on the basis of information from clinical records. Again the results showed a satisfactory interrater agreement (Mignolli et al, in preparation). For a recent review on the prevalence studies of schizophrenia published since 1948 see Torrey.[17]

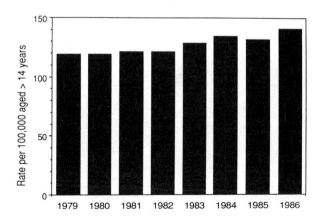

FIGURE 15.1. Prevalence of schizophrenic psychoses in South-Verona, 1979 to 1986. Rates per 100,000 adult population.

TABLE 15.2. Annual prevalence of schizophrenic psychoses (in case register areas).

Area	Rate per 10,000	Year
South-Verona (I)	13	1982–1986
Portogruaro (I)	25	1982–1986
Camberwell (UK)	34	1965
Mannheim (FRG)	23	1974–1980
Rochester (USA)	47	1980

Table 15.3 shows that incidence rates (first ever contacts) for schizophrenic and related disorders in South-Verona are similar to those reported in English case register areas and lower than those found in Germany and in the United States. The possible reasons for these differences between Europe and the United States have been discussed by Häfner and an der Heiden.[18] They stressed the importance of differences in diagnostic criteria and predicted that in the United States, after the introduction of DSM-III which uses a more narrow definition of schizophrenia as compared with ICD-9, the incidence rates and subsequently the prevalence rates of schizophrenia will decrease. Murphy[19] also discussed extensively the topic of variation between different people in the prevalence and incidence of schizophrenia.

One of the aims of the Italian psychiatric reform is to avoid, as much as possible, unnecessary hospitalization. Figure 15.2 shows that most of the South-Verona patients are treated outside the hospital only (Not IP). This consistently applies, in most recent years, also to patients with diagnoses of schizophrenic psychosis, probably in relation to the increasing community orientation of our programme.

Figure 15.3 shows that in South-Verona rates of long-stay inpatients (ie, those who remain in the hospital for 365 days or longer) are decreasing. However, rates of long-term patients outside the mental hospital (ie, those in continuous psychiatric care for 1 year, receiving treatment in the community by the various outpatient and day-patient facilities and in

TABLE 15.3. Annual incidence of schizophrenic psychoses (first-ever patients in case register areas).

Area	Rate per 10,000	Year
South-Verona (I)	1.0	1982–1986
Portogruaro (I)	2.5	1986
Camberwell (UK)	1.3	1971
Salford (UK)	1.1	1971
Mannheim (FRG)	5.9	1974–1980
Rochester (USA)	6.9	1970

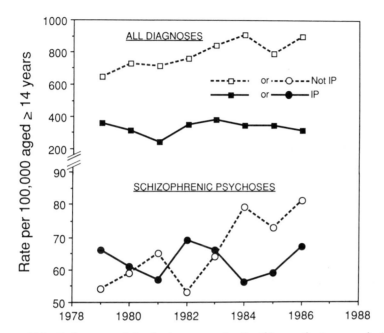

FIGURE 15.2. Patients receiving in the year outpatient/day-patient care only (*Not IP*) or both inpatient care and day/outpatient care or inpatient care only (*IP*). Patients in hospital on census day have been classified as IP. Rates per 100,000 adult population.

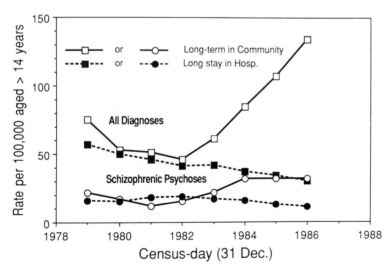

FIGURE 15.3. Patients who have been continuously in the hospital in the previous 365 days (long stay in hospital) and patients in continuous care in the previous 365 days, receiving treatment in the community by the various outpatient and day-patient facilities and in some cases short spells of inpatient care (long-term in the community). Continuous care means no breaks between psychiatric contacts of more than 90 days.

some cases short spells of inpatient care, without a break between contacts of more than 90 days) show an increasing trend. This means that the South-Verona CPS, the main psychiatric agency for South-Verona residents, is progressively taking over the functions previously undertaken by the mental hospital. It is now taking care of most psychiatric patients who before the reform would have been admitted to the mental hospital with a high risk of becoming long-term.

The clinical and social implications of the buildup of long-term patients in the community instead of long-stay inpatients in mental hospitals need to be considered. The hypothesis suggested by the results of a recent case register study[20] is that long-term community care by the South-Verona CPS is inducing to a lesser extent dependence on the services and chronicity of their use, as compared with the old hospital-centered system of care. This hypothesis needs to be confirmed by further longitudinal studies, using appropriate outcome measures.[10]

A Follow-up Study of Patients With a Diagnosis of Schizophrenic Psychosis

A survey of a cohort of all South-Verona patients with a diagnosis of schizophrenic psychosis (60 patients) who contacted the psychiatric services in 1979 (after the implementation of the psychiatric reform) was conducted 7 years later. Fifty-seven patients (93%) were traced and all those still alive ($N = 46$) were interviewed using Present State Examination (PSE-9), Disability Assessment Schedule (DAS-2), Social Skills and Psychological Impairments Rating Schedule (SS-PIRS), and other standardized instruments.

The results of this study will be reported in detail elsewhere (Mignolli et al, in preparation). In summary, they show that, when examining the whole sample, more than 50% of patients showed no change in clinical symptoms as well as in social performance. Moreover, 37% of patients improved in clinical symptomatology (and 9% got worse), whereas, as far as social performance is concerned, the corresponding figures were 20 and 24%. However, analysing separately the mental hospital subgroup ($N = 9$) (ie, those patients who have been long-stay in the state hospital through the 7-year study period) and the patients treated in the community ($N = 37$), a different picture emerges. From Figure 15.4 it may be seen that, in the mental hospital patients, clinical symptomatology remained unchanged (100% of cases), whereas social performance showed no change or a worsening. On the other hand, when considering the patients treated during the 7 years in the community, it may be seen that 50% of them showed an improvement in clinical symptoms (and 43% no change), and 24% of them showed an improvement in social performance (but 57% of them showed no change and 19% worsened).

On the same cohort of interviewed schizophrenic patients a parallel study was conducted to assess the needs for care. A standardized proce-

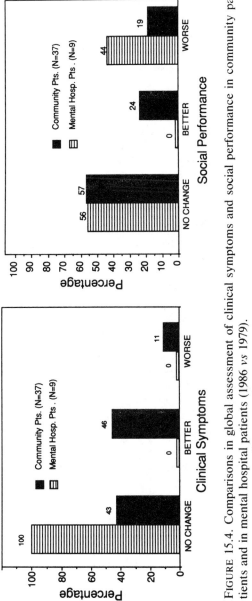

FIGURE 15.4. Comparisons in global assessment of clinical symptoms and social performance in community patients and in mental hospital patients (1986 vs 1979).

dure recently developed by Brewin et al[21] was used, the Need for Care Assessment Schedule (NFCAS), which covers 20 areas of clinical and social functioning and in each of these specifies appropriate interventions. Decision rules permit problems in functioning to be primarily classified as a met need, an unmet need, or as involving no needs, and allows the identification of various secondary needs. It was found that the South-Verona CPS was meeting the needs for care of its patients. The patients in contact with other services or with private practitioners were presenting few problems, particularly in the area of living skills, but they were more at risk of being rated under unmet needs. The patients out of contact with any psychiatric service were presenting the lowest number of problems and abandonment was not found among them. No patients were found in prison. On the other hand, the few long-stay inpatients still living in the mental hospital were poorly treated, with problems of institutionalization often encountered. Action to improve the conditions in the mental hospital was rated as unlikely to be undertaken (Lesage et al, in preparation).

This was a descriptive follow-up, not an experimental study with random assignment of patients to one of the two groups (community vs mental hospital treatment), so we cannot draw clearcut conclusions about the superiority of our alternative treatment programme over traditional hospital-based treatment. However, we have to consider that if we re-open the front doors of our mental hospitals those patients now treated by the community services who eventually enter these hospitals will be at risk of sharing the very poor outcome showed by the mental hospital patients. The risk of mortality of the above-mentioned cohort of schizophrenic patients also was assessed using three methods: case control with nonpsychotic patients and general population (matched for sex and age); indirect standardization using mortality tables; and indirect standardization with survival tables according to Sturt.[22] All methods yielded an excess mortality, that is, about the two-fold increase described in other studies. Moreover, the findings do not support the view that excess mortality in South-Verona schizophrenic patients is linked to suicide, but rather to natural causes (Lesage et al, in preparation.)

Is the Community-Based System More Suitable Than the Hospital-Based System of Care?

Kiesler and Sibulkin[23] recently reviewed 14 experimental studies, most of them with random allocations of patients, showing that community alternatives were more effective than hospitalization across a wide range of patient populations and treatment strategies. The Italian model of community care has distinctive features of "community priority" and a strong emphasis on integration, continuity, and social support. This model is based on the assumption that a comprehensive community service with a full range of facilities, including a few beds in the general hospital, is more effective than the traditional hospital-based psychiatric service. The reasons for the superiority of the community-based model may be outlined as follows: effective treatment of mental illness, especially of most severe forms, "involves not only the removal of florid symptoms of the disorder, but complete restoration of the social functioning of the patient"[24] (p 59) and also limiting of social impairments. Wing,[25] referring to schizophrenia, has defined four sources of social impairment: (1) the acute syndromes, which consist of florid symptoms; (2) the chronic syndromes, with withdrawal, slowness and underactivity; (3) secondary handicaps, which are not part of the disease process itself but include the attitudes, expectancy, and behavioural changes that hinder adequate community functioning; and (4) extrinsic disadvantages, that is, premorbid characteristics, such as lack of vocational competence, poor social supports, and low social skills.

Standard hospital treatment, especially that provided in large mental hospitals, which is mainly based on pharmacotherapy, in most cases has beneficial effects on only the first source of social impairment (improving social functioning through the reduction of acute symptoms[26]). Generally, it does not improve the chronic symptoms. On the contrary, it should be mentioned that an increasing severity of "negative symptoms" due to drugs often has been described.[27,28] On the other hand, effective community care, when provided by comprehensive, integrated, and responsible services, has beneficial effects not only on the first two but also on the third and fourth source of social impairment. Outside the hospital, in the "real world," it is possible to provide a more natural supportive interpersonal environment that promotes learning and practice of social and vocational skills.[29]

One question remains to be answered: what are the implications of the Italian experience for the organization of psychiatric care elsewhere? This topic has been discussed in an editorial by Williams and myself recently published in *Psychological Medicine*.[30]

First, the Italian experience confirms that the transition from a service that is predominantly hospital-based to one that is predominantly extramural cannot adequately be accomplished simply by closing mental hospitals. It is clear that appropriate alternative structures must be provided, and this requires adequate time for planning and implementation.

Second, commitment is necessary from the individuals running the service, as well from politicians and administrators. As stated in an editorial of the *British Medical Journal*, "Community care is not—and never will be—a cheap solution. Indeed, if it is to be effective, investment will have to be made in buildings, staff, and backup facilities."[31]

Third, monitoring and evaluation are important aspects of change; planning and evaluation should go hand in hand, and evaluation should, wherever possible, have an epidemiological basis.[32]

Finally, it should be noted that countries in which there exists a functioning and well-developed system of primary medical care are at a distinct advantage with regard to the provision of community psychiatric care.[30]

One point to be stressed here is that the Italian experience has to be considered in context, taking into account its social, cultural, and political background. It would be too simplistic to consider that the Italian model can be exported as such elsewhere or simply can be copied. There is in many countries a general trend of increasing community psychiatric care. However, each region and each country has to find its own way. Only the past can be copied, the future must be created.

Summary

In the past 2 decades mental health care has gradually shifted from hospital to community care. In a complementary model of community care new outpatient and community services are added to the existing hospital-based system of care.

Since the psychiatric reform of 1978 in Italy, a different model has been introduced in which new community services are developed as alternatives and hospital services are complementary to community care rather than vice versa—the "community priority." The goal has been an integration of care in outpatient facilities, day and residential training centres, residential accommodations in hostels, and sheltered workshops as well as inpatient units in general hospitals. Previous long-stay patients continue to be treated in mental hospitals, whose front doors have been closed without encouraging abrupt deinstitutionalization.

The South-Verona experience in treating patients with schizophrenic psychosis is an illustration of the "community priority." In South-Verona, an area of 75,000 inhabitants, a well-integrated, comprehensive service stressing multidisciplinary teamwork, extensive home support and home visiting, long-term continuous care, and social support began in July 1978. The area has been monitored since January 1979 by a psychiatric case register according to ICD-9 and by an epidemiological research team. The prevalence figures for schizophrenia and related disorders have been stable, 130 per 100,000 population. This is a low rate compared with other European towns or the United States using pre-DSM-III rates and was not found to be due to different diagnostic criteria. Since 1982 the numbers of long-term patients in the community are increasing, while rates of long-stay inpatients are decreasing. A 7-year follow-up study was done in 1986 for 60 patients with schizophrenia and related psychoses who originally contacted the psychiatric services in 1979 after the implementation of psychiatric reform. Results showed that patients treated with community alternatives fared much better than those in long-term hospital care. Their needs can be defined in two broad areas, clinical needs and living skills needs.

The community-based model is superior to hospital-based services because it is more effective in treating all four sources of social impairment including: (1) treatment of the acute syndromes or positive symptoms (hallucinations, delusions, and thought interference); (2) treatment of the chronic syndromes (withdrawal, slowness, and underactivity); (3) prevention or minimization of secondary handicaps (attitudes and behaviour preventing effective community functioning); and (4) correction of extrinsic disadvantages (inadequate social skills and lack of work).

The implications of the Italian experience must be considered in its own unique social context. Each region or country needs to develop its own unique plan; "only the past can be copied, the future must be created."

Acknowledgments: This study was supported by the Consiglio Nazionale delle Ricerche (CNR, Roma), Progetto Finalizzato Medicina Preventiva e Riabilitativa, Contracts no. 86.01962.56 and no. 87.00467.56, and by the Regione Veneto, Ricerca Sanitaria Finalizzata, Contract no. 134.03.86.

References

1. Tansella M, Zimmermann-Tansella CH: From mental hospitals to alternative community services, in Howells JG (ed): *Modern Perspectives in Clinical Psychiatry*. New York, Brunner-Mazel, 1988, pp 130–148.
2. Giel R: Care of chronic mental patients in The Netherlands. *Soc Psychiatry* 1986;21:25–32.
3. Fryers T, Wooff K: Il controllo dei servizi di salute mentale in una città inglese, in Tansella M (ed): *L'Approccio Epidemiologico in Psichiatria*. Torino, Boringhieri, 1985, pp 169–199.
4. Tranchina P, Archi G, Ferrara M: The new legislation in Italian psychiatry: an advanced law originating from alternative practice. *Int J Law Psychiatry* 1981;4:181–190.
5. Tansella M: Community psychiatry without mental hospitals. The Italian experience: a review. *J Royal Soc Med* 1986;79:664–669.
6. Mosher L: Italy's revolutionary mental health law: an assessment. *Am J Psychiatry* 1982;139:199–203.
7. Tansella M, De Salvia D, Williams P: The Italian psychiatric reform: some quantitative evidence. *Soc Psychiatry* 1987;22:37–48.
8. Mosher L: Radical deinstitutionalization: the Italian experience. *Int J Mental Health* 1983;11:129–136.
9. Mechanic D, Aiken LA: Improving the care of patients with chronic mental illness. *N Engl J Med* 1987;317:1634–1638.
10. Tansella M: Evaluating community psychiatric services, in Williams P, Wilkinson G, Rawnsley K (eds): *The Scope of Epidemiological Psychiatry*. London, Tavistock Publications, 1989, pp 386–403.

11. Williams P, De Salvia D, Tansella M: Suicide, psychiatric reform, and the provision of psychiatric services in Italy. *Soc Psychiatry* 1986;21:89–95.

12. World Health Organization: *Changing Patterns in Suicide Behavior*. Euro Report n. 74. Copenhagen, WHO Regional Office for Europe, 1982.

13. Williams P, De Salvia D, Tansella M: Suicide and the Italian psychiatric reform. An appraisal of two data collection systems. *Eur Arch Psychiatry Neurol Sci* 1987;236:237–240.

14. Burti L, Garzotto N, Siciliani O, et al: South-Verona's psychiatric service: an integrated system of community care. *Hosp Comm Psychiatry* 1986;37:809–813.

15. Tansella M, Faccincani C, Mignolli G, et al: Il registro psichiatrico di Verona-Sud. Epidemiologia per la valutazione dei nuovi servizi territoriali, in Tansella M (ed): *L 'Approccio Epidemiologico in Psichiatria*. Torino, Boringhieri, 1985, pp 225–259.

16. Sytema S, Giel R, ten Horn GHMM, et al: The reliability of diagnostic coding in psychiatric case registers. An interrater agreement study of the Nottingham, South-Verona, and Groningen PCRs. *Psychol Med* 1989 in press.

17. Torrey EF: Prevalence studies in schizophrenia. *Br J Psychiatry* 1987;150:598–608.

18. Häfner H, an der Heiden W: Registri psichiatrici e schizofrenia, in Tansella M (ed): *L 'Approccio Epidemiologico in Psichiatria*. Torino, Boringhieri, 1985, pp 260–299.

19. Murphy HBM: *Comparative Psychiatry. The International and Intercultural Distribution of Mental Illness*. Berlin, Springer-Verlag, 1982.

20. Balestrieri M, Micciolo R, Tansella M: Long-stay and long-term psychiatric patients in an area with a community-based system of care. A register follow-up study. *Int J Soc Psychiatry* 1987;33:251–263.

21. Brewin CR, Wing JK, Mangen SP, et al: Principles and practice of measuring needs in the long-term mentally ill: the MRC Needs for Care Assessment. *Psychol Med* 1987;17:971–981.

22. Sturt E: Mortality in a cohort of long-term users of community psychiatric services. *Psychol Med* 1983;13:441–446.

23. Kiesler CA, Sibulkin AE: *Mental Hospitalization: Myths and Facts about a National Crisis*. Newbury Park, California, Sage, 1987.

24. Falloon IRH, McGill ChW, Boyd JL, et al: Family management in the prevention of morbidity of schizophrenia: social outcome of two-year longitudinal study. *Psychol Med* 1987;17:59–66.

25. Wing JK: Social influence on the course of schizophrenia, in Wynne LC, Cromwell RL, Mahysse S (eds): *The Nature of Schizophrenia*. New York, John Wiley, 1978.

26. Falloon IRH, Watt DC, Shepherd M: The social outcome of patients in a trial of long-term continuation therapy in schizophrenia: pimozide *vs* fluphenazine. *Psychol Med* 1978;8:265–274.

27. Andrews WN: Long-acting tranquilizers and the amotivational syndrome in the treatment of schizophrenia, in King MH (ed): *Community Management of the Schizophrenic in Clinical Remission*. Amsterdam, Excerpta Medica, 1973, pp 1–4.

28. Van Putten T, May PRA: Subjective response as a predictor of outcome in pharmacotherapy. *Arch Gen Psychiatry* 1978;35:477–480.

29. Jacobs H, Donatroe P, Falloon IRH: Rehabilitation of the chronic schizophrenic, in Backer T, Pan L, Vash CL (eds): *Annual Review of Rehabilitation, 1983*. Berlin, Springer-Verlag, 1985, pp 83–113.
30. Tansella M, Williams P: The Italian experience and its implications. *Psychol Med* 1987;17:283–289.
31. British Medical Journal: Editorial: community care. *Br Med J* 1985;290:806.
32. Wing JK: The cycle of planning and evaluation, in Wilkinson G, Freeman H (eds): *Mental Health Services in Britain: the Way Forward*. London, Gaskell Books, 1986.

16
Mental Health Services and New Research in England: Implications for the Community Management of Schizophrenia

Nicholas Tarrier and Christine Barrowclough

The implications of recent research developments into the management of schizophrenia in Salford need to be placed in the context of the health and psychiatric services that exist within Great Britain. To achieve this, a short account of the British National Health Service (NHS) and of the role of the mental health services within the NHS, especially relating to community care policy, is given, with special reference to the Salford District Health Authority.

Mental Health Services in Great Britain

The National Health Service

The National Health Service Bill was published in March 1946 and received Royal Assent and became an Act of Parliament in November of the same year. The service itself began on July 5, 1948. The NHS, as created by the act of 1946, is a comprehensive service covering all forms of medical care which are freely available to all. It is funded from the general exchequer (ie, national taxes), and it is independent of insurance schemes or social security system.[1] The NHS is in effect part of a tripartite system of: (1) hospital and specialist services, (2) general practitioner services (who act as "independent contractors"), and (3) local authority services (funded and administered by local government).[1]

Community Care

Although there have been organisational, and more recently managerial changes, the NHS, including the mental health services, have largely continued in the spirit of the 1946 act. Especially pertinent for the care of the long-term mentally ill and for the development of innovation is the policy of care in the community as opposed to institutional hospital care. Community care began piecemeal in the 1950s and became increasingly embodied in official policy documents. For example, the 1959 Mental Health

Act emphasised the need to develop community-based care for mentally ill people. This policy has been restated and enlarged upon in subsequent documents, including Priorities for Health and Personal Social Services in England (1976), Care in the Community (1981), and Care in Action (1981). All these documents encourage Health Authorities to deemphasize large long-stay psychiatric institutions and develop smaller locally based services to meet the individual needs of mentally ill people.[2] The 1985 Parliamentary Social Services Committee's report on community care stated that services should be local, flexible, comprehensive, integrated, relevant, multidisciplinary, sensitive, and accessible. Community care, in the words of the then Secretary of State for the Department of Health and Social Services, Lord Glenarthur, ". . . means building up alternatives to care in the long-stay hospitals, providing care for people already in the community, and preventing unnecessary admissions to hospital."[3] However, even with extensive community mental health facilities, it is likely that family, friends, and neighbors will bear the brunt of caring in the community, and this situation may indeed be part of policy recommendations as suggested by the government-commissioned Griffiths report on community care.[4]

Salford District Health Authority: Mental Health Services

Acute Mental Health Services

England and Wales are divided into 15 Regional Health Authorities, which are further divided into 203 District Health Authorities. Salford District Health Authority is within the North West Regional Health Authority and has a catchment population of 244,000.[5] Salford is by many standards a deprived city; the rates of unemployment and permanent sickness are above the national average, and the population is highly dependent on local authority housing (47% of households live in council-owned property) mainly in the inner city area.

The mental health services have available four acute admission wards, one located at the district general hospital and three at the psychiatric hospital, of approximately 100 beds. Referral to the mental health services typically comes from the patients' general practitioners, who are responsible for the primary care function of the NHS. The medical staff are organized into six teams, each responsible for a geographical sector of the district and headed by a consultant psychiatrist. The medical staff are responsible for inpatient treatment and also hold outpatient clinics at both general and psychiatric hospitals and at community-based, health centres. The hospital-based acute services also have input from ward-based psychiatric nurses, psychiatric social workers, occupational therapists, and the department of clinical psychology. The latter department also runs outpatient clinics at both hospitals and at primary care health centres, but they deal mostly with nonpsychotic patients referred by their general practioners.[6]

Long-Stay Patients

The psychiatric hospital also accommodates approximately 800 long-stay beds. Under Regional Authority plans these will be reduced to 500 during the next 8 years. A resettlement team is presently implementing these policies by relocating chronic patients within the community.

Community Psychiatric Nurse Service

The provision of the community psychiatric nurse (CPN) service dates back to 1968 with three CPNs and rapidly expanded to 18 by 1982.[7] This service was initially aimed at following up psychotic patients who failed to attend treatment and by 1979 all CPNs were attached to primary care teams. The CPNs run depot injection clinics and are often the chronically mentally ill patients' most frequent contact with the services.

Day Services

There are day hospitals on both hospital sites and also a social services day centre and six "drop in" centres within the community.

Rehabilitation Services

The rehabilitation team consists of a specialist multidisciplinary team who work both with the long-stay population within the psychiatric hospital and in resettlement projects within the community. They have available a 22-bed rehabilitation hostel and a unit including seven supported flats, both administered by the social services department. There is also access to various "group homes" and lodgings.

Integration of Community Care

A recent review of mental health services for the long-term mentally ill within Salford concluded that the CPNs and the psychiatric team in their outpatient clinics were the two agencies who monitored the mental state and medication of the chronically psychotic population.[8] However, there were many obstacles to the liaison between these two services, including the CPNs having a primary care base and the psychiatrists being principally hospital based. Further, although the multidisciplinary coordination of patient management occurred through the ward round while the patient was in the hospital, no such facility or function existed for the management of the patient in the community.

In conclusion, although some mental health services exist within the community these services are largely uncoordinated and inadequate for the comprehensive community care of the psychotic patient. For acute relapses or other management problems care is largely still hospital based and consists of short-stay admissions. Little in the way of intervention within a community setting occurs other than monitoring and medication.

During the past 10 years there has been considerable interest in psychosocial interventions with families to reduce relapse in schizophrenia. A number of controlled studies have generated considerable excitement, with the possibility of preventing or reducing the frequency of schizophrenic relapse and improving the quality of life of patients and their relatives. This has coincided with a time when policies on care in the community are being implemented, and there is an increase in consumer demand for better services and support for the long-term mentally ill. The aim of the Salford Family Intervention Project was to evaluate the possibility of training relatives of schizophrenic patients in the management of schizophrenia and so reduce the rate of acute relapse.

Environmental Stress and its Effects on the Course of Schizophrenia

The development of neuroleptic medication produced great advances in the treatment of schizophrenia. However, even when patients are fully compliant, approximately 40% will relapse in the first year after discharge from the hospital.[9] Even patients who do not relapse may experience severe disabilities and deficits in functioning. These problems have led investigators to examine the environment, and especially the patients' social and familial environments, for factors that may help to explain relapse and poor recovery from the illness episode. The recent interest in psychosocial interventions with families has been the result of this research.

Stress Vulnerability Models of Schizophrenia

Two important influences, one theoretical, and one empirical, have created an impetus for the development of such psychosocial interventions. First, there has been the development of stress vulnerability models of schizophrenia which attempt to integrate both biological and environmental factors into an explanatory model of schizophrenia. The work of Joseph Zubin et al[10,11] has been especially influencial in this area. Zubin and his colleagues proposed a threshold model in which an inherent vulnerability to develop the illness interacts with the ambient environmental stress (see Figure 16.1).

According to the model, when the values of these two dimensions reach a certain cutoff point then the transition from "well" to "ill" occurs and

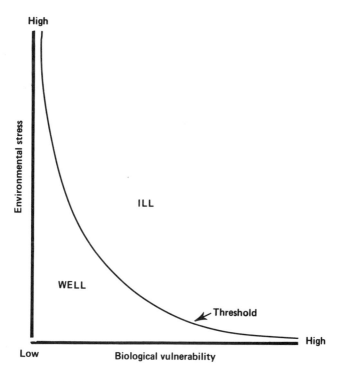

FIGURE 16.1. Relationship between biological vulnerability and environmental stress. (Adapted, with permision, from Zubin et al.[11])

positive symptoms appear. Although the simplicity of this model has appeal, there are also many inadequacies, such as the inability of the model to quantify either of the dimensions.

Originally the model proposed by Zubin was one of aetiology; however, it can also be used to explain relapse in someone who has already experienced an episode of the illness. In fact, this model can more profitably be applied to relapse because the biological predisposition to develop the illness has already been demonstrated as being present. Working from this simple prototype, other more complex models have been formulated that attempt to separate some of the different environmental and biological factors.[12,13]

The importance of these theoretical models is that schizophrenia, although a biological illness, is postulated to be stress related. The occurrence of symptomatic relapse is proposed to be an interaction between environmental and biological factors. Because this means that environmental factors can directly influence the course of the illness, they can at least in theory be identified and modified to improve prognosis. This psychobiological integration underlies the development of interventions designed to reduce relapse risk.

Expressed Emotion

Expressed Emotion and Schizophrenic Relapse

The second important factor that has given impetus to psychosocial interventions has been the development of the measure of expressed emotion (EE).[14] The conceptual and empirical origin and development of EE as a measure to investigate differing postdischarge relapse rates in schizophrenic patients has been described clearly elsewhere.[15] Expressed emotion is rated from an audiotaped semistructured interview (the Camberwell Family Interview, CFI) with the relative.[16] This interview is usually carried out at the time of the patient's hospitalisation. The relative is questioned about the onset of the recent illness episode, the patient's behaviour and symptoms, and the quality of the relationship between the patient and the relative. Five operationalised dimensions can be scored from the audiotaped interview: critical comments (a frequency count); hostility (a 4-point scale); emotional overinvolvement (a 6-point scale); warmth (a 6-point scale); and positive remarks (a frequency count). The scores on the first three dimensions are used to categorize the relative as high or low on EE. If the relative scores 6 or more critical comments, or 1 to 3 on hostility, or 3 to 5 on overinvolvement, then the relative is categorised as high EE. A score below all of these three thresholds results in a classification as low EE.

A number of studies (Table 16.1) have examined the relapse rates of patients returning to live with high or low EE relatives after their discharge from the hospital. In these 12 studies, 613 patients were observed during the postdischarge period of 9 or 12 months; of these 52.5% were

TABLE 16.1. Schizophrenic relapse and expressed emotion (EE): 9- to 12-month follow-up.

Study	N	Relapses			
		High EE		Low EE	
Brown et al, 1962[17]	97	38/50	(76%)	13/47	(28%) <.001
Brown et al, 1972[18]	101	26/45	(58%)	9/56	(16%) <.001
Vaughn & Leff, 1976[19]	37	10/21	(48%)	1/16	(6%) <.007
Vaughn et al, 1984[20]	54	20/36	(56%)	3/18	(17%) <.02
Kottgen et al, 1984[21]	50	12/29	(41%)	12/21	(57%) NS
Moline et al, 1985[22]	24	10/11	(91%)	4/13	(31%) <.004
Nuechterlein et al, 1986[23]	26	7/19	(37%)	0/7	(0%) <.03
Karno et al, 1987[24]	44	10/17	(59%)	7/27	(26%) <.03
Leff et al, 1987[25]	70	5/16	(31%)	5/54	(9%) <.05
Rostworowska et al, 1987[26]	36	15/25	(60%)	1/11	(9%) <.009
Tarrier et al, 1988[27]	48	14/29	(48%)	4/19	(21%) <.02
McCreadie & Phillips, 1988[28]	59	4/24	(17%)	7/35	(20%) NS
Total	613	171/322	(53%)	66/291	(23%)

living in high EE households. Fifty-three percent of patients living with a high EE relative relapsed compared with 23% of patients living with a low EE relative.

Cultural Factors and Expressed Emotion

The ratio of high to low EE households has not been constant in the studies. Examination of Table 16.2 indicates that the percentage of high EE households varies from 8% in rural India to 77% in Salford, England, and 74% in Sydney, Australia.

It is interesting to note that the percentage of high EE households appears higher in samples drawn from more westernised cultures and countries and lower in less developed and more traditional countries. For example, the sample from rural India has 8% high EE households compared with 30% in the urban Indian sample. Similarly, an Anglo-American sample from Los Angeles had 67% high EE households compared with 41% in a Mexican-American sample from the same location. Such differences in the ratio of EE households between westernised and more traditional societies may explain the more benign course of schizophrenia in underdeveloped countries.

Expressed Emotion as a Measure of Environmental Stress

Expressed emotion is an operationalised measure, albeit categorical, of environmental stress. Many patients will return to live with someone after hospital discharge, hence EE provides a measure of stress that the patient will experience after discharge. Therefore, EE is not a measure of "family pathology," nor would it be correct or appropriate to label high EE relatives as "bad" or "pathological." However, little is known about how EE, rated from an interview, contributes to the "emotional environment" of the home or how EE is related to the behaviour of the relatives

TABLE 16.2. Cultural variations in percentage of high expressed emotion households.

Study	Percent
India: rural, Wig et al, 1987[29]	8
India: urban, Wig et al, 1987[29]	30
Mexican-American: Karno et al, 1987[24]	41
Scotland: rural, McCreadie & Robinson, 1987[30]	42
Poland: Rostworowska et al, 1987[26]	44
London: Vaughn & Leff, 1976[19]	54
Denmark: Wig et al, 1987[29]	54
West Germany: Kottgen et al, 1984[21]	56
Anglo-American: Vaughn et al, 1984[20]	67
Sydney, Australia: Parker & Johnson, 1987[31]	74
Salford: Tarrier et al, 1988[27]	77

in the home situation. Some laboratory studies have demonstrated that EE ratings are correlated with interactional patterns of schizophrenic patients and their relatives.[32]

Expressed emotion is a useful measure of stress in a frequently occurring environment, the family home. The influence of different environmental stressors and EE is probably only one example of how a number of such factors probably act upon a common biological pathway involving the arousal system.[33] This formulation receives support from psychophysiological studies investigating the effect of the patient's relative on the patient's level of arousal.[33,34]

To summarise, the development and general acceptance of psychobiological models of schizophrenic relapse that emphasise the interaction of environmental and biological factors, sets the theoretical scene for interventions aimed at reducing relapse by reducing environmental stress. The development of the EE measure allowed an empirical demonstration of the effect of the home environment on relapse rates. If it is possible to decrease the level of the relatives' EE through psychosocial interventions, then relapse rates and hence relapse risk should also reduce.

Expressed emotion research also has demonstrated other factors, such as maintenance medication and face-to-face contact between the patient and relative as important in determining relapse.[19] Certainly, there appears little doubt that neuroleptic medication is superior to placebo in preventing relapse.[35] Hence, psychosocial interventions were never envisaged as an alternative to medication but as an adjunct. All the studies reviewed in this paper have implemented psychosocial interventions in combination with neuroleptic medication.

Psychosocial Family Intervention Studies

An Overview

The Camberwell Study

The first major controlled study of a psychosocial intervention was carried out by Leff and his colleagues[36,37] in London (Table 16.3). Twenty-four families were recruited into the study. Patients were hospitalised for an acute episode of schizophrenia and at least one relative was high EE and in high contact with the patient (more than 35 hours face-to-face contact per week). The patients and their families were randomly allocated on discharge to either the experimental group or the control group. The experimental group received a package of interventions including an educational programme to provide the relatives with information about the illness, a relatives' group, and individual family therapy. The control group received routine psychiatric aftercare as provided by the National Health Service. The experimental group showed significantly lower re-

TABLE 16.3. Relapse rates in family intervention studies based on expressed emotion.

Study	Relapse rates			
	9 or 12 months		24 months	
Camberwell[36,37]				
Family intervention	1/12	(8%)	2/10	(20%)
Routine treatment	6/12	(50%)	7/9	(78%)
California[38,39]				
Family intervention	1/18	(6%)	3/18	(17%)
Individual intervention	8/18	(44%)	14/18	(83%)
Hamburg[21]				
High EE intervention	5/15	(33%)		
High EE control	6/14	(43%)		
Low EE control	10/20	(20%)		
Pittsburgh[40]				
Family intervention	4/21	(19%)		
Social skills training	4/20	(20%)		
Combined intervention	0/20	(0%)		
Control	7/17	(41%)		
Salford[27,41]				
High EE groups				
Family intervention			8/24	(33%)
Enactive	2/13	(17%)		
Symbolic	1/12	(8%)		
Education only	6/14	(43%)		
Routine treatment	8/15	(53%)	17/29	(59%)
Low EE groups				
Education only	2/9	(22%)		
Routine treatment	2/10	(20%)	6/18	(33%)

lapse rates at 9 and 24 months compared with the control group (Table 16.3). Reassessment of the relatives' EE levels and contact time at 9 months indicated that the therapeutic goal of reducing either EE or contact time had been achieved in 75% of families in the experimental group. In drug-compliant patients whose relatives had had their EE or contact reduced to low levels there were no relapses in the first 9 months.

The California Study

In a study by Falloon and colleagues,[38,39] 36 patients and their families, who were identified as "high tension" families (33 were high EE households), were randomly allocated to an experimental family-focused intervention or to a control group. The experimental group received a behavioural family therapy package including an education programme, communication training when appropriate, and problem-solving training. The control intervention consisted of an education programme and individual psychotherapy. The experimental group showed significantly lower relapse rates at 9 and 24 months (Table 16.3). Falloon and his colleagues used numerous outcome measures, and demonstrated improvements in the patients' social functioning, a decrease in the burden of care experienced by relatives, an improvement in the families' problem-solving ability, and a significant advantage in economic cost, all for the behavioural family therapy group over the control group.[9]

The Hamburg Study

A study carried out in Germany[21] compared a high EE treatment group who received group psychotherapy separately for patients and relatives, with a high EE and a low EE no treatment control group. Unlike the other studies reviewed here which have adopted a behavioural and problem-solving approach, this study used group analytic methods. This intervention did not show any significant benefit over the no treatment control groups (Table 16.3).

The Pittsburgh Study

In a large study conducted in Pittsburgh by Hogarty and colleagues,[40] 78 high EE families were randomly allocated to one of four groups: family psychoeducation and management; social skills training for the patient; a combination of family management and social skills training; and a control group who received medication in the context of a supportive relationship. The relapse rates after 12 months were very impressive (Table 16.3). Both the individual treatment groups of family management and social skills alone were significantly superior to the control group. But in the combined group there were no relapses at all. It was further found that there were no relapses in households in which the relatives changed from high to low EE. Generally, relapse rates were elevated in households who remained high EE after 12 months, except in those in the combined treatment group.

   In light of the attention paid to family atmosphere and the emphasis on intervening with the family unit it may appear paradoxical that a patient-centred intervention such as social skills training could have an equivalent effect on family management. However, the skills training focused on how the patient interacted with his or her relative as opposed to generic skills training. Further, the explanation of the success of these interventions is probably better interpreted in terms of their functional effect (ie, stress reduction) rather than similarities in techniques.

The Salford Family Intervention Project

A study carried out in Salford by Tarrier and colleagues[27,41] attempted to evaluate a clinical service as well as treatment efficacy. The study aimed to evaluate a number of intervention programmes with both high EE and low EE families in terms of relapse rates, and to assess the viability of delivering family intervention as part of the regular psychology input to the mental health services.

Subjects

All patients who were admitted to the four acute psychiatric wards in Salford Health Authority were screened, and patients fulfilling the following four criteria were recruited into the study: (1) a diagnosis of schizophrenia using the PSE/Catego system; (2) between the ages of 16 and 64; (3) not suffering from any organic condition that could explain their psychopathology; and (4) having lived with their relative(s) for 3 months before admission and intending to return to the household.

Ninety-two families were identified as suitable for inclusion; of these, 9 families (10%) refused to be assessed. Of the 83 patients who were included, 30% were experiencing their first illness episode, and the overall mean duration of illness was 6.3 years (SD 7.4 years). Sixty-five percent of the patients were female, had a mean age of 35.3 years (SD 12.8 years), 54% were single, and 21% were unemployed. Fifty-one percent lived in parental homes and 35% in their marital homes. Seventy-five percent lived with one relative. Forty-two percent of the relatives were mothers, 24% fathers, 18% husbands, 6% wives, and 10% some other relation. The mean age of the relatives was 53 years (SD 15.2 years); 53% were female and 48% were in employment.

Study Design

Patients were divided into "high-risk" (ie, those who had a high EE relative) and "low risk" (those who did not) groups. Patients with high EE relatives ($N = 64$) were randomly allocated in a stratified manner (with first and multiple episodes, and presence or absence of residual symptoms as factors) to one of four groups: (1) a 9-month family behavioural intervention (enactive); (2) a 9-month family behavioural intervention (symbolic); (3) a short educational programme; and (4) routine National Health Service aftercare. The patients with low EE relatives only ($N = 19$) were allocated to one of two groups: (1) a short educational programme; and (2) routine treatment. Ten families did not take any further part in the study: four families refused to participate further; four patients did not return home; and two patients were transfered to long-stay rehabilitation wards.

Treatment Groups

The treatment offered to the different groups was as follows:

Routine Treatment: All patients were under the care of a multidisciplinary team during admission and after discharge. The research team maintained contact with the family for assessment purposes, and acted as a link with the clinical team when necessary, but no specialist intervention was offered.

Education Only: Families allocated to this group received a standardised two-session educational programme, designed to give patients and relatives extensive and individualised information about schizophrenia and how to manage it in the home environment. This programme has been described elsewhere.[42]

Behavioural Intervention: These were two 9-month behavioural interventions of similar content but of different levels (enactive and symbolic). Initially the family received the educational programme of two sessions, followed by three sessions of stress management within the family environment with the relatives. This programme was designed to teach the relatives to monitor sources of stress and their reactions to it, and then learn more appropriate methods of coping. Finally, there was an 8-session programme of goal setting, in which patients and relatives were taught to identify areas of change or need, to set goals to meet these needs, and to operationalise procedures to achieve the goals. These treatment methods have been described in detail elsewhere.[43,44] The difference between the enactive and the symbolic groups is in the level of intervention and not in content. Both interventions are didactic, in that families are taught skills with which to manage schizophrenia, the difference is in how these skills are taught. The enactive group was taught management and coping skills through participation methods, such as role playing, guided practice, recordkeeping, and corroborated active participation in the programme. The symbolic group received similar instruction, but through discussion and instruction only (ie, through the symbolic mode of language rather than the enactive mode of participation). It was hypothesised that the enactive group would more readily learn management skills and should, therefore, be more effective at reducing stress in the home environment. This in turn should result in less relapses in this group.

Assessment

A battery of assessment measures were applied at admission and at 4.5 months and 9 months after discharge. These included: the Camberwell Family Interview (CFI) and an assessment of the relatives' level of EE, the level of the relatives' personal distress and the relatives' perception of the patients' problem behaviour; and assessment of the patients' level of social functioning, and the patients' psychophysiological reactions to their relative. Only some of these data are presented in this account. The patients' clinical condition was assessed at least on a monthly basis. If there was any suggestion of a relapse, either through a recurrence or worsening of symptoms, then a Present State Examination (PSE) was carried out by a psychiatrist who was blind to the patient's treatment allocation. Detailed records of medication, independent life events, and patient contacts with the psychiatric services during the 9-month follow-up period were kept.

Results

The relapse rates for the 9-month and 2-year follow-up periods are presented in Table 16.3. At 9 months the high EE routine treatment and education only groups had significantly higher relapse rates than the comparable low EE groups. Further, the two high EE behavioural intervention groups had significantly lower relapse rates than the high EE education only and routine treatment groups. In both the high EE and low EE groups the group who received the education programme did not show any significant differences in terms of relapse rates than the routine treatment group. However, it is quite possible that education may have benefits other than in terms of relapse rates. There were no significant differences between the enactive and symbolic behavioural interventions. This is surprising as it was predicted that the enactive intervention would teach the relatives management skills to a higher level, which would be translated into clinical benefit.

The fact that the high EE groups who received the 9-month behavioural intervention with families had significantly lower relapse rates than the two high EE groups who did not is not in itself proof that the intervention itself was responsible for the reduced relapse rate. It is necessary to rule out other alternative explanations where possible.

One alternative explanation is that the behavioural intervention group differed in the dose of medication they received or in their compliance with medication during the 9-month period. Comparisons were made between the treatment groups in terms of medication compliance, number of months without medication, whether the patient was receiving oral medication or depot injection, and the total dose of medication in neuroleptic equivalents. No significant differences between the groups was evident, indicating that differences in medication did not explain the difference in relapse rates. A second alternative explanation was that the intervention resulted in the patient having more contact with the psychiatric services and hence better care, and this resulted in the relapse rate difference rather than the intervention itself. A comparison was made between treatment groups in terms of number of outpatient appointments, compliance with appointments, attendance at injection clinics, contact with community psychiatric nurses, attendance at daycare, duration of daycare, contact with social workers, and contact of relatives with community psychiatric nurses and social workers. None of these comparisons were significant, which indicated that contact with the psychiatric services did not explain the difference in relapse results. Lastly, a comparison was made between the treatment groups in terms of the number of independent life events experienced by patients in each group. It was possible that the higher relapse rates in the high EE routine treatment and education only group could be explained by a higher incidence of life events experienced by this group. A comparison of the number of events experienced by patients in each group in fact indicated that patients in the behavioural family intervention groups experienced significantly more events. Certainly, the frequency of life events did not explain the difference in relapse rates and may indicate that the behavioural intervention increased the patients' functioning so that they experienced more events and increased the patients' abilities to cope with them.

Examination of the changes in the relatives' EE produced interesting results. Significant changes from high to low EE were found to occur generally in the high EE groups, but greater changes were found in the two behavioural intervention groups. The behavioural intervention groups had significantly less high EE relatives at 9 months than the high EE education and routine treatment groups. Significant decreases in criticism and emotional overinvolvement (EOI) were found generally, but to a significantly greater magnitude in the behavioural intervention groups. Significant decreases in hostility were only found in the behavioural intervention groups. The behavioural intervention groups had significantly fewer critical comments than the high EE education and routine treatment groups at 9 months. Relatives in the low EE routine treatment group showed a tendency to be rated high EE at 9 months, although this trend was not significant. These changes in levels of EE and its constituent dimensions suggest that reduced relapse rates are associated with changes in relatives from high to low EE and reductions in criticism, EOI, and hostility. Although such changes did occur in the high EE education and routine treatment groups, they were of significantly smaller magnitude than those that occurred in the behavioural intervention groups. This indicates that the behavioural family intervention is effective in reducing relapse rates by reducing the EE levels of the relative. A cautionary point that should be noted is that low EE families who do not receive any specialist service (ie, those in the low EE routine treatment group) tend to become high EE, and therefore there is a potential increase in relapse risk in these families. This was not apparent in the low EE families who received education. Hence, low EE families need specialist intervention to keep the risk of relapse low, but this input may not need to be extensive.

The 2-year follow-up results show that the benefit of the behavioural intervention is maintained.[41] The combined behavioural intervention group showed a 33% relapse rate compared with 59% in the combined high EE education and routine treatment group. The combined low EE group also showed a 33% relapse rate. These differences are significant. However, the relapse rate in the behavioural intervention group increased from 9 to 24 months, suggesting that in some patients relapse is not prevented but delayed. This suggests the need of some patients and their families for continuous and not time-limited intervention.

Mechanisms of Intervention Effectiveness

Four controlled studies have demonstrated the efficacy of psychosocial interventions in reducing schizophrenic relapse.[36,38,40,27] What are the common elements in these interventions that result in a successful reduction in relapse rates? There are probably many similarities in these successful interventions, but it may be more productive to examine the functional effects of the intervention rather than to compare a description of techniques. If the core deficits of the schizophrenic illness result from an interaction between a dysfunction in information processing and in arousal regulation,[12] then an environment that exacerbates these dysfunctions will precipitate and maintain symptoms of the illness. Hence, an environment that has a stimulus input that is complex, vague and ambiguous, emotionally charged, and unpredictable will result in an overload of the information-processing abilities of the individual. continuous exposure to this stressful environment will result in increased arousal levels and positive symptoms reappearing. If, however, the environmental input becomes clear, simple, predictable, and defused of excess emotion then relapse is less likely to occur. Hence, stress reduction within the home environment is the key to effective intervention. Family interventions will be effective and beneficial if they result in reducing behaviours that are characteristic of high EE relatives. Social skills training alone will also be effective, as has been demonstrated,[40] if it improves the patient's perception of the social behaviour of others and allows him or her to select and implement the correct and appropriate responses.

If the levels of stress reach a certain threshold, then schizophrenic symptoms are likely to recur. To be effective, any intervention must perform the function of reducing the ambient stress experienced by the patient in his or her environment. Future efforts must be made to refine assessment and intervention methods, so that environmental stressors can be carefully monitored and effectively reduced.

Implications for Service Provision

Finally, it is important to draw conclusions from the empirical research on psychosocial interventions with families of schizophrenic patients into statements about psychiatric services for the long-term mentally ill and the community management of schizophrenia. To do this it is necessary to examine some of the comments we made previously concerning the mental health services within Salford, and to describe some of the present and projected developments within these services.

First, it is apparent that although quite extensive services may exist within the community, if these are poorly coordinated they will not provide effective community care. During the years from 1968, extensive community psychiatric services were built up within Salford mainly through the provision of community psychiatric nurse (CPN) and psychiatric social work (PSW) services.[45] The CPN service especially was designed to extend the community management of the long-term mentally ill, especially schizophrenic patients, and reduce the need for hospitalisation. However, data from the Salford case register indicated that between 1968 and 1978 when community services were active, far from decreasing hospital populations, these populations actually increased.[45] Further investigation of the CPN service demonstrated that although more patients were receiving care, this actually reflected an increase in patients suffering from minor psychological disorders rather than the long-term mentally ill.[7] This latter group were also receiving far less in CPN time than those suffering from anxiety or depression.[46] The lesson from these studies is that providing and extending community psychiatric services does not necessarily reduce the demands on the traditional services nor meet the needs of the most severely disabled.

Second, traditional psychiatric services may have ''out reach'' and aftercare services within the community, but they are still hospital based and biased toward treatment of acute episodes. This results in clinical reviews of patients while they are inpatients but no such multidisciplinary review for patients once they return to the community or for those who remain in the community for long periods.

Third, a well organised and coordinated service needs to incorporate therapeutic interventions of proven efficacy and employ staff with the appropriate skills and training to deliver them.

A comprehensive community mental health service should be community based and provide clinical reviews for patients while they are in the community. Although hospital backup for acute relapses and special medium-stay units may be required for ''difficult to manage'' patients, the focus of the service and resource allocation should be within a community setting. In an attempt to achieve a comprehensive community-based and high-quality mental health service, the Mental Health Unit of Salford District Health Authority has embarked on a programme to relocate the locus of its service. The acute admission wards at the psychiatric hospital are to be closed down along with the majority of services of the institution. These wards will be relocated in a new inpatient unit of four wards at the district general hospital. The majority of day hospital and outpatient facilities will be integrated within an initiative of four new community mental health centres (CMHCs), one of which will serve each of four geographic sectors of the district. The CMHCs will function at a number of different levels and provide service input from the case of the chronically mentally ill through to health promotion. To coordinate the community management of schizophrenia, each CMHC will have a clinical review procedure that will provide initial detailed medical and social assessments, assessment updates, and formulate individual care plans (ICPs) for each patient. Figure 16.2 presents a diagrammatic representation of this case management system.

The CMHC's multidisciplinary team will implement the case management system but will be able to liaise closely with primary care teams, hospital services, and social services and draw on their resources where

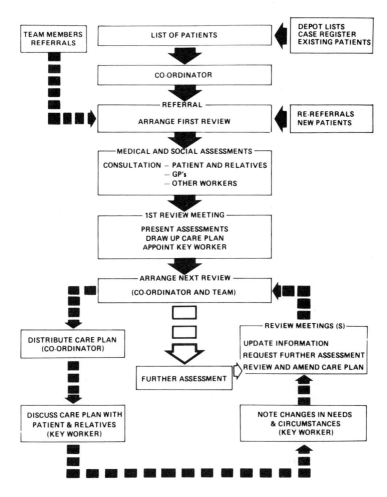

FIGURE 16.2. Diagram of case management system. (Reprinted, with permission, from Whitehead.[8])

necessary. An important function of the case management procedure is to involve both the patient and his or her relatives in consultation concerning that patient's intensive care management. In this manner the family intervention implemented in the Salford Family Intervention Project, where the relatives are taught the skills to reduce environmental stress and identify and meet the patient's needs, can be incorporated into a mental health service for the management of schizophrenia. This service is community based, comprehensive, and involves cooperation between both service providers and service receivers.

At this point one CMHC has been operational for 12 months and a second under construction and will become operational at the end of

1989. The case management system including family intervention under the direction and supervision of the team's senior clinical psychologist is now being implemented.

Summary

This chapter reviews the research on psychosocial family interventions and relapse prevention in schizophrenia and describes the Salford Family Intervention Project carried out by the authors. The project's aim was to evaluate the effect of training the relatives of schizophrenic patients in the management of schizophrenia to reduce acute relapse and the need for hospitalisation. The project was carried out within a British National Health Service health district and was, in part, a test of providing such an intervention as part of a comprehensive mental health service based on the policy of community care.

The authors briefly describe the British NHS as a system of comprehensive medical care and the place of mental health services within it, with specific reference to the Salford District Health Authority.

The research on family interventions is reviewed within the context of the development of stress vulnerability models of schizophrenia and the research on expressed emotion as an indicator of environmental stress. Of the studies reviewed, significant improvement in functioning and reduced relapse rate were obtained in the Camberwell, California, and Pittsburg studies. This success is attributed to the behavioural and problem-solving techniques used in these studies in combination with neuroleptic medication, which focused on reducing environmental stress and the level of expressed emotion in family members.

The Salford Family Intervention Project evaluated both the clinical service and treatment outcome in a number of intervention programmes with both high and low EE families. Relapse rates were found to be significantly lower in high-risk patients who received a 9-month behavioural family intervention compared with appropriate control groups. Follow-up after 2 years showed that the benefits of the behavioural intervention were maintained for some patients; however, the relapse rate increased. This finding indicates that, for some patients and families, intervention needs to be continuous. The common factor identified as being important in the efficacy of these psychosocial interventions is stress reduction within the home environment. Thus, the primary focus must be on: enhancing clear, simple, and predictable input from the environment; reducing high expressed emotion in relatives; improving the patient's social skills; and providing continuous monitoring of the level of ambient stress in the home.

Finally, the potential implications of this empirical research for community management of schizophrenia are discussed with reference to the present and projected mental health services within Salford required to meet the needs of the most seriously disabled.

References

1. Willcocks AJ: *The creation of the National Health Service*. London, Routledge and Kegan Paul, 1967.
2. *National Health Service Handbook*. Birmingham, National Association of Health Authorities, 1988.
3. Lord Glenarthur: Introduction and current developments, in Wilkinson G, Freeman H (eds): *The Provision of Mental Health Services in Britain: The Way Ahead*. Oxford, Gaskell, 1986.
4. Griffiths R: *Community Care: Agenda for Action*. London, HMSO, 1988.
5. Office of Population Censuses and Surveys: Census 1981. County reports Greater Manchester, parts I & II. London, HMSO, 1981.
6. Tarrier N, Wooff K: Psychologists in primary care and their effects on general practitioner referrals to psychiatry. *Br J Clin Soc Psych* 1983;2:85–87.
7. Wooff K, Goldberg D, Fryers T: Patients in receipt of community psychiatric nurse care in Salford, 1976–82. *Psychol Med* 1986;16:407–414.
8. Whitehead C: Coordinated aftercare for schizophrenia: report of a pilot project. Final report for DHSS Mental Health Division, Salford Health Authority, 1987.
9. Falloon IRH, Boyd JL, McGill CW: *Family Care of Schizophrenia*. New York, Guilford Press, 1984.
10. Zubin J, Spring B: Vulnerability: a new view of schizophrenia. *J Abn Psychol* 1977;86:103–126.
11. Zubin J, Magaziner J, Steinhauer SR: The metamorphosis of schizophrenia: from chronicity to vulnerability. *Psychol Med* 1983;13:551–571.
12. Nuechterlein KH, Dawson ME: A heuristic vulnerability stress model of schizophrenic episodes. *Schizophr Bull* 1984;10:300–312.
13. Nuechterlein KH: Vulnerability models of schizophrenia: state of the art, in Hafner H, Gattaz WF, Jangarik W (eds): *Searches for the Causes of Schizophrenia*. Berlin, Springer–Verlag, 1987.
14. Leff J, Vaughn C: *Expressed Emotion in Families*. New York, Guilford Press, 1985.
15. Brown G: The discovery of expressed emotion: induction or deduction, in Leff J, Vaughn C (eds): *Expressed Emotion in Families*. New York, Guilford Press, 1985.
16. Vaughn C, Leff J: The measurement of expressed emotion in the families of psychiatric patients. *Br J Soc Clin Psychol* 1976;15:157–165.
17. Brown G, Monck EM, Carstairs GM, et al: Influence of family life on the course of schizophrenic illness. *Br J Prevent Soc Med* 1962;16:55–68.
18. Brown G, Birley JLT, Wing JK: Influence of family life on the course of schizophrenic disorder, a replication. *Br J Psych* 1972;121:241–258.
19. Vaughn C, Leff J: Influence of family and social factors on the course of psychiatric illness. *Br J Psych* 1976;129:125–137.
20. Vaughn C, Snyder KS, Jones S, et al: Family factors in schizophrenic relapse:

replication in California of British research on expressed emotion. *Arc Gen Psych* 1984;41:1169–1177.

21. Kottgen C, Sonnichsen I, Mollenhauer K, et al: Results of the Hamburg Camberwell Family Interview study I, II, III. *Int J Fam Psych* 1984;5:61–94.

22. Moline RA, Singh S, Morris A, et al: Family expressed emotion and relapse in schizophrenia in 24 urban American patients. *Am J Psych* 1985;142:1078–1081.

23. Nuechterlein KH, Snyder KS, Dawson ME, et al: Expressed emotion, fixed dose fluphenazine decanoate maintenance, and relapse in recent onset schizophrenia. *Psychopharma Bull* 1986;22:633–639.

24. Karno M, Jenkins JH, de la Silva A, et al: Expressed emotion and schizophrenic outcome among Mexican-American families. *J Nerv Ment Dis* 1987;175:143–151.

25. Leff J, Wig NN, Ghosh A, et al: Influence of relatives' expressed emotion on the course of schizophrenia in Chandigarh. *Br J Psych* 1987;151:166–173.

26. Rostworowska M, Barbaro B, Cechnicki A: The influence of expressed emotion on the course of schizophrenia: a Polish replication. Poster presented at 17th Congress of the European Association for Behaviour Therapy, Amsterdam, 26–29th August 1987. Published in the abstracts.

27. Tarrier N, Barrowclough C, Vaughn C, et al: The community management of schizophrenia: a controlled trial of a behavioural intervention with families to reduce relapse. *Br J Psych* 1988;153:532–542.

28. McCreadie RG, Phillips K: The Nithsdale schizophrenia survey: VII Does relatives' high expressed emotion predict relapse? *Br J Psych* 1988;152:477–81.

29. Wig NN, Menon DK, Bedi H, et al: Distribution of expressed emotion components among relatives of schizophrenic patients in Aarhus and Chandigarh. *Br J Psych* 1987;151:160–165.

30. McCreadie RG, Robinson ADT: The Nithsdale schizophrenia survey: VI. Relatives' expressed emotion: prevalence, patterns, and clinical assessment. *Br J Psych* 1987;150:640–644.

31. Parker G, Johnson P: Parenting and schizophrenia: an Australian study of expressed emotion. *Austr NZ J Psych* 1987;21:60–66.

32. Miklowitz DJ, Goldstein MJ, Falloon IRH, et al: Interactional correlates of expressed emotion in the families of schizophrenics. *Br J Psych* 1984;144:482–487.

33. Turpin G, Tarrier N, Sturgeon D: Social psychophysiology and the study of biopsychosocial models of schizophrenia, in Wagner H (ed): *Social Psychophysiology: Perspectives on Theory and Clinical Application.* Chichester, Wiley, 1988.

34. Tarrier N: Arousal levels and relatives' expressed emotion in remitted schizophrenic patients. *Br J Clin Psychol* 1989;28:177–180.

35. Davis JM: Overview: maintenance therapy in psychiatry: I schizophrenia. *Am J Psych* 1975;13:1237–1254.

36. Leff J, Kuipers L, Berkowitz R, et al: A controlled trial of social intervention in the families of schizophrenic patients. *Br J Psych* 1982;141:121–134.

37. Leff J, Kuipers L, Berkowitz R, et al: A controlled study of social intervention in families of schizophrenic patients: A two-year follow-up. *Br J Psych* 1985;146:594–600.

38. Falloon IRH, Boyd JL, McGill CW, et al: Family management in the prevention of exacerbation of schizophrenia. *N Eng J Med* 1982;306:1437–1440.

39. Falloon IRH, Boyd JL, McGill CW, et al: Family management in the prevention of morbidity of schizophrenia: clinical outcome of a two year longitudinal study. *Arch Gen Psych* 1985;42:887–896.

40. Hogarty GE, Anderson CM, Reiss DJ, et al: Family psychoeducation, social skills training and maintenance chemotherapy in the aftercare treatment of schizophrenia. *Arch Gen Psych* 1986;43:633–642.

41. Tarrier N, Barrowclough C, Vaughn C, et al: Community management of schizophrenia: A two-year follow-up of a behavioural intervention with families. *Br J Psych* 1989;154:625–628.

42. Barrowclough C, Tarrier N, Watts S, et al: Assessing the functional value of relatives' knowledge about schizophrenia: a preliminary report. *Br J Psych* 1987;151:1–8.

43. Barrowclough C, Tarrier N: A behavioural family intervention with a schizophrenic patient: a case study. *Behav Psychother* 1987;15:252–271.

44. Barrowclough C, Tarrier N: Recovery from mental illness: following it through with a family, in Patmore C (ed): *Living After Mental Illness: Innovations in Services.* London, Croom Helm, 1987.

45. Wooff K, Freeman HL, Fryers T: Psychiatric service use in Salford: a comparison of point-prevalence ratios 1968–1978. *Br J Psych* 1983;142:588–597.

46. Wooff K, Goldberg DP, Fryers T: The practice of community psychiatric nursing and mental health social work in Salford: some implications for community care. *Br J Psych* 1988;152:783–792.

17
Delivery Systems for the Care of Schizophrenic Patients in Africa—Sub-Sahara

GHULAM MUSTAFA

This chapter is primarily concerned with reviewing the ways and means whereby psychiatric care is currently made available to schizophrenic patients in Africa (sub-Sahara), in a fashion that maximally uses rare specialist skills as well as other limited resources that are available.

General Background

In most African countries, psychiatry lags a long way behind other medical facilities. This is due to the rightful preoccupation in the past, with urgent problems in the field of nutrition, maternal and child health, and the prevention of infectious diseases. Only more recently has consideration been given to the effects of psychiatric illness on a community's well-being and its economic efficiency. Approximately 10% of the population in any 1 year is likely to be handicapped by some sort of psychiatric symptomatology, either mild or severe. Although common, these psychiatric diseases rarely cause death directly and in some way this reduces the degree of concern about them.

Two types of schizophrenic psychoses among Africans have been described, the "short schizophrenic episodes" with favorable prognosis and the "chronic schizophrenic psychosis" with an unrelenting and debilitating course.[1] The former is characterized by confusion, excitement, unsystematized delusions, transient hallucinations, and often massive anxiety and conversion symptoms; it is common in illiterate, socially underprivileged Africans.[2] The latter, also called "true schizophrenia," is characterized by classical symptoms and signs and is seen in Africans of all socioeconomic groups.[1]

There are no large-scale epidemologic data regarding the prevalence of schizophrenia in African countries.[1] However, in a survey of 100 households in a small Ethiopian town, 33 individuals had a psychiatric diagnosis and of them, one was diagnosed as schizophrenic.[3] In another study of a rural population of Ugandans over 50 years of age the prevalence of chronic schizophrenia was estimated at 2.3%.[4] Thus, the prevalence of "true schizophrenia" in Africa does not seem to be that different than for chronic schizophrenia in Western countries.

The symptoms of schizophrenia also appear to be generally similar between African and European schizophrenic patients[5]; however, a cross-cultural study suggested that hallucinations in general are more frequent among African, West Indian, and Asian patients than among English patients and other groups.[6] Also, olfactory hallucinations[7,8] and subcultural delusions and hallucinations[9] were found to be more frequent among black patients than among "white and colored patients."

Self-mutilation in response to delusions has been rarely reported from Africa and underdeveloped areas and is thought to be rare in contrast with reported cases in the West.[10] However, a series of four cases within a period of 1 year described in Nairobi suggests that self-mutilization in schizophrenic patients is probably as common in Africa though underreported.[11]

By having an almost normal life expectancy, the schizophrenic patient often becomes a potential burden to his community over many years. Not only are he and his relatives unhappy, and their home life disrupted, but the patient also is frequently nonproductive in his society. However, with modern psychiatric treatment, this long-term erosion of health, happiness, and productivity can be greatly reduced, but only if treatment facilities are readily available, efficient, and adequate.

It is not enough to lock the patient in an asylum. This is merely an expensive way of keeping him out of sight. Efficient psychiatric care must concern itself with prevention where practical. Rapid, effective intervention and treatment must be provided where necessary, with minimal disruption to the patient's family so that the patient can return to a normal life as soon as possible. Preventive measures in treatment, supervision, and follow-up are required to prevent further relapses and increasing incapacitation. Unfortunately, facilities in African countries are inadequate to provide such comprehensive care.

In developing societies all sorts of people at different stages of development are to be found, who tend to adopt the habits and lifestyle of the Western society.[12] In some ways, developing societies are more varied and complex than developed ones. It is true that in Africa one finds a large, traditional, and stable family-centered group; however, this is changing rapidly and may not be the case for very much longer.

The development of mental health facilities in African countries has been out of step. At one end there are no modern comprehensive psychiatric facilities, and at the other extreme, highly specialized services are available. In between these two extremes the prisons and closed houses with chained and starved patients pose the most challenging problems to the psychiatrist working in Africa.

Until recently, psychiatry was not given its due importance by many of the African Health Ministries.[13] The care of the mentally ill was the least concern even of the medical profession, and therefore many psychological problems were cared for outside the medical profession. Still in many of the less developed societies, even medical problems are dealt with at two levels, those which are the concern of the hospital, and those which fall within the domain of the traditional healers. Not surprisingly, psychiatric problems belong to the latter group. Consequently, the extent of psychiatric problems was unknown, and the paucity of knowledge left many gaps. The primary objective of mental health workers was to bridge these gaps and to improvise ways and means to meet the needs of patients and prevent the occurrence of disease. Many African countries are now reaching the stage of selecting the patterns for development of psychiatric services, and psychiatry has gradually developed to a point where a relatively good service is provided to many patients.

Personnel, finance, and psychiatric facilities in African countries are very sparse.[1] Long distances are involved to reach the rural settlements, and means of transport are poor. These are some of the difficulties present in almost all the African countries. The growth of the psychiatric services, therefore, has a relatively similar pattern. The delivery systems for the care of schizophrenic patients described in this chapter relate by and large to the situation in Kenya. Most of the African countries have very similar problems, and where differences are found, these are mentioned accordingly to show the comparison. Besides, the delivery systems stated are for psychiatric patients in general. In African countries there are no separate facilities for different psychiatric disease entities. Schizophrenia, however, forms the bulk of psychiatric morbidity. While discussing the delivery system for the care of schizophrenic patients in African countries, one has to keep in mind that although the problems may vary from country to country, there are general features that cross all national boundaries.

To study the topic effectively it would be convenient to discuss it under the following headings:

1. Personnel
2. Psychiatric hospitals
3. Psychiatric units in general hospitals
4. Psychiatric wards in general hospitals
5. Outpatient services
6. Community-based psychiatric services
7. Traditional healers
8. Forensic issues and facilities for the criminal schizophrenics

Personnel

An effective delivery system for the care of schizophrenic patients is dependent largely upon skilled personnel more than on extensive technical equipment. Whereas there is a worldwide need to deploy personnel to the best advantage, this need is even greater in African countries where skilled personnel are very limited, and greater still in specialities such as psychiatry which tend to be neglected when developing other services in the efforts to promote progress. The numbers of skilled and trained psychiatric staff are currently not enough to give any adequate service to the many psychiatrically ill, and this situation is likely to prevail for many years.[5] Not long ago many African countries had only one or two trained psychiatrists to render psychiatric services to the entire nation. There has, however, been a gradual increase in the number of mental health workers in the African countries. But the number available is still very far from the optimum needed to provide the minimum of psychiatric services. Thus, the delivery of mental health services, which is handled by only a few psychiatrists, necessitates concerted effort to deal with the many difficult issues. With the new pattern and expansion of delivery systems, the traditional psychiatric team has to join hands with other health workers to provide the necessary coverage for the growing needs of the community.[14]

Psychiatrists, therefore, often have to make use of the existing general health services, which have not been fully used, and to train general health workers (eg, the general nurse) to participate in the needed mental health activities.[14] When trained, these nurses play a major role in providing rural psychiatric services, and they often work in an independent and responsible capacity. These nurses give the frontline service of psychiatric care in rural areas. At present and as awareness increases, the general population will learn to view psychiatric symptoms as illness. There will be a greater need for trained personnel, who can provide leadership in psychiatric care programs.

It requires considerable effort and hard work to design and develop good systems of integration between psychiatric and general medical personnel. Mental health training programs that are an investment in the future may even impair initially the present medical services by diverting skilled personnel from their full-time work. In every country, however, there are other opportunities possible for organizing training in mental health activities. When skilled personnel is limited, one turns to the less skilled and relatively unskilled to carry out the services, while deploying the skilled in leading, organizing, and coordinating the services to the best level possible. Such delegation of skills, techniques, responsibilities, and authority is perhaps the only way to run the services in the absence of adequate numbers of trained staff.

In view of the small number of qualified psychiatric personnel who could be employed for teaching, some countries organize courses of training for the nurse tutor with the view that these tutors in turn will teach psychiatric nursing to pupils in their respective schools. This has brought about a better orientation in mental health activities, and psychiatric nursing has become an integral part of the general curriculum in most nursing schools in Africa.[15]

Psychiatric Services

Psychiatric Hospitals

It is still not uncommon to find the insane confined in jails in some African countries. Fortunately, nowadays this happens when the only psychiatric hospital is more overcrowded than normal. The building of psychiatric hospitals in most African countries dates back to the second decade of this century. The basic idea was to build one large mental hospital to serve the whole country. These hospitals are mostly situated some miles outside the cities and are a considerable distance away from communities and residential areas. This presents traveling difficulties and barriers to cooperation with other medical facilities.

In many African countries, all the psychiatric services have been restricted to one archaic mental hospital that has no facilities for community-based services or other such responsibilities outside the hospital walls. The majority of these hospitals are unplanned and have grown haphazardly to their present size—wards being added as the needs became greater. This resulted in the gross lack of the basic amenities, such as adequate facilities for catering, laundry, bathrooms and toilets within the wards, and other similar services. In addition, the maintenance of these hospitals was neglected due to lack of resources, which resulted in the poor state of the buildings. Many of these buildings have been condemned, and a complete rebuilding has been recommended. But, again, such projects are many times held in abeyance due to a lack of resources. As these hospitals were established during the era when only custodial care was available, the administration that evolved had a strong hierarchical structure. This type of administration permits very limited delegation of responsibility and allows the flow of little real information, other than commands. Whereas this system of administration perhaps has its uses, it is questionable whether such a system can fully support the structure of a therapeutic hospital. Unfortunately, the hospital organization has not undergone an essential change in keeping with the modern therapies, which to a great extent have outmoded the old custodial care. Whereas the role of the hospital may have changed with therapeutic progress, the role of the staff has often remained almost unchanged. No new information, understanding, or new role has been given to the established nurse and ward worker.

In a developing country it is appropriate to question closely the function of the existing psychiatric hospitals, so as to modify the present ones to a greater effectiveness in the light of local needs and to establish principles for the planning of much needed new psychiatric facilities. This is particularly true when a developing country has inherited a hospital based on an outdated Western model, as may often be the case in Africa. While the hospital buildings still may be appropriate for local conditions, it is therefore not so much the building that requires close scrutiny as the established organization and internal structure of the hospital and the role of its staff.

The principal function of a hospital is to treat its patients efficiently and effectively, using whatever resources are available. This, however, can easily be overlooked. In the setting of a developing country the emphasis is often put on treating as many patients as possible because there are never enough hospital places to cater to all. This means extending the available services, around the clock, at their maximum therapeutic efficiency. The patients' needs, however, must come first. The organization of the hospital must focus around the needs of a large number of patients. The larger the number of patients, the greater the need for skilled staff, much more than are presently available.

Excellent treatment does not mean simply receiving the schizophrenic patient in the hospital to protect society from his presence and to look after his physical needs. Even if this were the best possible treatment it would not be possible to look after as large a number of patients as required because inpatient beds would be blocked permanently. To provide relatively good treatment for the individual and to care for as many patients as possible, the service should therefore be geared to the rapid treatment of illness and speedy rehabilitation of the patient to community life outside the hospital. There is a clear need for providing early effective physical methods of treatment coupled with psychological and social therapy techniques to restore the patient in all ways possible to normality or near normality in daily living. All too often, the organization of psychiatric hospitals seems to be actually antitherapeutic in applying psychological and social techniques that are destructive to the patients' well-being (eg, the patient is stripped of dignity and individuality and clad in a hospital uniform, for administrative convenience). The phenomenon of institutionalization, the archetype of antitherapy, has its roots in the admission procedure. There is a clear need to avoid these harmful techniques and to substitute therapeutic ones in their place. This calls for a close examination of all procedures in the ward, which, instead of processing patients, might be given a new, more therapeutic role.

Psychiatric Units in General Hospitals

Until recently all the psychiatric services throughout Africa were concentrated in one large psychiatric referral hospital, generally situated at the outskirts of the capital city. The outpatient services in countries where medical schools have been established have been rendered by the department of psychiatry. These services were inadequate and too centralized, giving rise to difficulties in transportation, communication, and follow-up of patients. The obvious need was to decentralize and to establish adequate peripheral services. Keeping this in mind, a number of African countries have built mental health centers or units attached to provincial general hospitals. These units have facilities for both inpatients and out-patients. It was envisaged that each of these centers would eventually have a psychiatrist, a trained psychiatric nurse, and a psychiatric social worker. Where trained psychiatrists were not available to be stationed in the center, provisions were made that the psychiatrists would visit the center at intervals. During such visits the psychiatrist would not only see inpatients but also conduct outpatient clinics for new cases and follow-up. Cases which for some reason could not be admitted to these centers and could not be given ambulatory treatment were transferred to the main referral psychiatric hospital of the country.

Schizophrenic patients treated and discharged from the referral hospital are sent to the outpatient clinics of the psychiatric units in the provincial general hospital nearest to them for follow-up. The psychiatric social worker and the community nurses stationed at the provincial general hospital make home visits to ensure follow-up and thereby reduce the relapse rate.

By doing so, efforts are made to ensure that psychiatric services are more evenly spread throughout the country. These centers reduce the need for building large psychiatric hospitals and facilitate follow-up attendance. It has been observed that one of the main reasons for patients' failure to attend for follow-up is the distance and the consequent expense and trouble involved in traveling. Patients who had to be restrained, hands and feet, for hours or days to get to the referral psychiatric hospital, are spared this pain and agony for any length of time, as these units are nearer their homes and they can get immediate attention. Furthermore, these centers have encouraged the acceptance of psychiatry as part of medicine not only by the community at large, but also and particularly by other members of the medical profession.

Despite the fact that these centers were established with correct and clear aims and objectives, in most countries they have not functioned effectively. Some of the reasons are that these centers were too small and their catchment area was too large. Hence, the need for beds was too great and the centers remained constantly overcrowded, and thereby their efficacy and treatment suffered. The upkeep of the building was neglected due to lack of funds, and so the facilities deteriorated rapidly and many centers had to be closed. Lack of personnel, particularly trained psychiatrists, was one of their major difficulties and the effective care of the patients suffered. General lack of supplies of equipment and drugs further worsened the problem. Although these centers are far from providing adequate services to patients, they are still proving to be very useful because they take a service load and in turn reduce the pressure on the beds of the main psychiatric referral hospital. It is hoped that in the future the plight of the centers will get better as the personnel situation in each developing country improves and, hopefully, the financial and administrative difficulties abate. Additionally, the plans to build more of these units will reduce the size of the catchment area, and the pressure for the available beds will ease. It is also hoped that each of the centers will have mobile units so that a large number of patients could be seen and cared for nearer to their homes.

Psychiatric Wards in General Hospitals

Psychiatric wards in general hospitals differ from country to country, but the basic principles are the same all over Africa. Generally, these wards are run by the Department of Psychiatry of the local medical school, and everywhere effort is made such that the teaching potential of the ward is fully used. In many African countries the need for the establishment of such psychiatric wards in general hospitals is apparent. Medical and public acceptance is also high. But a lack of personnel, space, and resources is the biggest constraint. Although the establishment of psychiatric wards in general hospitals has proven to be rewarding and encouraging, their construction in most African countries is only possible when a new hospital is being proposed, an old hospital is planning to add a new wing, or a hospital is moving to a new site. These wards certainly bring psychiatry closer to medicine. Efforts are made to ensure that the construction of these psychiatric wards is such that all forms of accepted psychiatric treatment are offered. Usually the ward occupies a wing of the main hospital and is often similar to the other medical or surgical wards as far as the basic amenities and facilities are concerned. Emphasis is placed on avoiding steel bars and metal doors. Certain security features, although present, are not conspicuous. These wards usually contain 30 to 50 beds with facilities to segregate disturbed patients, and seclusion rooms with special security features to care for very disturbed or uncooperative patients.

Occupational therapy plays an increasingly important role in psychiatric treatment programs in general hospitals. Consequently, occupational therapy departments should be well equipped and of an adequate size. But, unfortunately, most of these psychiatric wards lack the basic occupational therapy needs. Because these wards are improvised and not specially constructed for psychiatric use, many basic requirements are missing. Despite these difficulties, these wards many times offer the whole range of modern psychiatric therapies. Patients in these wards are admitted without the process of law, which makes the admission and discharge of patients easier and avoids much inconvenience of their patients and relatives. Besides, it is also a useful setting for professional training and research. All categories of psychiatric patients are admitted to these psychiatric wards and there is no limitation on their length of stay.

Drug therapy, due to recent advances in psychopharmacology, has had most gratifying results in these psychiatric wards, partly because the patient's illness is usually acute and of short duration. This advance also has made it possible to treat schizophrenic patients in an open ward of a general hospital, side by side with patients suffering from physical diseases. However, similar to findings in many other countries throughout the world, serious side effects such as tardive dyskinesia occur with neuroleptic drugs. One study in Nigeria of 70 schizophrenic patients found a prevalence of tardive dyskinesia of 37%[16] as compared with an average prevalence of 15 to 20% in the United States across numerous studies.[17-19]

Electroconvulsive therapy (ECT) remains one of the most rapid and effective techniques of treating acutely psychotic patients. This is now done under general anesthesia in most African countries. Electroconvulsive therapy is also provided on an outpatient basis to selected patients.

It is noted that the majority of admissions fall in the group of psychoneuroses, schizophrenia, and toxic psychoses. But on the whole, these psychiatric wards tend to accept the entire range of psychiatric disorders. The majority of patients stay less than 1 month on an average. Life in the wards within general hospitals as compared with psychiatric hospitals is easy, simple, and relaxed. Since admission is without the process of law, no rigid restrictions are laid. Patients are allowed to leave the ward at any convenient time. Relatives are encouraged to visit and a cheerful, friendly, and homelike atmosphere is created.

Outpatient Services

If outpatient services were effective, the demands on inpatient treatment would be reduced and perhaps there would be a lesser need to build large mental hospitals. Unfortunately, the establishment of psychiatric outpatient and other similar services in Africa did not coincide with the shift from institutional treatment to the free and open community care, as was the case in the developed countries. When the move in Europe and America was for breaking down the walls of archaic mental hospitals and unlocking their wards, in Africa the need was badly felt for giving some kind of psychiatric care, institutional or otherwise.

The establishment of psychiatric outpatient services even in the absence of adequate inpatient facilities was a necessity to provide some initial care to the mentally ill. Many times the situation was so desperate that there was no time to wait for a carefully planned building but to commence service with whatever was available. Outpatient services are more effective when there is a sufficient concentration of population. Even in urban areas patients may have to travel long distances to attend an outpatient clinic. This is very expensive for patients especially when they are out of work and frequent attendance is required at the clinic. Whenever possible, outpatient services were established within easy reach of the patients so that they formed an integral part of the normal social environment. Many times the public viewed the location with doubt and fear.

The deeply rooted stigma adversely prejudiced the community against centrally located psychiatric outpatient services. They could not accept agitated patients visiting the outpatient department. Education and rewarding results subsequently dispelled their false beliefs and fear.

Despite the intention to treat as many patients as possible at outpatient clinics, the backup inpatient facilities are never sufficient. Additionally, the outpatient facilities faced many other problems, especially the scarcity of skilled personnel. Ideally, the psychiatric team in an outpatient unit should be composed of a psychiatrist, a clinical psychologist, a psychiatric social worker, a psychiatric nurse, a community nurse, and an occupational therapist. This psychiatric team, however, is often not possible to obtain and one has to make use of the available human resources. The pioneer staff in most of these outpatient units was not more than a few general trained nurses and aides, headed by a psychiatrist, when available.

These outpatient units serve as the main centers to provide active treatment for schizophrenic patients, before their admission and after discharge from various inpatient facilities. Here, treatment is available with none of the rigid administrative procedures of the psychiatric hospital. The patients generally feel at ease and often tend to accept the treatment easily. The newer psychotropic drugs have made it possible to treat a schizophrenic patient effectively as an outpatient.

Outpatient services are the first link between the hospital and the community.[3] The active participation of the family in treatment is of central importance. In the outpatient setup, the family is encouraged to take part in whatever therapeutic program is prescribed for the patient. Fortunately, in Africa the families are still closely knit, and relatives are ready to give time and support to their patients. This strong human relationship helps in the treatment. As the outpatient services generally have no occupational therapy facilities within their premises, the family is advised and the patients are encouraged to engage in doing some useful work. Wherever possible, domiciliary visits are made by the psychiatric social worker.

With the availability and awareness of the outpatient services, the relatives bring their patients early for treatment. The referral from general practitioners and other hospitals has also increased rapidly. This increased the workload both on outpatient and inpatient services. Records show that 5 to 10% of the general psychiatric outpatients find their way into the inpatient facilities. In the case of schizophrenic patients, admission is restricted to only acutely excited patients or those who have responded poorly to outpatient treatment and therefore intensive inpatient therapy is indicated.

In developing countries with their well-known limitations of services, one of the most difficult problems is how to strike a balance between the capacity of a psychiatric outpatient service and the increasing number of psychiatric patients. It is difficult to send patients away. The patients seek treatment and they must get it, but the facilities are very limited. Despite their limitations, psychiatric outpatient services have proven to be a very vital development in providing care to schizophrenics.

Community-Based Psychiatric Services

The well-being of any community is largely dependent on reliable health and social services. Psychiatric services form a vital component of this complex. Their specific task is to bring to the public the benefit of available mental health knowledge and skills that, unfortunately, have not reached the rural poor in African countries. Whenever a developing country attempts to expand its health and social services it has to first look into the available resources, personnel, and other service facilities. Therefore, while planning mental health services in African countries, one has to use the utmost care because of the multifaceted difficulties. One important factor is the rapid urbanization, which is gradually disorganizing the traditional family structure with consequent disruption of traditional values and lifestyle. Therefore, while developing these community-based mental health services, due importance has to be paid to understanding the culture of the region, because the sociocultural and ecological factors have a great influence on the mental health of a community.

Almost all African countries face a common difficulty of lack of integration between the central psychiatric services and the meager community mental health services available. In other words, there is hardly any organized rehabilitation of schizophrenic patients. Apart from the outpatient services, other facilities such as rehabilitation centers, day or night care centers, sheltered workshops, and welfare services, are totally absent.

Some countries in the past made efforts to establish some kind of community-based mental health services. This was again an attempt to decentralize the care of psychiatric patients, and to reduce the overcrowding of the central psychiatric hospitals. In some African countries these efforts resulted in the development of village settlements. These village settlements in most cases were supervised by assistant nurses. The underlying concept of the village fit in with the national emphasis on self-reliance and on improving the image of the care of psychiatric patients in the eyes of the general population. This enabled selected patients to move from the psychiatric hospitals to the village, after the acute period of emotional disturbance was over. In this manner the patient took a big step toward more normal living. These village settlements are like "halfway homes" in the West. The patient is able to maintain contact with his family, builds self-confidence, and prepares himself to take his place with his family and neighbors again. Such village settlements, however, did not prove very successful as they lacked proper planning and there was not enough integration with the general medical delivery system.

After the initial failure, some countries like Kenya have been trying to reorganize the community-based psychiatric services. The new approach taken is that mental health forms an integral part of primary health care. The community, it is hoped, will eventually be involved in the recognition of mental illness, treatment, rehabilitation of the mentally sick, and reintegrating them back to their families and social folds. The community will also participate in preventive programs as well as promotion of good mental hygiene.

Currently, there are three pilot districts providing primary mental health care in Kenya (Okonji MO, personal communication, 1988). This will eventually lead to the involvement of the multipurpose village health worker, health supervisor, community health worker, and doctor. These personnel would be trained to provide mental health care. The aim here is to lower the incidence of mental disorders by improving quality of life and enhancing the tolerance of the community to life stresses. The health workers are given basic mental health education so as to understand that mental illness has identifiable causes and that these can sometimes be modified to prevent illnesses. Health workers are also given education to recognize mental illnesses, their early management, and referral. They are also given basic training for supervision of continued medication. A group of villages have been organized to form health committees. The function of village health committees is to identify health problems in the village and devise methods of solving them.

The success of these community-based psychiatric services is certainly dependent on how effectively health education is imparted to the rural people.

Traditional Healers

While discussing the delivery systems for managing the care of schizophrenic patients in Africa, one cannot leave out the role of the traditional healers. Every society has ways of dealing with problems. In many less developed societies, psychiatric problems at times still fall within the domain of traditional healers. Among these less developed societies in Africa, people still believe that witchcraft is the cause of all sickness and particularly mental sickness. Violent and uncontrolled outbursts and apathy and indifference are all brought about because someone, somewhere had cursed the unfortunate victim. As witchcraft is the cause, traditional healers are first consulted for cure. One particular tribe in Kenya, the Kamba, had and still have a highly specialized clique to deal with these cases. After a tribal dance the patient is led to undergo exorcism. The Luo were known also to be extra efficacious in curing mental illness, and people from several tribes consulted their traditional healers. Non-Luos carried a white chicken into Luo territory when they were on such visits so that they would not be mistaken for enemy raiders. Probably the strangest cure was the "Kisii" operation! Kisii tribal doctors listened to their patients' explanation of where the noises in their heads were coming from, made them drunk, and then cut out the offending piece of scalp and scraped the skull with a sharp knife until the bone became paper thin and gave way. Inasmuch as tribal specialists are efficient psychologists, exorcism is many times successful. But mentally sick people are generally grouped with epileptics and the deaf and dumb, and are regarded as not fit members of society.

Traditional healers have a very powerful image in the community. Their methods of healing largely depend upon the common beliefs and attitudes of the community. The biggest problem is how to integrate traditional healers with the modern methods of today's psychiatry. Attempts have been made but the two systems are based on completely opposite philosophies. Traditional healers many times use minerals, animal organs, and very potent herbs. Efforts have been made to analyze these herbs but nothing specific has been found. A proper pharmacological analysis of the herbs is long overdue.

To consult a traditional healer is usually a terrifying experience, because the methods used by them cause a great deal of fear and pain in the patient. They often use psychotherapeutic techniques which are not very different from modern psychotherapy of the superficial type. The effect on the patient, however, is much more due to the fear reaction produced by the entire procedure.

The traditional healers almost always find some scapegoat for the ills and misfortunes of their patients. The most painful aspect of the treatment is that many times the patient is tied down to a tree or locked in a hut for days. This results in septic wounds, dehydration, and a severe risk of tetanus. The condition of the patient becomes further deteriorated by the suffocation resulting from the smoke that is created around him and by painful flagellation.[20]

Traditional healers are better able to understand the patient's language and they employ techniques handed down from generation to generation. They cannot be ignored because they are important people in their communities. Moreover, they may be helping some mentally ill patents, especially the psychoneurotics. But the value of their work in treating schizophrenic patients is not only doubtful, but sometimes tragic.

Forensic Issues and Facilities for the Criminal Schizophrenics

Forensic issues involve both the design of a theoretical framework for understanding the process of criminal behavior and the various interventions of psychiatrists who treat the criminal offender. The latter effort involves the application of traditional psychiatric therapies to the schizophrenic criminal, as well as the commitment to assist the community in the administration of correctional justice.

Criminology has been a field of special interest to psychiatrists almost from the time that psychiatry became an organized profession. Penrose[21] stated that society's concern with mental health would result in the diminution of serious crime, particularly homicide. Although legal and administrative regulations form an integral part of the social and cultural context in which they are enforced, these laws very often lag behind social, medical, and scientific progress. In Kenya and many other African countries there is still old legislation in force concerning the status and confinement of schizophrenic patients and outmoded laws that perpetuate outdated practices in mental hospitals. The McNaughton rule,[22] a formula propounded by English judges in 1843, has been found to be the greatest obstacle of all to any real compromise between scientific medicine and law. The rule is the accepted yardstick for deciding whether or not the accused is legally sane and so fully responsible at the time of committing the offense with which he is charged. Difficult situations still sometimes occur when psychiatrists offer medical evidence in an attempt to free the schizophrenic criminal patient for required mental treatment. The patient may be quite mentally ill, but unless he is found "unfit to plead" under the McNaughton rule, he will be considered to be fully responsible. "Diminished responsibility" is not an acceptable legal plea in Kenya. However, the psychiatrist has an important contribution to make in this regard. For example, when the psychiatrist is called into the courtroom to testify in a criminal insanity trial, he is in effect, asked to answer questions that will help the judge to decide if the mentally disturbed offender should be fully responsible for his act and therefore punished. Until the late 1960s (sometimes even now), the Kenyan prison authorities were reluctant to transfer sentenced psychiatric patients to Mathari Hospital, fearing these patients would escape from the wards, where emphasis is on therapeutic care and treatment rather than on custodial surveillance.

In most African countries the main psychiatric hospital has a criminal section or unit. This is where psychiatric patients who have committed a criminal offense are housed. At Mathari Hospital in Kenya, a maximum security unit was built in 1978. Since then, there has been a remarkable change in the facilities offered to criminal schizophrenic patients.[23] Before the construction of the maximum security unit, criminal schizophrenic patients were distributed in prisons as well as in general and psychiatric hospitals (ie, Mathari Hospital). When these patients were kept in general hospitals it was the usual practice of the law-enforcing authorities to handcuff the patients to their beds. At the Mathari Hospital only two small wards were allocated to very disturbed criminal psychiatric patients, and others were kept with civil patients. It was during 1969 when 10 patients escaped from these wards that the problem was publicized in the press. The authorities then started thinking seriously that a maximum security unit must be built at Mathari Hospital. The title was a mistake as it trapped some administrators into believing that what was required was a miniprison which would have locks, bars, and high walls guarded by prison wardens. It was not easy to persuade authorities to build this unit according to medical needs and thereby remove all the psychiatric patients from the prison. The unit had to be closely linked to Mathari Hospital where a whole network of other facilities already existed. Duplication of these facilities at that time was impossible, both financially and due to lack of personnel. In addition, that was the time when many developed countries were trying to amalgamate the prison hospitals and the Ministry of Health hospitals. However, the feeling still prevailed that highly dangerous patients for whom maximum security was required should continue to go to the special hospitals. Nevertheless, the maximum security unit is at present coping with some noncriminal patients who tend to run away or are disruptive in other ways.

Scott[24] has very rightly said, "Security is a highly skilled process; like medicine, it is something of a science and something of an art. It is by no means a mechanical process but very much concerned with group interrelationship." To achieve anything near to that apart from proper buildings, a specially trained staff consisting of psychiatrists, nurses, psychiatric social workers, clinical psychologists, occupational therapists, ward attendants, hospital guards, and other staff skilled at managing impulsive and disruptive patients was required urgently. Training schemes were not yet available in Kenya even on a small scale, except for nurses training. Therefore, all the skilled personnel had to be derived from the existing staff of Mathari Hospital. The biggest problem was that even the increase in staff of Mathari Hospital was not considered. The maximum security unit was built at one end of Mathari Hospital and designed in such a way that the wards and infirmary would be situated along a central spine of the hospital. Separated from wards by open space are the administration, therapy, and outpatient departments. Staff facilities and social hall are located along the main access road. Two play fields and more formal open space activity areas are located on either side of the central spine.

Managing an intensive security unit of 350 beds functioning as part of a large psychiatric hospital posed a multifaceted problem. Newly admitted patients, mostly transferred from prisons, needed affection, friendship, and medical care as well as discipline. This required a high staff ratio, which was not available. This unit went through a very difficult time, but by transferring from Mathari Hospital the more senior and more experienced nurses, occupational therapists, and understanding subordinate staff, all of whom had leadership abilities, the situation gradually improved and was later improved further by increasing the staff ratio. Today the unit is functioning at a relatively warm, happy, and friendly level, and is a more human environment than a prison.

Many times psychiatrists are forced to keep a schizophrenic patient in the hospital when they know institutionalization is not needed. The gratifying medical experience of treating a patient, seeing him improve, and return to the community is diluted or prevented by restrictive laws and punitive correctional practices. The psychiatrist in such security hospitals cannot function as in civil hospitals nor can he perform his duties like other psychiatrists.

Schizophrenic patients treated in the maximum security unit are either those found incompetent to stand trial, those found guilty but insane, or those who become disturbed while serving a prison sentence. Releasing this patient from the hospital is not entirely in the hands of the psychiatrist. Once the patient is better he is returned to prison either to stand trial or to finish his prison sentence. Those who face trial and are found guilty but insane at the time of committing the offense are returned to the hospital as special category criminals, and are made to stay in the maximum security unit for a further period. They are discharged through a special category criminal board, chaired by the Office of the Attorney General. Usually they are discharged on probation only when they have completed a symptom-free period of 3 to 5 years. However, efforts are now being made to provide some level of service outside the hospital to meet the need of these patients to help them toward a more independent life. It is hoped that in the future other less institutionalizing environments will be available.

Conclusions

The incidence of schizophrenia is no less in rural and remote parts of Africa than in developed countries.[25] The type of facilities available in African countries for schizophrenic patients has been described. These facilities do not meet the general requirements and cannot be termed comprehensive. There is a gross lack of personnel, physical facilities, and financing. The services, however, are under pressure to gradually become countrywide in all parts of Africa. The aim can be focused either to provide an excellent service for a limited part of the population, or better, to provide a reasonably good service for a wide section of the population. Development of mental health facilities is largely dependent on the medical, social, and political action, which is influenced by the culture of the country. Therefore, any effort in the development of mental health care facilities should take into account the culture and the medical needs of the community. To define the exact requirement of any nation's mental health care need is a very difficult task facing health planners everywhere. Unfortunately, there are no defined and clearcut guidelines. The need for mental health facilities in all African countries is enormous. It is encouraging to note that overall there is a great deal of activity going on, and the image of psychiatry in most of these countries has taken a definite shape.

Recommendations

Perhaps one approach would be to take psychiatric services inside the pattern of general medical services. In other words, the emphasis should be placed on the community-based services. This requires integration and coordination of mental health services, with total health care at all levels of the health care program. Here I would like to quote Robert Ellis, Jr.[26] who said, "when disease cannot be prevented, it is necessary to ensure that the patient's needs are satisfied by providing care and treatment. This implies that the health educator must start by making known to consumers all existing health care delivery systems available to them. Secondly, health education and information must serve as key partners in the planning and implementation of training programs for all categories of health care workers by assisting professionals to develop skills, knowledge, and attitudes for effective communication in all areas of health."

African countries must refine their mental health sector priorities, sharpen their goals, and increase their efforts to realize the goal of health for all by the year 2000. Emphasis must be placed on the rural sectors, wherein the bulk of the population currently resides and will continue to reside for many decades to come.

Summary

The problems of delivery systems for the care of schizophrenic patients in Africa are multifaceted yet the incidence of schizophrenia is equal in rural Africa to that of more developed countries. Major difficulties encountered in providing care include a lack of mental health personnel and facilities and a decentralized service. Psychiatric care lags behind other medical programs in Africa. The primary concerns are nutrition, maternal and child care, and infectious disease control. However, 10% of the population per year are handicapped by psychiatric illness. Available decentralized services are not adequate to cope with the large catchment areas due to either the dense population in the cities or to the large distances involved in the sparsely populated rural areas.

Within developing societies, there is a very complex structure. With rapid urbanization, the traditional stable family structure is changing. There are few individuals trained in mental illness care and an excessive use of the prisons because of the overcrowding of psychiatric hospitals. Previously, the care of the mentally ill was of low priority among African health ministries. In less developed parts of the society, most mental illness has been treated by traditional healers. Furthermore, in large rural areas, transportation is inadequate or nonexistent. There is a scarcity of existing appropriate physical facilities and problems related to the insufficient number of skilled personnel. Too often the hospital environment itself is antitherapeutic in that the focus is on keeping the patient confined rather than returning him to the community. Supplies and medications are often lacking. Mobile units are needed for these centers, and there is a need to train the general health nurse to provide frontline rural mental health care. The population also needs to be educated to view the symptoms of psychiatric disorders as illness.

To overcome the chronic problem of overcrowding in mental hospitals of some countries in Africa, psychiatric units have been built in peripheral general hospitals. These decentralized psychiatric units in general hospitals provide both inpatient and outpatient care. Drug therapy has made it possible to treat schizophrenic patients in these psychiatric units. In Kenya there is a need to use village health workers who receive education in the recognition of mental illnesses, treatment, and referral.

Difficult forensic issues involving criminal schizophrenics are created by the outmoded legal systems. In certain countries where there are no special facilities for the criminal schizophrenic, these patients are still incarcerated. The McNaughton rule is the greatest obstacle to treatment of the patient who has criminal behavior. There is no acceptance of diminished responsibility, and the restrictive laws may prevent the return of an improved patient into the community.

There is now more pressure to provide reasonably good mental health services for more people as opposed to providing excellent services for only a few. There is a concensus and a recognition of need to achieve the goal of mental health for all by the year 2000.

References

1. German A: Aspects of clinical psychiatry in sub-Saharan Africa. *Br J Psych* 1972;121:461–479.
2. Lambo TA: *Schizophrenia, its Features and Prognosis in Africa.* Deuxieme Colloque African de Psychiatrie, Paris. Paris: Association Universitaire pour le Developpement de I 'Enseignement et de la Culture en Afrique et a Madegascar, 1968.
3. Giel R, Vanluijk JN: Psychiatric morbidity in a small Ethiopia town. *Br J Psych* 1969;115:149–162.
4. Muhangi J: The nature and prevalence of psychotic states in elderly people in a rural area in Uganda. Paper read to Third Pan-African Psychiatric Workshop, Abeokuta, Nigeria. Mimeographed proceedings available from Department of Psychiatry, Makerere University, Kampala, 1971.
5. Boroffka A: Psychiatrie in Nigeria. *Zbl F Neur Psychiat* 1964;176:103–104.

6. Ndetei DM, Vadher A: A comparitive cross-cultural study of the frequencies of hallucinations in schizophrenia. *Acta Psychiatr Scand* 1984;70:545–549.

7. Teggin AF, Elk R, Ben-Arie O, et al: A comparison of catego class 'S' schizophrenia in three ethnic groups: psychiatric manifestations. *Br J Psych* 1985;147:683–687.

8. Ndetei DM, Singh A: Hallucinations in Kenyan schizophrenic patients. *Acta Psychiatr Scand* 1983;67:144–147.

9. Swartz L, Ben-Arie O, Teggin AF: Subcultural delusions and hallucinations: comments on the Present State Examination in a multicultural context. *Br J Psych* 1985;146:391–394.

10. Greilsheimer H, Groves JE: Male genital self-mutilation. *Arch Gen Psych* 1979;36:441–446.

11. Muluka EAP: Severe self-mutilation among Kenyan psychotics. *Br J Psych* 1986;149:778–780.

12. Diop M: La depression chez la noir african. *Psychopath Afric* 1967;3:183–194.

13. Baasher T: The influence of culture on psychiatric manifestations. *Transcultural Review and News Letter* 1963.

14. Baasher T: Survey of mental illness, Wadi Haifa. *World Mental Health* 1961; 13 (4):181–185

15. Wood JF: A half century of growth in Ugandan psychiatry, in Hall, Langlands (eds): *Uganda Atlas of Disease Distribution*. Kampala, Uganda: Makerere University College, 1968.

16. Gureje O: Tardive dyskinesia in schizophrenics. *Acta Psychiatr Scand* 1987;76:523–528.

17. Jeste DV, Wyatt RJ: *Understanding and Treating Tardive Dyskinesia*. New York, Guilford Press, 1982.

18. Kane JM, Woerner M, Lieberman JA, et al: The prevalence of tardive dyskinesia. *Psychopharmacol Bull* 1984; 21:136–139.

19. Kane JM, Woerner M, Weinhold P, et al: Incidence of tardive dyskinesia: five year data from a prospective study. *Psychopharmacol Bull* 1984; 20:387–389.

20. Asuni T: Methods of delivering mental health care. Reports on workshops on mental health. The Commonwealth Foundation Paper 1969, IV, (11):1–47.

21. Penrose LS: Mental diseases and crime outline of a comparative study of European statistics. *Br J Med Psychol* 1938;18:1–15.

22. McNaughton's case (1843), 10 Clark and Finnelly, 200. Series H. L. Vol 12 (1831–1846) Eng. Rep. 6–8:203–211.

23. Mustafa G: Development of a forensic unit. *Am J Forensic Psych* 1987;viii(1):31–35.

24. Scott PD: *The Disease of Crime*. London, Royal Society of Medicine, Edwin Stevens Lecture, 1972.

25. Leighton AM, Lambo AT, Hughes CC, et al: Psychiatric disorders among the Yoruba. *Transcultural Psychiatric Research Review and News Letter* April 1964

26. Ellis R, Jr: Community health information and education. Afro Technical Papers no. 16. Regional Office for Africa. Brazzaville, World Health Organization, 1979.

18
Delivery Systems and Research for Schizophrenia in China

ZHANG MINGDAO AND XIA ZHENYI

China is a multinationality country with a total population of 1 billion. Administratively it has 23 provinces, 5 autonomous regions, and 3 municipalities directly under the central government.

China's first psychiatric hospital was set up in Guangzhou in 1897, and modern psychiatry developed since the beginning of the twentieth century, particularly the last three decades.

In Chinese psychiatric practice, schizophrenia is the most frequent diagnosis both in different regions of the country and at the different levels of mental health care. This chapter presents an outline of the mental health delivery system and also reviews the epidemiology, diagnostic criteria and treatment of schizophrenia as well as the laboratory studies of this disorder in China.

Epidemiology

In the late 1950s and early 1960s, there were several cities and regions that conducted epidemiological surveys locally. Because of the lack of standardization and the inconsistency of the investigation methods, criteria, and instruments used in these studies, China did not have its own accurate national epidemiological data on mental disorders until the early 1980s. To obtain a figure of the frequency of mental illness in the whole nation as part of a blueprint for developing mental health services, the Ministry of Public Health of the Chinese Central Government initiated, in July 1982, a nationwide epidemiological investigation on mental disorders in 12 regions,[1,2] namely, Beijing (Anding), Beijing (BMU), Shanghai, Sichuan, Hunan, Nanjing, Guangzhou, Lanzhou, Liaoning, Jilin, Daqing, and Xinjiang. The investigation instruments used in this survey were: (1) Major Psychoses Screening Schedule, (2) Neuroses Screening Schedule, (3) Intelligence Scale for Children, (4) Social Disability Screening Schedule (SDSS), and (5) Present State Examination (PSE).

Of these (1), (2), (4), and (5) were from the World Health Organization

(WHO), whereas (3) was modified from the Wechsler Intelligence Test for Children—Revised (WISC-R). The sample included 38,136 people aged 15 years and over from 12,000 households (6,000 from urban areas and 6,000 from rural areas). The results are summarized as follows (Table 18.1)[1]:

1. The general prevalence of various mental disorders was 12.69 per thousand within the total population investigated.
2. The prevalence of schizophrenia ranked first as 5.69 per thousand (6.06 in urban districts; 3.42 in rural areas).

According to these statistics, at the time of the survey, there presumably were 12 million psychiatric patients (5.6 million schizophrenics) in China. Clearly, it is a tremendously difficult task to develop the mental health services necessary to meet the country's mental health needs and demands.

Diagnostic Criteria and Treatment

Diagnostic Criteria of Schizophrenia

The Society of Neurology and Psychiatry of the Chinese Medical Association (CMA) proposed the first draft of the "Chinese Classification of

TABLE 18.1. Prevalence of mental disorders.

Disorders	Prevalence*
Schizophrenia	5.69
Mental retardation	2.88
Affective psychoses	0.76
Reactive psychosis	0.68
Cerebrovascular disease associated with mental disorders	0.50
Epileptic psychosis	0.42
Drug dependence	0.39
Paranoid psychosis	0.29
Senile dementia	0.29
Head injury associated with mental disorders	0.21
Alcoholism	0.16
Personality disorder	0.13
Schizoaffective psychosis	0.10
Physical diseases associated with mental disorders	0.10
Alcohol-induced mental disorders	0.03
Intracranial infection associated with mental disorders	0.03
Intoxication-induced mental disorders	0.03
Total	12.69

*per thousand
Reprinted, with permission, from Chen.[1]

Mental Disorders'' at the First National Conference for the Prevention and Treatment of Mental Diseases in Nanjing in 1958. Since the late 1970s and early 1980s, Chinese psychiatrists have been devoting much more of their attention to the classification of mental disorders and the working diagnostic criteria for schizophrenia. The Suzhou seminar (1981) was a special occasion on these issues. Again, in 1984, the society held another conference in Anhui province where revisions of the "Chinese Classification of Mental Disorders" and "Working Diagnostic Criteria of Schizophrenia" were adopted. Three years later, the Society convened another meeting discussing diagnostic criteria and classification of mental disorders in Xinxiang county, Henan province (August, 1987), where the members introduced the DSM-III-R and ICD-10 (draft), and developed a new draft for the "Working Diagnostic Criteria of Schizophrenia" that was re-revised in 1988 in Jinan.

Because the 1988's draft is still in the process of discussion, it has not yet been adopted by the Society of Neurology and Psychiatry, so in current Chinese psychiatric practice psychiatists are using the 1984 draft. Thus, we describe in detail "The Working Diagnostic Criteria of Schizophrenia" from the 1984 draft.[3]

Clinical Working Diagnostic Criteria of Schizophrenia (CMA, October 1984)

Definition:
Schizophrenia is a common psychosis in which the cause is still uncertain. It mainly occurs in adolescence and adulthood and is characterized by disturbance of thought, emotion, perception, and behavior, which so often results in distintegration of mental functioning. Usually there is no disturbance in consciousness and intelligence. The course may be persistent.

A. Criteria of symptomatology

Presence of at least two of the following symptoms. If the symptoms are uncertain or atypical, at least three of the following:

1. Disorders of association: loosening of association, thought splitting, paralogic thinking, pathological symbolic thought or poverty of thought.
2. Delusion: primary delusion, delusional hallucination or delusions with bizarre, autistic, unsystematic content.
3. Disturbance of affect: apathy, parathymia or silly laughing (cachinnation).
4. Hallucination: voices commenting on one's action, arguing among people or imperative hallucination, or echo of thought.
5. Disturbance of behavior: catatonic syndrome, mannerism or odd behavior.
6. Feeling of being controlled.

7. Feeling of being exposed or thought broadcasted.
8. Thought insertion, thought deprivation or thought blocking.

B. Criteria of severity

Meet the following three criteria:

1. Withdrawal from reality and loss of the ability of being in contact with or evaluating the environment appropriately.
2. Decline in function of social adjustment (including social activity, daily life, work or school functioning).
3. Lack of insight.

C. Criteria of course

The course of illness has persisted for at least 3 months, during which period there was an active psychotic phase for at least 1 month.

D. Criteria of exclusion

The psychotic disturbance does not meet the criteria of the following mental disorders:

1. affective psychoses
2. brain organic psychoses
3. physical illness associated with mental disorders
4. reactive psychosis
5. paranoid psychosis
6. schizoaffective psychosis

Treatment of Schizophrenia

There are mainly five forms of treatment for dealing with schizophrenics in our practice. They are: (1) drug therapy, (2) electroconvulsive therapy (ECT) and insulin shock therapy (IST), (3) psychotherapy, (4) traditional herbs and acupuncture, and (5) occupational and recreational therapy.

The first psychotropic drug, chlorpromazine, was introduced into Chinese psychiatry in the first half of the 1950s.[4] At present, there are more than 15 antipsychotic drugs being used for schizophrenic patients. Most of these drugs are domestically manufactured. A survey conducted on June 1, 1987, in the Shanghai Mental Health Center revealed that 98.7% of inpatients took antipsychotic drugs (including lithium).[5] The frequency of use of these drugs was ranked in order as follows: (1) chlorpromazine (55.1% of inpatients), (2) clozapine (39.4%), (3) perphenazine (14.0), (4) sulpiride (11.2), (5) lithium (8.4%), (6) haloperidol (6.4%), (7) stelazine (6.2%), (8) taractan (3.2%), (9) fluphenazine (2.2%), and (10) penfluridol (0.3%). The average dosage (mg/day) was: chlorpromazine 350, clozapine 275, perphenazine 24, sulpiride 600, haloperidol 24, and lithium 1050.

Electroconvulsive therapy and IST are being used in only a minority of psychiatric patients. Most mental hospitals stopped using IST years ago, whereas ECT still maintains its place (about 5 to 8% of inpatients, usually combined with drugs) in the treatment of schizophrenia.

Psychotherapy, both individual and group, is a part of the treatment program for schizophrenics, mainly for those patients who have remitted from severe mental disturbance.

Traditional herbal medicine and acupuncture in combination with western chemotherapy are tried on some schizophrenics (about 7 to 9% of inpatients). The aims of this combination are to make them mutually supplemental of each other in their effects, reduce the dosage of psychotropic drugs to alleviate side effects, and enhance patients' rehabilitation.[6]

In addition, occupational and recreational therapy have been adopted to rehabilitate schizophrenic patients and enrich their daily lives.

Sociocultural Aspects of Developing Mental Health Delivery Systems

Before 1949 (preliberation), there were only nine psychiatric hospitals with a total number of 1,100 beds (454 in Shanghai) staffed with about 50 psychiatrists (12 in Shanghai) for all of China, with nearly 450 million people. Needless to say, the majority of psychiatric patients were neglected by insufficient medical care.

Since 1949, under the great support and auspices of the government, mental health services have been rapidly developed throughout the country. In 1958 when the First National Conference on Mental Health Services (ie, The First National Conference for the Prevention and Treatment of Mental Diseases) was held in Nanjing, the number of psychiatric hospitals had increased to 58 staffed with 450 psychiatrists who were in charge of 12,000 beds.[7]

The Nanjing conference was an extremely important beginning for the developing mental health delivery system in China. Shanghai, Nanjing, and other cities were the pioneers in carrying out psychiatric census surveys to obtain epidemiological figures for planning the development of mental health services. A tremendous increase in development has occurred since 1958, although we encountered a difficult period during the Cultural Revolution (1966 to 1976). By 1986 when the Second National Conference on Mental Health Services convened in Shanghai, there were 348 psychiatric hospitals equipped with 60,000 beds and staffed with 6,000 psychiatrists. Concomitantly, various models and programs of mental health delivery systems were horizontally established throughout the country. In the following section, these models and programs are described in detail.[8]

However, it is worth noting that it is important to make an appropriate plan directed toward the development of mental health services which fits the needs of our own society. Every society has its own unique sociocultural background. We have had to create a system that lies on a foundation of our own philosophical, political, economical and cultural conditions. There are five major sociocultural issues that we have considered in developing our mental health delivery system:

(1) As stated before, the number of psychiatric hospitals is still far from adequately meeting the needs of the people. Even now, we have about 70,000 psychiatric beds, but this provides only a ratio of 0.70 beds to 10,000 people, although the ratio is 13.3 to 10,000 in the United States, 27.8 in Japan, and 30.0 in Denmark.

(2) The number of schizophrenic patients needing psychiatric service is markedly increasing. Taking Shanghai as an example, in 1958 the prevalence of mental disorders was 2.8 per thousand (schizophrenia 0.98 per thousand). Twenty years later, in 1978 it had reached 7.3 per thousand (schizophrenia 4.0), whereas in 1986 it was as high as 12.2 per thousand (schizophrenia 6.6). This increase in prevalence rate is actually not all due to an increase in incidence rate (prevalence rate refers to the total number of cases at the time of investigation, whereas incidence rate refers to the number of new cases found within a year). The increase of prevalence of schizophrenia is related to two facts: (1) the extension of lifespan in schizophrenics, because of better health care than before, and (2) the accumulation of relapsed cases.

(3) As a developing country, a very limited budget is available for developing psychiatric facilities. Obviously, the supply of psychiatric hospitals never meets the needs of the ever increasing number of psychiatric patients in a country with so huge a population. A rational and practical decision to solve our dilemma is to use the nonpsychiatry resources available in our society to develop a community mental health delivery system.

(4) The most essential issue is that our design of a mental health delivery system closely follows the government's political policy, namely: (1) a primary concern for laborers, farmers, and soldiers; (2) an emphasis on prevention; (3) integration of Chinese traditional medicine and western medicine; and (4) combined health work and mass movements. Our proposed mental health system certainly extends mental health services to the level of factories, villages, and neighborhoods, so that ordinary people, most of them laborers and farmers, will benefit from such community-oriented care. The mental health delivery system we have in mind is aimed at the early detection and timely treatment of psychiatric patients as well as the promotion of better rehabilitation for patients in the community, which obviously relates to the policy of emphasis on prevention. Furthermore, to convince people to share jointly in the concern for psychotic patients is a part of combining health work with mass movements. In this case, we have obtained the government's enthusiastic support.

(5) The sociocultural structure of China is a foundation for developing a family– and community-based mental health delivery system. Chinese people have traditionally maintained a strong family concept, even

though there has been some recent change in family structure. If anyone in the family becomes mentally ill, then the rest of the family members feel a strong responsibility to care for the sick member. Therefore, the family members welcome and accept care from the mental health delivery system and join in the care of their sick member.

In China, there exists not only a strong family concept, but also traditionally, close neighborhood relationships. The offical neighborhood organization (neighborhood committee) established in the 1950s further promotes these close relationships. To provide assistance in caring for old, weak, sick, and handicapped persons is one of the committee's functions. The existence of a strong family concept, good neighborhood relationships, and tight neighborhood organization are all assets for developing community-based mental health services in China.

Different Schemes of the Mental Health Care System

Since the First National Conference on Mental Health Services, psychiatry in China has been undergoing profound development. Beginning in the 1960s, there has been a unique development of the mental health delivery system that provides community services at the neighborhood, factory, and village levels throughout the country. Owing to 1 billion people living in such a huge geographic territory, it is apparently impossible to have one model fitting all the demands of the different areas. As a matter of fact, there have been various schemes of the mental health delivery system created in this country within the past 2 decades. Following is a description of those models representative of different parts of China.[9,10]

Shanghai Model—A Three-Level Scheme

Shanghai, one of the three municipalities directly under the Central Government of China, is situated in the middle of the east coast. The total population is 11.94 million. The city itself is international, industrial, and the largest municipality in China. Shanghai has 12 urban administration districts and 10 rural counties. According to statistics for 1986, the prevalence of schizophrenia was 6.6 per thousand (12.2 per thousand for the general prevalence of various mental disorders) in Shanghai.[2] There were 27 psychiatric hospitals staffed with 491 psychiatrists, with a total bed capacity of 5,789 (4.8 beds per 10,000 population). In the early 1960s, Shanghai developed a system of mental health care in a three-level scheme, namely municipal, district (or county), and grass roots levels (Fig. 18.1).

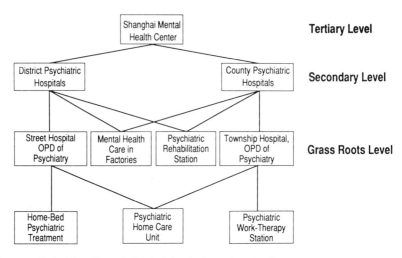

FIGURE 18.1. The Shanghai Model—A three-level scheme.

Municipal Level (Third or Tertiary Level)

At the municipal level, a coordinating committee organized by the representatives from the Municipal Health Bureau, the Civil Welfare Agency, and the Bureau of Public Security has the responsibility to:

1. Draw up the policies, blueprint, and coordinate the plan for mental health care in the whole city.
2. Coordinate projects and programs created by different agencies and organizations.
3. Mobilize and organize medical, paramedical, and nonmedical personnel to implement mental health work.
4. Supervise the district or county coordinating committee and psychiatric facilities to carry out various programs of primary mental health care.

With the assistance of this municipal coordinating committee, the Shanghai Mental Health Center (1,860 beds), three civil welfare psychiatric sanatoriums (1,520 beds total), and one public security mental hospital (254 beds) function as the municipal psychiatric facilities. The Shanghai Mental Health Center, sponsored by the Municipal Health Bureau, plays the leading role for overall municipal mental health services.

The Shanghai Mental Health Center (formerly the Shanghai Psychiatric Hospital founded in 1958) consists of three parts—the main hospital (980 beds with 124 psychiatrists), the branch hospital (set up in 1935, 880 beds, 65 psychiatrists), and the research institute called the Shanghai Institute of Mental Health. This center has been named the executive institution which functions to:

1. Provide psychiatric treatment and rehabilitation (inpatient and outpatient services), medical training in psychiatry, scientific research, and medical consultation.
2. Train medical personnel and provide consultation services downward to the district—county and grass roots levels.
3. Assist the municipal coordinating committee to establish policies, create methods, and mobilize medical personnel to advance the development of mental health work.
4. Take responsibility to gather epidemiological data and relevant information, register psychiatric patients, and analyze those materials for promoting mental health services in the whole city.

The three civil welfare psychiatric sanatoriums basically are taking care of chronically ill patients who have no family members. The public security mental hospital is a special facility that is only for psychotic patients who commit crimes.

District or County Level (Second Level)

In Shanghai, the number of inhabitants of each district in the city proper ranges from 200,000 to 850,000, with a total population of 6,391,000 for 12 districts; while each county in the rural area has 450,000 to 750,000 people, for a total of 5,549,000 in 10 counties. During the 1960s, each district or county established its own psychiatric hospital equipped with 60 to 200 beds. According to the complete figures for 1986, there are 2,155 psychiatric beds with 269 psychiatrists at the district or county level. In addition, at the district and county level, there also have been established coordinating committees, which have their own definite functions as well as responsibilities to relate upward and downward to the corresponding coordinating committees.

The district or county psychiatric hospital that provides inpatient and outpatient care is assigned as the key agency, and the local mental health center is at the second level. The district or county psychiatric hospital train nonpsychiatric medical staff and paramedical personnel locally, publicize the knowledge of mental health to the general public, and supervise the various mental health services at the grass roots level. One simple statistical figure will illustrate the importance of the district psychiatric hospitals in conducting community mental health services. In 1985, the total number of visits of psychiatric patients to outpatient departments or clinics in the city of Shanghai was 365,385. Of these, 126,280 visits (34.6%) were received in the district or county psychiatric hospitals, whereas 40.8% of the total number were in the Shanghai Mental Health Center, and the rest at the grass roots level. Apparently, the second-level psychiatric facilities cover more than one third of all mental health services.

Grass Roots Level

There are mainly five forms of community mental health programs at the grass roots level in Shanghai. These programs include: (1) psychiatric outpatient services of the street hospital or township hospital, (2) the psychiatric work-therapy station, (3) the psychiatric home care unit, (4) care of mental patients in factories, and (5) the psychiatric rehabilitation station.

(1) Psychiatric outpatient services of the street hospital or township hospital: To date, there are 107 street hospitals in the city proper and 222 township hospitals in the rural area of Shanghai. Of these, 101 (94.4%) street hospitals and 222 (100%) township hospitals have provided a psychiatric outpatient program. They received 55,195 (15.1%) visits of psychiatric outpatients in Shanghai in 1985.

(2) Psychiatric work-therapy station: The psychiatric work-therapy stations are, in certain ways, similar to what are referred to as day hospitals in the western countries. At present, there is a total of 118 psychiatric work-therapy stations staffed with 826 personnel, providing care for 3,227 patients, the majority of whom are schizophrenics. The stations are organized under the auspices of the community administrations, that is, the neighborhood committees, villages, or factories. The staff of the stations is composed of paramedical personnel from the community. Occupational work, supplemented with drug therapy and recreational therapy, is the primary mode of therapy. The number of patients in each station varies from 10 to 100 with an average of 28 cases. Each patient works 6 hours a day, 6 days a week. Most of the work is light handwork, such as sewing, making boxes, assembling notebooks, and other kinds of handicrafts. Patients can receive some subsidy from their work. The majority of the mental patients being seen in stations are partially recovered from the illness but are not yet capable of returning to their previous jobs or are patients who have had no previous job. In each station, there are one or two paramedical personnel and more retired laborers. They supervise patients' medications, observe patients' mental conditions, and keep contact with local psychiatrists for professional advice. They also try to help patients whenever there is some acute life event that disturbs the patients. This assistance, in a sense, is similar to the service of crisis intervention.

By participating in the work-therapy stations, the patients are able to take medication regularly, which makes the drug therapy more effective and reduces remarkably the relapse rate. Additionally, patients can participate in social activities, undertake work, obtain some income, and decrease their insecurity. So far, this program has been beneficial to the patients' rehabilitation by preventing them from deteriorating. Thus, the psychiatric work-therapy station certainly has been welcomed by the patients and their families as well as the government.

(3) Psychiatric home care unit: The statistics (1986)[9] show that in Shanghai, 79.6% (2,162 of 2,717) of the neighborhood committees have established psychiatric home care units, which were staffed by 36,625 volun-

teers taking care of 29,574 psychiatric cases. The psychiatric home care units are composed of patients' family members (49.9%), retired workers and neighborhood residents (34.8%), and health workers in the street health stations (15.3%). Their responsibilities are to supervise patients in taking drugs, to observe the patient's psychiatric conditions, to provide guidance and education, and to help the patient in solving any psychological problems that may arise. A member of the home care team acts as a bridge and mediator among patient, family, hospital, and society.

Having established the psychiatric home care system, there have been great improvements in follow-up care and efficient prevention of relapse and disturbing behavior by psychotic patients.

(4) Care of mental patients in factories: The care of mental patients in factories is provided by the factory's health station as part of the health care system. The factory health stations function similarly to other community-level health clinics to provide outpatient service programs and to treat psychiatric patients either at the clinic or at the patient's home. In each factory station, there are usually one or two medical doctors or health workers who have received short-term psychiatric training from the psychiatrists in the district psychiatric hospitals, or even in the Shanghai Mental Health Center. In Shanghai 514 factories have established a primary mental health program serving 4,918 patients for a total of 34,928 outpatient visits in 1986.[9]

(5) Psychiatric rehabilitation station: In carrying out the economic reform policy, the first psychiatric rehabilitation station run by a private owner emerged in 1983 in the rural area of Shanghai. Up to now 2,500 beds have been set up in 20 psychiatric rehabilitation stations (eight have private ownership, eight collective ownership, and four are public). Among them, 16 are located in rural areas, and four in the city proper. The appearance of psychiatric rehabilitation stations increased the total number of psychiatric beds in Shanghai from 5,789 to more than 8,200 in 1988. The psychiatric rehabilitation station is a new program in the mental health delivery system. It is still too early for conclusions about its real value for providing better mental health services in the community. Nevertheless, it has released, to some degree, the stress resulting from a shortage of psychiatric beds in such a densely populated city.

Training of Mental Health Workers

Psychiatrists are one of the important components in running mental health services, but the presence of the psychiatrists alone is not enough. Providing mental health services also requires a considerable number of nonpsychiatric medical staff as well as paramedical personnel. In the past, we have provided psychiatric training for 1,156 basic medical staff from neighborhood health stations, township or street hospitals, and factory health stations, as well as a large number of paramedical personnel, in order to build a network and organize a large task force to provide mental health services. The training course lasts about 4 to 6 weeks including theoretical lectures and clinical practice. The content of such training includes psychiatric symptomatology, diagnosis, psychopharmacology, and psychiatric care. Several studies evaluating medical staff who completed the training course revealed that most trainees can accurately identify most of the psychotic symptoms. Nearly 90% of them are able to function satisfactorily and more than 40% are very satisfactory as judged by psychiatrists. Our experience illustrates that if medical and paramedical personnel are properly trained, they can become a vital asset in providing primary mental health care.

Other Models of Mental Health Care

At the Second National Conference on Mental Health Services (1986), several other models, besides Shanghai, also were introduced.[9] Of them the following models were most impressive.

Mental Health Services in the General Hospital

Providing mental health services in general hospitals is another essential model. In some cities and regions, the department of psychiatry of the medical university plays the leadership role in mental health work. The Institute of Mental Health of Beijing Medical University in Beijing, is a well equipped psychiatric facility functioning as a full-service care institution. In Chengdu (the capital of Sichuan province), West China University of Medical Sciences has an excellent psychiatric department which provides mental health services to the whole city of 4 million people, while also providing teaching and research tasks. The departments of psychiatry at Hunan Medical University in Changhsha and Zhongshan Medical University in Guangzhou provide excellent medical consultation, treatment for minor mental disorders, and acute psychiatric inpatient care as well as aftercare of discharged patients.

Because of the shift from the biomedical approach alone to the biopsychosocial medical model and the urgent demands of mental health care from the people, the need for us to develop the model of mental health services in general hospitals is great.

Statistics[11] from the Chinese Ministry of Public Health showed that in 1985 China had 60,000 hospitals with 2.2 million beds and 127,000 clinics. However, in the field of psychiatry, as stated previously, we only have 348 psychiatric hospitals (0.6%, 348 per 60,000) with 60,000 beds (2.7%, 60,000 per 2,200,000). Obviously, the psychiatric facility is merely a tiny minority of the entire health care framework in this country. The substantive involvement of general hospitals would not only dramatically build a huge network to facilitate the mental health care for the people's needs, but would also reintegrate psychiatry into general medicine and intensify the medical foundation of psychiatry.

Home-Bed Treatment of Community Services

The home-bed treatment program closely relates to the home care unit described in the Shanghai model. The difference is that more treatment and professional counseling than simple care is given by psychiatrists or medical staff from county or district mental hospitals in the home-bed treatment program. The experience of Yantai prefecture in Shangdong province is a representative case in the rural area, and Zhengyang district in Shengyang, Liaoning province is a typical one in the city. At the end of 1985, there was a total of 4,865 home beds in Yantai. Home-bed treatment is an effective and economical program, which not only makes it convenient to treat actively sick patients, but also directly solves the problems of the scarcity of psychiatric hospital beds.

Other Types of Mental Health Care Programs

Shashi Veteran's Hospital in Shashi (Hubei province) and affiliated with the welfare agency is another model of the mental health care system. This kind of civil welfare hospital, usually equipped with 300 to 800 beds, serves the chronic psychiatric patients who are veterans or have no family members.

In some oilfields, mine stopes, and collieries, such as Daqing oilfield and Tongchuan area, there is a special mental health program provided by the government which is different from others. In some provinces, particularly in remote areas in China, there may be only one or two mental hospitals serving the entire population and operating only at one level (province) or two levels (province and city, without district–county and grass roots levels).

General Conduct of Clinical and Laboratory Research

In the late 1950s and early 1960s, researchers in Shanghai, Beijing, Changsha, Chengdu, Nanjing, and other areas of the country began research in biological psychiatry in the fields of biochemistry, genetics, psychopharmacology, and electrophysiology. During the last 2 decades, these research fields have been remarkably expanded to a much wider scope. Moreover, since 1976 international psychiatric exchange and collaboration have developed rapidly. These activities keep us in touch with the trends and developments in world psychiatry. In this section, a brief review of psychiatric research work in this country during the past years is presented.

Genetic Studies

The genetic study of schizophrenia has been directed toward the following approaches: (1) family studies, (2) twin studies, (3) adoption studies, and (4) cytogenetic studies.

Family Studies

The first systematic family study of schizophrenia was carried out in Shanghai (1964) and investigated 1,196 probands of schizophrenia with 54,576 relatives. It showed that the risk rate of schizophrenia was 6.2 times higher among the relatives of probands than in the general population.[12] The frequency of morbidity risks in sequence, according to family relationship, was as follows: parents, 3.3%; siblings, 3.0%; uncles and aunts, 1.4%; grandparents, 1.3%; and nephews or nieces, 0.6%. This result was confirmed by later findings.

The rate of positive family history of mental disorders in schizophrenic patients reported in subsequent studies ranged from 20 to 30%.[13,14]

The recent family studies on the heritability rate of schizophrenia in China showed that the lowest rate was 63.0%[15,16] and the highest 82.9%.[17]

The results reported from Nanjing[18] showed that negative symptoms were more likely to be inherited than positive symptoms. The authors speculated that the hereditary predisposition seems to be related to the negative symptoms.

A study carried out in Inner Mongolia (1987) revealed that the rate of positive family history in the Hui minority was 50% in schizophrenics, which was significantly higher than Han (21.1%) and Mongolian (33.8%) in the same region.[19]

Twin Studies

Twin studies were first reported in 1961 in China when Lou Huanming reported on the concordance rate for schizophrenia in five pairs of twins.[20] Recent more extensive twin studies of schizophrenia were implemented in Shanghai and Shan Dong.[20-22] The results showed that the concordance rate in monozygotic twins was 46.4% and in dizygotic twins 18.2%. These findings are similar to the results presented by Gottesman and Shields.[23] Fang et al[24] also reported a case of triplets who were all diagnosed as schizophrenic.

Adoption Studies

Zha[25] conducted a study of the prevalence of schizophrenia in 89 cases of adopted children. The findings suggested that environmental factors were not as important as genetic factors. Further evidence has come from a series of studies. One of these was carried out by Lou Kailing in 1986,[26] in which two groups of adoptees were identified: 31 who had schizophrenia, and 24 as a matched group who were not schizophrenic. Both their biological and adoptive parents and relatives were investigated. The results as shown in Table 18.2 illustrate that the highest psychiatric morbidity rate (PMR) is in biologic parents and relatives of schizophrenic adoptees compared with the other groups.

TABLE 18.2. Psychiatric morbidity rate (PMR) in biological and adopted families.[26]

Disorders	B1* N(PMR)	B2† N(PMR)	A1‡ N(PMR)	A2§ N(PMR)
Schizophrenia	13	2	0	4
Other mental illnesses	24	5	8	9
Total	37	7	8	13
	(25.17%)	(7.86%)	(6.20%)	(12.50%)

*B1: Biological parents and relatives being psychotic in the group of schizo-phrenic adoptees.
†B2: Biological parents and relatives being psychotic in the group of normal control adoptees.
‡A1: Adopted parents and relatives being psychotic in the group of schizo-phrenic adoptees.
§A2: Adopted parents and relatives being psychotic in the group of normal control adoptees.

Cytogenetic Studies

A study of cytogenetics in 48 cases of schizophrenia and 37 control cases recently was made in Shengyang.[27] The finding showed that the pericentric inversion of chromosome 9 was confirmed by C band and G band techniques in 10 cases in the schizophrenic group, but in only one case in the control group ($P < 0.05$). These results were close to the findings reported by Axelsson and Wahlström[28].

Zhang et al[29] found that the rate of sister chromatid exchange (SCE) of peripheral lymphocytes in schizophrenics was significantly higher than that in the control group. This result was similar to the findings of Crosses and Morgan.[30] In addition, some linkage marker studies and studies of drug-induced mutation also were conducted recently.

One of the most exciting research projects in the world today on the molecular genetics of schizophrenia is the gene marker study of restriction fragment length polymorphism (RFLP). We have a strong interest in this research field. An international collaboration of the molecular genetic study of schizophrenia with the United States is being discussed and planned.

Biochemical Investigations

The biochemical study of schizophrenia was started in the late 1950s in China. Recent biochemical studies have focused on aspects of bioamines, cyclic adenosine monophosphate (cAMP), brain peptides, enzymes, and trace elements.

Chen et al[31] found that the mean value of CSF 3-methoxy-4-hydroxy-phenethyleneglycol (MHPG) in 102 schizophrenics was significantly lower than that in the control group. During neuroleptic treatment, the levels of CSF homovanillic acid (HVA) were remarkably increased, whereas MHPG decreased. Before Chen's report, Zhang et al[32] and Shen et al[33] found that the level of 5-HT and 5-HIAA were lower in schizophrenics.

In 1982, Shen et al[34] presented a paper in which they indicated that CSF GABA and glutamic acid levels were considerably reduced in schizophrenics. Recently, Li et al[35] carried out a study and reported that both prostaglandin (PGA2, PGE1, PGE2) and cAMP in CSF and plasma of schizophrenics were lower than that in normal adults.

The studies of trace elements (Cu, Zn, Fe, Li, Mn) in serum and hair of schizophrenic patients were conducted by Wang et al[36] and Zhang and Huang[37] who found that Cu, Zn, Fe, and Li in schizophrenics were slightly higher than in normal subjects, whereas Mn was lower in schizophrenics.

Some attention has been paid to enzyme change in schizophrenics. Huang et al[38] reported that the activity level of platelet MAO was lower in schizophrenics, particularly in chronic cases. Huang's finding confirmed the results presented by Murphy and Wyatt.[39] However, Sun[40] could not find any significant differences in platelet MAO activity between schizophrenics and normal subjects in her subsequent study. Plasma dopamine-β-hydroxylase (DBH) activity was assayed in 100 schizophrenics by Kuang et al.[41] Although the mean level of DBH in plasma was lower in schizophrenics, it did not reach statistical significance. Low activity of lactate dehydrogenase (LDH) and its analogues in schizophrenics was reported by Huang et al.[42] Unfortunately, there were no further LDH studies reported.

Psychopharmacological Studies

In November 1987 in Shenzhen, five major psychopharmacological issues in our psychiatric practice were discussed at the Conference of Reasonable Usage of Psychotropic Drugs. Gu et al[43] reported the results of the pharmacokinetics of clozapine when used in 50 cases of schizophrenia. The mean half-life of clozapine was 9 hours, and the optimal plasma concentration might be more than 400 mg/ml. Shu et al[44] concluded the optimal plasma level of haloperidol for Chinese schizophrenics was 4.2 to 20.0 mg/ml in her report.

When antipsychotic drugs were administered to schizophrenic patients, Chen and Lu[45] and Jiao et al[46] revealed some abnormalities in their EEGs and EKGs.

As described previously, clozapine and sulpiride are commonly used in the treatment of schizophrenia in China (see treatment section of this chapter). We started using clozapine in 1976. The clinical effectiveness rate of clozapine in schizophrenics is about 80%. Xu and Zhang[47] reported the prevalence of agranulocytosis with clozapine used in 2,096 cases was only 1.9 per thousand (4 cases).

Drug-induced tardive dyskinesia (TD) and neuroleptic malignant syndrome also were reported in our clinical practice. A study found that the prevalence of TD was 8.6%[48], which was lower than that in some western countries (17.5%; Jeste and Wyatt[49]).

Studies of Immunology and Endocrinology

Recently, the study of immunology in mental illnesses has become a more active research field in Chinese psychiatry. A great number of papers related to this field have been published. Table 18.3 shows their findings in detail.[50–63]

TABLE 18.3. Immunological findings in schizophrenia.[50–63]

Authors	N	Celluar immunity	Humoral immunity	Complement	Autoantibody, immune complex
Wang et al[50] (1987)	40	NK ↑, HLA-B22 ↑			
Ni et al[51] (1986)	44	ANAE ↓ LTT(PHA) ↓	IgG ↑,IgA ↑, IgM ↑	CH50 ↓ AP CH50 C3 ↓,C4 ↓	ANA 13.6% Anti-ds DNA(−) RE 2.3% ATA ↑,CIC59.1%
Wang et al[52] (1986)	20	ExRFC ↓ EaRFC ↓	IgG ↑,IgA ↑, IgM ↑	C3 ↓	CIC ↑
Guo et al[53] (1985)	80		IgG ↑,IgA ↑, IgM ↑		
Wang et al[54] (1984)	47	HLA-B15 ↑, A9 ↑			
Yan et al[55] (1984)	42				Anti-DNA ↑
Chi et al[56] (1983)	86	ANAE ↓			
Guo et al[57] (1983)	54		IgG ↑,IgA ↑		
Lou et al[58] (1982)	100		IgG ↑,IgA ↑, IgM ↑		
Li et al[59] (1982)	169	PHA ↓			
Weng et al[60] (1980)	184		IgG ↑,IgA ↑, IgM ↑		
Huo et al[61] (1979)	36		IgG ↑,IgA ↑, IgM ↑		
Qiou et al[62] (1979)	20		IgG ↑,IgM ↑		
Gu et al[63] (1979)	100	PHA ↓ OT ↓			

Some comparative studies[64,65] of the dexamethasone suppression test (DST) in depression and schizophrenia were carried out. The results showed that the positive rate (nonsuppression) was about 40 to 43% in depression, 20 to 22% in chronic schizophrenia, and 5 to 6% in acute schizophrenia, whereas in normal control subjects it was 8 to 28%. The authors found that symptoms of "lack of initiation (apathy, withdrawal, etc)" in schizophrenics might be related to a DST nonsuppression reaction.

Zhang et al[66] found that serum prolactin (PRL) was higher in schizophrenics who were treated with antipsychotic drugs than in normal subjects. This suggests that neuroleptics block the dopamine system, which may be a part of the mechanism for treating schizophrenia.

Research in Neuropathology and Physiology

Ventricular enlargement in schizophrenia was reported previously[67] in China from studies using air encephalography. The introduction of computed tomography (CT) scanning has provided a noninvasive method for investigating the brain size in schizophrenic patients. Yu et al[68] found evidence in schizophrenics of significant ventricular enlargement, widening of the sulci, and atrophy of the brain. These changes seemed to correlated with the length of hospital stay and the course of the illness. There was some evidence that patients with enlarged ventricles had more "negative symptoms," such as indifference, lack of drive, and poverty of speech. Subsequent reports[69,70] confirmed the above findings.

Electroencephalogram and evoked potentials (EP) abnormalities in schizophrenic patients have been reported. Zhang et al[71-74] found some significant differences in the EP between schizophrenics and normal subjects in studies using the summation technique of auditory evoked potentials (AEP), visual evoked potentials (VEP), and contingent negative variation (CNV). The results showed the wave patterns of AEP and VEP were more variable and their amplitude was markedly decreased in the schizophrenics. Further statistical analysis revealed that the P2 latency of VEP and AEP in the schizophrenics with recent onset were significantly shorter than those of normal adults. The CNV study showed that the amplitude of CNV declined, and the latency of CNV, especially PINV (postimperative negative variation), was considerably prolonged in schizophrenics.

Recently, Hou et al[75,76] carried out some EEG studies using computerized spectrum analysis and information flow analysis. The results have confirmed that the power of delta waves and beta waves were increased and alpha waves decreased in schizophrenics, but these findings did not present a specific abnormality that appears in all schizophrenics.

Summary

Chinese psychiatry is crucially challenged by the fact that an extreme scarcity of mental health facilities and psychiatrists exists, particularly in rural and remote areas. Therefore, there is an urgent need to develop and extend mental health care, research, and training programs to meet the demands required by the one billion people living in an immense land with very limited economic resources.

Of 12 million psychiatric patients in China, nearly half of them are diagnosed with schizophrenia. Chinese mental health professionals are still in the process of developing specific diagnostic criteria for this prevalent disorder; the current Clinical Working Diagnostic Criteria of Schizophrenia are based on a 1984 draft of the Chinese Classification of Mental Disorders and have not as yet incorporated material from the DSM-III-R or ICD-9.

The treatment of schizophrenia in China encompasses five major treatment modalities: drug therapy; electroconvulsive and insulin shock therapies; psychotherapy; traditional herbs and acupuncture; and occupational and recreational therapies. Over 98% of hospitalized patients are administered antipsychotic medications, while about 8% receive electroconvulsive therapy. Occupational and recreational therapies are applied to most patients whereas psychotherapies, both individual and group, are reserved for those patients who are in remission from their illness. Traditional herbal medicine and acupuncture are administered to about 7–9% of inpatients; the primary aim of these treatments is to reduce the dosage of antipsychotic medications.

Beginning in 1949, mental health services developed rapidly throughout China with the number of psychiatric beds increasing 60-fold over this 40-year period. Over the last two decades, various models and programs of mental health delivery systems were established throughout the country, with the unique development of a system that provides community services at the municipal, district (or county), and grass roots levels, that is, the Shanghai Model—a "three-level scheme."

As depicted in the Shanghai Model, the municipal level functions primarily to develop mental health policies and coordinate programs geared for the city. At the district level, mental health professionals train nonpsychiatric medical staff and paramedical personnel locally, and supervise mental health services at the grass roots level. There are mainly five forms of community mental health programs at the grass roots level: (1) psychiatric outpatient services of the street or township hospital; (2) the psychiatric work-therapy station; (3) the psychiatric home care unit; (4) care of mental patients in factories; and (5) the psychiatric rehabilitation station.

The chapter concludes with a review of the major areas of schizophrenia research in China. These areas include: genetics; biochemistry; psychopharmacology; and neuropathology and physiology.

References

1. Chen CG, Zhang WX, Shen YC: Data analysis of an epidemiological study on mental disorders, drug and alcoholic dependencies, and personality disorders. *Chinese J Neurol Psychiat* 1986;19:70–71.
2. Chen CG, Zhang WX, Shen YC: Analysis of epidemiological data of schizophrenia. *Chinese J Neurol Psychiat* 1986;19:73–76.
3. CMA: The clinical working diagnostic criteria of schizophrenia. *Chinese J Neurol Psychiat* 1985;18:317.
4. Jia YC, Shu ZH: Chlorpromazine treatment in mental disorders. *Chinese J Neurol Psychiat* 1956;2:89–100.
5. Da ZM, Gu NF, Bo SK, et al: The prescribing trend of psychotropic medication during the past 10 years as observed at the SMHC. *Shanghai Arch Psychiat* 1988;6:1–4.
6. Yan HQ, Xu, SH: Traditional Chinese medicine and psychiatry.
7. Xia ZY, Zhang MY: History and present status of modern psychiatry in China. *Chinese Med J* 1981;94:277–282.
8. Xia ZY: The mental health delivery system in Shanghai, in Tseng WS (ed): *Chinese Culture and Mental Health*. Orlando, FL Academic Press, Inc, 1985, pp 341–355.
9. SMHC/MPH: Proceedings of The Second National Conference on Mental Health Services, China. 1986, unpublished.
10. Lin TY: The shaping of Chinese psychiatry in the content of politics and public health, in Lin TY, Eisenberg L (eds): *Mental Health Planning for One Billion People. A Chinese Perspective*. Vancouver, UBC Press, 1985, pp 3–37.
11. The Ministry of Public Health, PRC: A brief introduction on China's medical and health services. China. 1986, unpublished.
12. Ji M, Xu JJ, Xia ZY, et al: Genetic investigation on 1196 cases of schizophrenia in Shanghai. *Chinese J Neurol Psychiat* 1964;8:80–81.
13. Zhu XX, Yao JX, Yang JF, et al: Heredofamilial analysis of 2,000 cases of schizophrenic inpatients. *Chinese J Nerv Ment Dis* 1978;4:254–255.
14. Lei S: Heredofamilial and treatment effectiveness investigation on 1932 cases of schizophrenia. *Chinese J Nerv Ment Dis* 1983;9:5.
15. Wang TX, Wang M, Yang KY, et al: Nonmatched pedigree investigation on 150 schizophrenics. *Chinese J Nerv Ment Dis* 1985;11:269–271.
16. Lou HM, Wu YB, Zhao YZ. An investigation of the heritability of schizophrenia in northeast China. *Chinese J Neurol Psychiat* 1983;16:49–50.
17. Xia ZY, Giang SD, Bei GP et al: Genetic factors and mode of inheritance in childhood schizophrenia. *Chinese J Nerv Ment Dis* 1982;8:18–21.
18. Wang WY, Yu DS, Zhe ST: The clinical symptomatological concordance in the first degree relatives of schizophrenic patients. *Chinese J Neurol Psychiat* 1987;20:219–220.
19. Gang YQ: Difference in the familial and kinsfolk morbidity of schizophrenia among different nationalities. *Chinese J Neurol Psychiat* 1987;20:95–96.

20. Fang HT, Giang SD, Li CF, et al: Preliminary report on schizophrenic twins. *Chinese J Nerv Ment Dis* 1980;6:216–220.
21. Bei GP, Ling ZG, Fong GQ: A study of genetic marker in a schizophrenic twin pedigree. *Chinese J Nerv Ment Dis* 1983;9:30–31.
22. Deng ZY, Wu LX, Wang YG: A case report on concordance of monozygotic twins. *Chinese J Neurol Psychiat* 1987;20:191.
23. Gottesman I, Shields J (eds): *Schizophrenia and Genetics. A Twin Study Vantage Point*. New York, Academic Press, 1972, pp 51–68.
24. Fang HT, Ling ZG, Li CF, et al: A report of triplet siblings all suffering from schizophrenia. *Chinese J Neurol Psychiat* 1982;15:49–50.
25. Zha FS: A preliminary report of study on schizophrenia in adopted children. *Chinese J Nerv Ment Dis* 1984;10:32–34.
26. Luo KL: A study on 31 cases of schizophrenic adoptees. *Chinese J Neurol Psychiat* 1986;19:32–33.
27. Hong ML, Mei ZY, Tan Y, et al: Cytogenetic changes in 48 cases of schizophrenia. *Chinese J Neurol Psychiat* 1986;19:188–191.
28. Axelsson R, Wahlström J: Mental disorder and inversion on chromosome 9. *Hereditas* 1981;95:337.
29. Zhang ZL, Shen WJ, Chen YM: Preliminary study of SCE frequency in the patients with schizophrenia. *Chinese J Nerv Ment Dis* 1986;12:292–293.
30. Crosses PE, Morgan WF: The effect of chlorpromazine on SCE frequency in human chromosomes. *Mutation Research* 1982;96:225–232.
31. Chen YF, Shen YC, Li XX, et al: Changes of the levels of CSF monoamine metabolites in 102 chronic schizophrenic patients following probenecid before and after neuroleptic medication. *Chinese J Neurol Psychiat* 1984;17:273–277.
32. Zhang WH, Shu L, Shen YC: Metabolism of 5-hydroxytryptamine in schizophrenia. *Chinese J Neurol Psychiat* 1978;11:45–49.
33. Shen YC, Zhang WH, Shun LL, et al: A study of renovation rate of dopamine and 5-hydroxytryptamine in brain in chronic schizophrenics. *Chinese J Neurol Psychiat* 1979;12:158–160.
34. Shen QJ, Ling ZW, Xie GR, et al: Quantitative analysis of γ-aminobutyric acid and glutamic acid in the CSF in schizophrenics. *Chinese J Neurol Psychiat* 1982:15:98–102.
35. Li E, Song GY, Ling XB, et al: Study on pathogenesis of schizophrenia: Assay of PG and cAMP in CSF and plasma in 25 cases. *Chinese J Neurol Psychiat* 1987;20:81–83.
36. Wang SB, Chen GF, Zhao BZ, et al: A preliminary study on the measurements of microelements in the serum of schizophrenics. *Chinese J Neurol Psychiat* 1987;20:217–218.
37. Zhang DR, Huang RG: Pilot study of Mn in hair in schizophrenics. *Chinese J Neurol Psychiat* 1987;20:187.
38. Huang MS, Liou XH, Dong YH, et al: Preliminary study on platelet monoamine oxidase in schizophrenic patients. *Chinese J Neurol Psychiat* 1980;13:193–196.
39. Murphy DL, Wyatt RJ: Reduced monoamine oxidase activity in blood platelets from schizophrenic patients. *Nature* 1972;238:225–226.
40. Sun HR: Preliminary studies of platelets monoamine oxidase in chronic schizophrenia. *Chinese J Nerv Ment Dis* 1982;8:224–226.

41. Kuang PG, Xu B, Dai CL, et al: A study of plasma dopamine-β-hydroxylase activity in patients with schizophrenia. *Chinese J Neurol Psychiat* 1982;15:193–197.

42. Huang MS, Lion XH, Dong YH, et al: A preliminary study on lactate dehydrogenase and its analogues in schizophrenics. *Chinese J Neurol Psychiat* 1980;13:154–156.

43. Gu NF, Ying JL, Zhang C, et al: Pharmacokinetic study of clozapine. *Chinese J Neurol Psychiat*. 1988;21:259–262.

44. Shu L, Shen YC, Zhou DF, et al: Comparison of therapeutic effects between haloperidol and insulin coma for schizophrenia and the optimal blood level of haloperidol. *Chinese J Neurol Psychiat* 1987;20:43–48.

45. Chen YF, Lu XW: Changes of EEG in 84 schizophrenic patients treated with haloperidol or chlorpromazine. *J Electroencephalography Nerv Ment Dis* 1988;4:22–23.

46. Jiao HQ, Li SL, Yu SC, et al: Complications in antipsychotic drug treatment. *Chinese J Nerv Ment Dis* 1981;7:29–31.

47. Xu SH, Zhang YH: Clozapine and agranulocytosis. *Chinese J Neurol Psychiat* 1984;17:271–272.

48. Zhang LD, Yan WW, Zhang EL, et al: A tardive dyskinesia study of psychiatric inpatients. *Chinese J Neurol Psychiat* 1988;21:232–235.

49. Jeste DV, Wyatt RJ: Changing epidemiology of tardive dyskinesia. *Am J Psychiatry* 1981;138:297–309.

50. Wang QD, Jiang SD, Feng GC, et al: Preliminary study on NK activity in peripheral blood lymphocytes of schizophrenic patients. *Chinese J Neurol Psychiat* 1987;20:215–216.

51. Ni CY, Xu H, Xia JZ: A preliminary study on the immunological changes in schizophrenics. *Chinese J Neurol Psychiat* 1986;19:34–37.

52. Wang WS, Han YZ, Jin H: Autoimmunity in schizophrenic patients. *Chinese J Neurol Psychiat* 1986;19:332–334.

53. Guo ZH, Zhen GZ, Lu XD, et al: Assay of serum immunoglobulin in 80 cases of schizophrenics. *Chinese J Nerv Ment Dis* 1985;11:179–180.

54. Wang WS, Jing SZ, Mu CH, et al: Human leukocyte antigen and schizophrenia. *Chinese J Neurol Psychiat* 1984;17:284–286.

55. Yan JS, Pu Q, Li YL: Positive reaction of serum anti-DNA antibody induced by phenothiazines in schizophrenic patients. *Chinese J Neurol Psychiat* 1984;17:333–335.

56. Chi ZZ, Jiang SY, Liou XZ, et al: Preliminary observation on changes of T-lymphocytes labelled with non-specific esterase in schizophrenics. *Chinese J Neurol Psychiat* 1983;16:242–243.

57. Guo ZH, Zheng GZ, Men XD, et al: A controlled study of cerebrospinal fluid immonoglobulins in 54 chronic schizophrenic patients. *Chinese J Nerv Ment Dis* 1983;9:85–87.

58. Lou WW, Xiao GM, Chen MG: Preliminary study of Serum immunoglobulin in 100 cases of schizophrenia. *Chinese J Nerv Ment Dis* 1982;8:103

59. Li LX, Qiou Y, Muo GM: Cellular immunity of schizophrenics. *Chinese J Nerv Ment Dis* 1982;8:261–263.

60. Weng Z, Li BY, Hou YY, et al: Preliminary study of serum immunological globulin in schizophrenics. *Chinese J Nerv Ment Dis* 1980;6:260–263.

61. Huo KJ, Yan SJ, Liou XH, et al: Preliminary observations on immunoglobulins in schizophrenics. *Chinese J Neurol Psychiat* 1979;12:161–163.

62. Qiou Y, Luo ZK, He XQ: Study on serum immunoglobulin in schizophrenia. *Chinese J Neurol Psychiat* 1979;12:241–242.
63. Gu JS, Xu CL, Yan HQ, et al: Preliminary study on lymphocytic transformation test and intracutaneous tuberculin test in schizophrenics. *Chinese J Neurol Psychiat* 1979;12:193–195.
64. Gu NF, Zhang MY, Ren FM, et al: A comparative study on the dexamethesone suppression test in acute and chronic schizophrenia. *Chinese J Neurol Psychiat* 1985;18:287–290.
65. Fan MH, Chen GQ, Muo GM: A preliminary report of dexamethasone test in depressive, manic, schizophrenic patients, and control subjects. *Chinese J Nerv Ment Dis* 1985;11:23–25.
66. Zhang FC, Zhang JF, Wang DN, et al: Study on the effect of antipsychotic drugs on serum prolactin in schizophrenic patients. *Chinese J Nerv Ment Dis* 1986;12:80–82.
67. Wu EH, Mo BC, Zhuo HY: A study of air encephalography on 384 cases. *Chinese J Neurol Psychiat* 1960;6:42–44.
68. Yu QH, Chen PZ, Liu TS, et al: Cognitive function and computerized tomography of the brain in deteriorated schizophrenics. *Chinese J Neurol Psychiat* 1983;16:42–45.
69. Zhang TP, Len JP: CT observations on the morphological changes of the brain in schizophrenics. *Chinese J Neurol Psychiat* 1985;18:158–161.
70. Wang XY, Li WD, Hu JR, et al: Comparative study of the brain CT scan and clinical manifestation in schizophrenia of 73 cases. *Chinese J Nerv Ment Dis* 1986;12:345–347.
71. Zhang MD, Xia ZY, Li ZD, et al: A preliminary study of evoked brain potentials on schizophrenics. *Chinese J Neurol Psychiat* 1983;16:274–277.
72. Zhang MD, Chen XS, Li ZD, et al: A comparative study of evoked potentials on clinical symptoms and treatment effectiveness in acute schizophrenics. *Chinese J Neurol Psychiat* 1988;21:178–182.
73. Zhang MD, Chen XS, Li ZD, et al: Clinical study of AEP and VEP on acute schizophrenics. *Shanghai Arch Psychiat* 1987:5:47–51.
74. Xia ZY, Zhang MD, Jiang KD, et al: A clinical study on schizophrenics with contingent negative variation. *Chinese J Neurol Psychiat* 1983;16:321–324.
75. Hou Y, Di S: A preliminary report on EEG spectrum analysis of schizophrenia. *Chinese J Neurol Psychiat* 1984;17:129–130.
76. Yang ZJ, Hou Y, Shu L, et al: Computerized analysis of spontaneous EEG in schizophrenics. *Chinese J Neurol Psychiat* 1987;20:87–91.

Author Index

Subject Index

DATE DUE

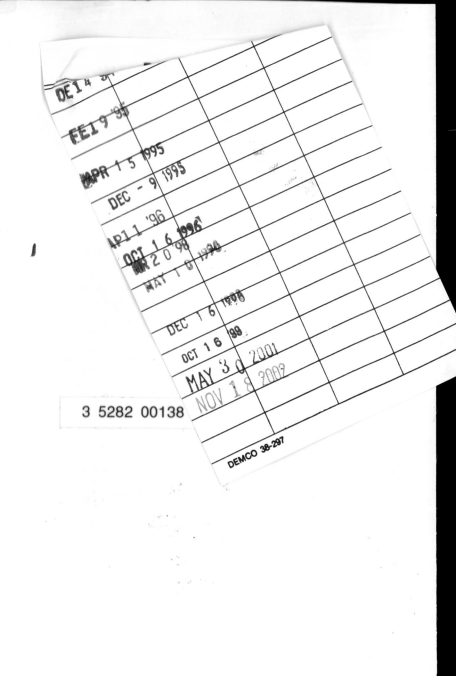